Endocrine Imaging

Guest Editor

MITCHELL E. TUBLIN, MD

RADIOLOGIC CLINICS
OF NORTH AMERICA

www.radiologic.theclinics.com

Consulting Editor
FRANK H. MILLER, MD

May 2011 • Volume 49 • Number 3

SAUNDERS an imprint of ELSEVIER, Inc.

W.B. SAUNDERS COMPANY
A Division of Elsevier Inc.

1600 John F. Kennedy Boulevard • Suite 1800 • Philadelphia, Pennsylvania 19103-2899

http://www.theclinics.com

RADIOLOGIC CLINICS OF NORTH AMERICA Volume 49, Number 3
May 2011 ISSN 0033-8389, ISBN 13: 978-1-4557-1149-9

Editor: Barton Dudlick
Developmental Editor: Eva Kulig

Radiologic Clinics of North America (ISSN 0033-8389) is published bimonthly by Elsevier Inc., 360 Park Avenue South, New York, NY 10010-1710. Months of issue are January, March, May, July, September, and November. Periodicals postage paid at New York, NY and additional mailing offices. Subscription prices are USD 386 per year for US individuals, USD 610 per year for US institutions, USD 185 per year for US students and residents, USD 450 per year for Canadian individuals, USD 766 per year for Canadian institutions, USD 556 per year for international individuals, USD 766 per year for international institutions, and USD 266 per year for Canadian and foreign students/residents. To receive student and resident rate, orders must be accompanied by name of affiliated institution, date of term and the signature of program/residency coordinatior on institution letterhead. Orders will be billed at individual rate until proof of status is received. Foreign air speed delivery is included in all *Clinics* subscription prices. All prices are subject to change without notice. **POSTMASTER:** Send address changes to *Radiologic Clinics of North America*, Elsevier Health Sciences Division, Subscription Customer Service, 3251 Riverport Lane, Maryland Heights, MO63043. **Customer Service: Telephone: 1-800-654-2452** (U.S. and Canada); **1-314-447-8871** (outside U.S. and Canada). **Fax: 1-314-447-8029. E-mail: journalscustomerservice-usa@ elsevier.com** (for print support); **journalsonlinesupport-usa@elsevier.com** (for online support).

Reprints. For copies of 100 or more of articles in this publication, please contact the Commercial Reprints Department, Elsevier Inc., 360 Park Avenue South, New York, New York 10010-1710. Tel.: (+1) 212-633-3812; Fax: (+1) 212-462-1935; E-mail: reprints@elsevier.com.

Radiologic Clinics of North America also published in Greek Paschalidis Medical Publications, Athens, Greece.

Radiologic Clinics of North America is covered in *MEDLINE/PubMed (Index Medicus), EMBASE/Excerpta Medica, Current Contents/Life Sciences, Current Contents/Clinical Medicine, RSNA Index to Imaging Literature, BIOSIS, Science Citation Index,* and *ISI/BIOMED*.

Printed in the United States of America.

Contributors

CONSULTING EDITOR

FRANK H. MILLER, MD
Professor of Radiology; Chief, Body Imaging
Section and Fellowship Program and GI
Radiology, Medical Director MRI,
Department of Radiology, Northwestern
University Feinberg School of Medicine,
Chicago, Illinois

GUEST EDITOR

MITCHELL E. TUBLIN, MD
Professor of Radiology; Chief, Abdominal
Imaging Section, Division of Abdominal
Imaging, Department of Radiology, University
of Pittsburgh School of Medicine, Pittsburgh,
Pennsylvania

AUTHORS

GILES W.L. BOLAND, MD
Vice Chair of Radiology, Department of
Radiology, Massachusetts General Hospital,
Associate Professor, Harvard Medical School,
Boston, Massachusetts

AMIR A. BORHANI, MD
Radiology Resident, Department of Radiology,
University of Pittsburgh Medical Center,
Pittsburgh, Pennsylvania

SALLY E. CARTY, MD, FACS
Professor of Surgery, Section of Endocrine
Surgery, Department of Surgery, University of
Pittsburgh School of Medicine, Pittsburgh,
Pennsylvania

SUE M. CHALLINOR, MD
Associate Professor of Medicine, Division of
Endocrinology and Metabolism, Department
of Medicine, University of Pittsburgh Medical
Center, Pittsburgh, Pennsylvania

AMY E. COX, MD
Fellow, Division of Endocrinology and
Metabolism, University of Pittsburgh Medical
Center, Pittsburgh, Pennsylvania

MATTHEW T. HELLER, MD
Assistant Professor of Radiology, Division
of Abdominal Imaging, Department of
Radiology, University of Pittsburgh Medical
Center, Pittsburgh, Pennsylvania

TARA L. HENRICHSEN, MD
Assistant Professor, Department of Radiology,
Mayo Clinic, Rochester, Minnesota

NATHAN A. JOHNSON, MD
Assistant Professor, Department of Radiology,
Division of Abdominal Imaging, University of
Pittsburgh School of Medicine, Pittsburgh,
Pennsylvania

JUDITH M. JOYCE, MD
Clinical Associate Professor, Clinical Director
Nuclear Medicine, Division of Nuclear
Medicine, Department of Radiology, University
of Pittsburgh Medical Center, Pittsburgh,
Pennsylvania

SHANE O. LEBEAU, MD
Clinical Assistant Professor of Medicine,
Division of Endocrinology and Metabolism,
University of Pittsburgh Medical Center,
Pittsburgh, Pennsylvania

JASON M. NG, MD
Research Fellow, Division of Endocrinology
and Metabolism, Department of Medicine,
University of Pittsburgh Medical Center,
Pittsburgh, Pennsylvania

N. PAUL OHORI, MD
Professor of Pathology, Medical Director of
Cytopathology, Department of Pathology,
University of Pittsburgh Medical
Center-Presbyterian, Pittsburgh, Pennsylvania

TAO OUYANG, MD
Assistant Professor of Radiology, Division of
Neuroradiology, Department of Radiology,
Penn State Hershey Medical Center, Hershey,
Pennsylvania

CARL C. READING, MD
Professor, Department of Radiology, Mayo
Clinic, Rochester, Minnesota

WILLIAM E. ROTHFUS, MD, FACR
Professor of Radiology and Neurosurgery;
Chief, Division of Neuroradiology, Department
of Radiology, University of Pittsburgh Medical
Center, Pittsburgh, Pennsylvania

KAREN E. SCHOEDEL, MD
Associate Professor of Pathology, Department
of Pathology, University of Pittsburgh
Medical Center-Presbyterian, Pittsburgh,
Pennsylvania

AMAR B. SHAH, MD
Assistant Professor of Radiology, Division
of Body Imaging, Department of Radiology,
New York Medical College, Valhalla, New York

BIATTA SHOLOSH, MD
Assistant Professor, Division of Abdominal
Imaging, Department of Radiology, University
of Pittsburgh Medical Center, Pittsburgh,
Pennsylvania

MICHAEL T. STANG, MD
Section of Endocrine Surgery, Department of
Surgery, University of Pittsburgh, Pittsburgh,
Pennsylvania

ANDREW SWIHART, MD
Diagnostic Radiology Resident, Department
of Radiology, University of Pittsburgh Medical
Center, Pittsburgh, Pennsylvania

MITCHELL E. TUBLIN, MD
Professor of Radiology; Chief, Abdominal
Imaging Section, Division of Abdominal
Imaging, Department of Radiology, University
of Pittsburgh School of Medicine, Pittsburgh,
Pennsylvania

LINWAH YIP, MD, FACS
Section of Endocrine Surgery, Department of
Surgery, University of Pittsburgh, Pittsburgh,
Pennsylvania

Contents

classification system for thyroid cytopathology. The role of molecular and other ancillary studies in refining diagnostic practice is also examined.

Thyroid cancer is the most common endocrine malignancy. Historically, the diagnosis has been made via fine-needle aspiration cytology; however, molecular marker analysis, particularly in indeterminate specimens, is beginning to play a more prominent role. Once the diagnosis of thyroid cancer is established, patients should undergo preoperative ultrasound evaluation followed by appropriate surgical resection, radioiodine ablation, and thyrotropin suppression. After the initial treatment, patients must be monitored regularly for recurrent disease utilizing clinical examination, thyroglobulin measurement, and radiological imaging.

Surgery is often needed to diagnose thyroid cancer, but is also the initial therapeutic modality. Several current imaging techniques are important for preoperative risk stratification. By optimizing initial thyroidectomy and lymphadenectomy, accurate and appropriate imaging can help minimize operative morbidity and potentially reduce the risk of recurrent disease.

Intensive imaging surveillance has resulted in the ability to detect small-volume, often clinically occult, residual or recurrent disease. For most patients with differentiated thyroid cancer (DTC), such findings are unlikely to have an impact on disease-specific survival but our ability to predict which patients are at greatest risk and should receive the most aggressive therapies is surpassed by our ability to detect recurrence. Thus, the optimal treatment and surveillance regimens will surely continue to evolve as our ability to predict tumor behavior and aggressiveness improves. This article explains the rationale underlying current surveillance strategies and the utility and implications of imaging findings that are critical for the appropriate care of patients with DTC.

Primary hyperparathyroidism is a common endocrine disorder caused by the overproduction of parathyroid hormone either by a single adenomatous gland or by multiple adenomatous or hyperplastic glands. Surgical resection of the abnormal parathyroid glands is the standard treatment, the goal of initial parathyroidectomy being durable biochemical cure. Surgeons have recently shifted to more minimally invasive and selective techniques for parathyroid exploration. More selective surgical approaches rely on accurate preoperative imaging techniques to localize abnormal parathyroid glands. It is imperative that radiologists are familiar with imaging features of parathyroid glands as well as the role of imaging in patient care.

Despite their small size, pathologic condition of the adrenal glands is often far from insignificant. Imagers should therefore be familiar with the principles and techniques that underpin the ability of imaging to characterize most lesions. Ignorance of these techniques fails to deliver the necessary imaging value to referrers and patients alike. This article, outlines the range of possible abnormalities encountered in the adrenal gland, the imaging modalities and specialized techniques used to detect and characterize them, the principles based on which these techniques are used, and finally a working imaging algorithm that can be readily used in daily practice.

Neuroendocrine tumors (NETs) constitute a large group of diverse neoplasms with a wide spectrum of clinical, imaging, and pathologic findings. Imaging diagnosis of NETs can be challenging, and several complementary imaging modalities may be needed during the diagnostic workup. Accurate interpretation of the imaging findings is important to facilitate diagnosis and contribute to patient management. This article discusses the gastrointestinal site-specific features and the tumor-specific features of several NETs and the role of several imaging modalities such as computed tomography, MR imaging, ultrasonography, and positron emission tomography in the evaluation of these NETs.

In the appropriate clinical setting of pituitary hyperfunction or hypofunction, visual field deficit, or cranial nerve palsy, imaging of the pituitary is necessary. This article reviews the normal appearance of the pituitary and its surroundings, emphasizing magnetic resonance imaging. Typical and variant appearances of pituitary pathology are discussed. Because growth of adenoma into surrounding structures is important to surgical management, cavernous sinus invasion and suprasellar spread as well as adenoma mimics are illustrated. Typical examples of pituitary dysfunction from other entities that secondarily affect the gland, hypophysis, or third ventricle are discussed. Some common errors of interpretation are listed.

GOAL STATEMENT

The goal of the *Radiologic Clinics of North America* is to keep practicing radiologists and radiology residents up to date with current clinical practice in radiology by providing timely articles reviewing the state of the art in patient care.

ACCREDITATION

The *Radiologic Clinics of North America* is planned and implemented in accordance with the Essential Areas and Policies of the Accreditation Council for Continuing Medical Education (ACCME) through the joint sponsorship of the University of Virginia School of Medicine and Elsevier. The University of Virginia School of Medicine is accredited by the ACCME to provide continuing medical education for physicians.

The University of Virginia School of Medicine designates this educational activity for a maximum of 15 *AMA PRA Category 1 Credits*™ for each issue, 90 credits per year. Physicians should only claim credit commensurate with the extent of their participation in the activity.

The American Medical Association has determined that physicians not licensed in the US who participate in this CME activity are eligible for a maximum of *15 AMA PRA Category 1 Credits*™ for each issue, 90 credits per year.

Credit can be earned by reading the text material, taking the CME examination online at http://www.theclinics.com/home/cme, and completing the evaluation. After taking the test, you will be required to review any and all incorrect answers. Following completion of the test and evaluation, your credit will be awarded and you may print your certificate.

FACULTY DISCLOSURE/CONFLICT OF INTEREST

The University of Virginia School of Medicine, as an ACCME accredited provider, endorses and strives to comply with the Accreditation Council for Continuing Medical Education (ACCME) Standards of Commercial Support, Commonwealth of Virginia statutes, University of Virginia policies and procedures, and associated federal and private regulations and guidelines on the need for disclosure and monitoring of proprietary and financial interests that may affect the scientific integrity and balance of content delivered in continuing medical education activities under our auspices.

The University of Virginia School of Medicine requires that all CME activities accredited through this institution be developed independently and be scientifically rigorous, balanced and objective in the presentation/discussion of its content, theories and practices.

All authors/editors participating in an accredited CME activity are expected to disclose to the readers relevant financial relationships with commercial entities occurring within the past 12 months (such as grants or research support, employee, consultant, stock holder, member of speakers bureau, etc.). The University of Virginia School of Medicine will employ appropriate mechanisms to resolve potential conflicts of interest to maintain the standards of fair and balanced education to the reader. Questions about specific strategies can be directed to the Office of Continuing Medical Education, University of Virginia School of Medicine, Charlottesville, Virginia.

The faculty and staff of the University of Virginia Office of Continuing Medical Education have no financial affiliations to disclose.

The authors/editors listed below have identified no financial or professional relationships for themselves or their spouse/partner:

Giles W. L. Boland, MD; Amir A. Borhani, MD; Sally E. Carty, MD, FACS; Sue M. Challinor, MD; Amy E. Cox, MD; Barton Dudlick, (Acquisitions Editor); Matthew T. Heller, MD; Tara L. Henrichsen, MD; Nathan A. Johnson, MD; Judith M. Joyce, MD; Shane O. LeBeau, MD; Frank H. Miller, MD (Consulting Editor); Jason M. Ng, MD; N. Paul Ohori, MD; Tao Ouyang, MD; Carl C. Reading, MD; William E. Rothfus, MD, FACR; Karen E. Schoedel, MD; Amar B. Shah, MD; Biatta Sholosh, MD; Michael T. Stang, MD; Mitchell E. Tublin, MD (Guest Editor); Andrew Swihart, MD; and Linwah Yip, MD.

The authors/editors listed below have identified the following financial or professional relationships for themselves or their spouse/partner:

Klaus D. Hagspiel, MD (Test Author) is an industry funded research/investigator for Siemens Medical Solutions.

Disclosure of Discussion of Non-FDA Approved Uses for Pharmaceutical Products and/or Medical Devices.

The University of Virginia School of Medicine, as an ACCME provider, requires that all faculty presenters identify and disclose any off-label uses for pharmaceutical and medical device products. The University of Virginia School of Medicine recommends that each physician fully review all the available data on new products or procedures prior to clinical use.

TO ENROLL

To enroll in the Radiologic Clinics of North America Continuing Medical Education program, call customer service at 1-800-654-2452 or sign up online at http://www.theclinics.com/home/cme. The CME program is available to subscribers for an additional annual fee USD 245.

Radiologic Clinics of North America

THE CLINICS ARE NOW AVAILABLE ONLINE!

Access your subscription at:
www.theclinics.com

Preface
Endocrine Imaging

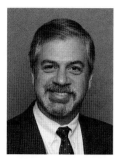

Mitchell E. Tublin, MD
Guest Editor

The central role of imaging in the diagnosis and management of patients with diseases of the endocrine system has been highlighted in the recent radiology, endocrine, and endocrine surgery literature. Imaging is the common link between the many specialties that take care of these often complicated and debilitated patients. In the first sections of this issue of *Radiologic Clinics*, an expert panel of specialists—many from a multidisciplinary group at the University of Pittsburgh—discusses the utility of imaging in the diagnosis and management of thyroid and parathyroid diseases. The impact of imaging upon clinical decision-making by the endocrinologist and the endocrine surgeon is highlighted. The importance of fine-needle aspiration technique, the potential benefits of refined cytology grading schemes, and the potential of molecular markers to triage the countless thyroid nodules encountered in clinical practice are assessed. The differential diagnosis of adrenal lesions, a tailored approach for the characterization of the incidental adrenal nodule, and the imaging manifestations of neuroendocrine tumors are described in the following articles. The imaging workup of pituitary lesions and other sellar lesions are addressed in a final review of neuroendocrinology.

The expertise of all of the contributors and their common sense approach to endocrinology and imaging are apparent in each of the articles. The care provided by the University of Pittsburgh multidisciplinary endocrinology group and the camaraderie of its members are unparalleled. It is an honor to be considered one of their peers. I also continue to learn from my colleagues and friends from the Mayo Clinic and Massachusetts General Hospital. I'm most indebted, however, for the love, support, and care given to me by the home team: my wonderful wife, Mary, and my sons, Daniel, Joshua, and Andrew.

Mitchell E. Tublin, MD
Division of Abdominal Imaging
Department of Radiology
University of Pittsburgh School of Medicine
200 Lothrop Street
Suite 3950 PST
Pittsburgh, PA 15213, USA

E-mail address:
tublme@UPMC.EDU

Radiol Clin N Am 49 (2011) xi
doi:10.1016/j.rcl.2011.04.001

Thyroid Ultrasound Part 1: Technique and Diffuse Disease

Biatta Sholosh, MD[a],*, Amir A. Borhani, MD[b]

KEYWORDS

- Thyroid • Ultrasound • Thyroiditis • Hashimoto's thyroiditis

Dramatic improvements in ultrasound resolution, coupled with the superficial location of the thyroid gland, have made ultrasound the primary imaging modality in the evaluation of focal and diffuse thyroid disease. Ultrasound is widely available, relatively inexpensive, painless, free of ionizing radiation, and does not require intravenous contrast. High-resolution transducers allow ultrasound penetration up to 5 cm and create high-definition images with a spatial resolution of 0.7 to 1.0 mm.[1]

A wide spectrum of diffuse diseases affects the thyroid gland (**Table 1**). The most common cause of diffuse thyroid disease is autoimmune thyroid disease (AITD): Hashimoto's thyroiditis and Graves disease are the most common autoimmune diseases, but the rarer subacute lymphocytic thyroiditis is also placed within the AITD spectrum. Thyroiditis is a generic term referring to a group of several common inflammatory conditions of the thyroid gland; it is characterized by lymphocytic infiltration of the gland leading to parenchymal destruction. If the thyroid follicles are destroyed slowly, as in Hashimoto's thyroiditis, hypothyroidism eventually results. If follicles are rapidly destroyed, as in subacute granulomatous and subacute lymphocytic thyroiditis, the release of preformed thyroid hormone stores into the blood stream causes transient thyrotoxicosis. Thyrotoxicosis is followed by a period of hypothyroidism until the thyroid recovers and thyroid hormone production resumes. On the other hand, hyperthyroidism in the setting of Graves disease and hyperfunctioning autonomous adenoma is caused by increased production of thyroid hormone. It is important to distinguish between these entities because they may have similar clinical presentation but their treatment varies. Graves disease must be treated with antithyroid drugs, radioisotope therapy, or subtotal thyroidectomy, whereas patients with destruction-induced thyrotoxicosis are treated conservatively.

The histology of autoimmune disease (lymphocytic parenchymal infiltration and follicular destruction) results in fewer sound reflectors, and thus accounts for the characteristic decreased echogenicity of the thyroid at ultrasound.[2,3] The clinical diagnosis is usually based on an algorithm of presenting symptoms, laboratory analysis of thyroid function, immunology, and occasionally radioactive iodine uptake scans.[4] Ultrasound is not generally required for the diagnosis of diffuse thyroid diseases; however, Hashimoto's thyroiditis is primarily a subclinical disease,[5] and ultrasound can detect this subset of patients before they come to clinical attention, when typical ultrasound findings are present. In addition, ultrasound has a role in excluding focal thyroid disease and in assessing the size of the thyroid.

In the classic imaging paradigm, ultrasound is useful to evaluate structure and radionuclide thyroid scintigraphy is used to assess function. Recently, color and spectral Doppler have also been used to assess function by measuring thyroid vascularity. Despite the seeming similarity in the imaging

The authors have nothing to disclose.

[a] Division of Abdominal Imaging, Department of Radiology, University of Pittsburgh Medical Center, 200 Lothrop Street, Pittsburgh, PA 15213, USA

[b] Department of Radiology, University of Pittsburgh Medical Center, 200 Lothrop Street, Pittsburgh, PA 15213, USA

* Corresponding author.

E-mail address: sholoshb@upmc.edu

Table 1
Diffuse thyroid disease (typical appearances are listed)

Thyroid Disorder	Grayscale Ultrasound	Color Doppler	Key Features
Graves thyroiditis	Enlarged, mildly hypoechoic, and heterogeneous	Markedly ↑	Markedly hyperemic; proptosis; hyperthyroid; +antithyroid antibodies
Hashimoto's thyroiditis	Enlarged, heterogeneous with lobular margins; hypoechoic and micronodular, septal lines	Highly variable: both ↑ and ↓ flow possible	+Antithyroid antibodies, hypothyroidism; cervical adenopathy
Subacute lymphocytic thyroiditis (painless)	Hypoechoic	*	+Antithyroid antibodies; postpartum; transient
De Quervain thyroiditis (subacute granulomatous)	Painful patchy areas of hypoechogenicity	↓ in the hypoechoic patch	Thyroid pain over area of hypoechogenicity; ↑ ESR
Acute suppurative thyroiditis	Abscess or infected linear tract in the thyroid	Normal background; no flow within an abscess	Acute presentation with signs of infection and pain; ↑ ESR; possible pyriform sinus fistula
Riedel thyroiditis	Large hypoechoic thyroid with course parenchyma	*	Large, rock-hard gland; encases adjacent structures
Medication-induced (ie, amiodarone) (AIT)	Type 1: abnormal thyroid Type 2: normal thyroid	Type 1: ↑ Type 2: absent	History of current or recent amiodarone use; hyperthyroid
Atrophic thyroiditis	Small, hypoechoic thyroid	↓	+Antithyroid antibodies; usually hypothyroid
Radiation thyroiditis	Small, hypoechoic thyroid	Variable	Known external beam or ^{131}I administration
Thyroid lymphoma	Large, ill-defined markedly hypoechoic nodules or masses with ↑ through transmission on background of Hashimoto's thyroiditis	↓ in the hypoechoic mass	Rapidly enlarging neck mass in patient with history of Hashimoto, ± adenopathy
Multinodular goiter	Closely opposed or interspersed, similar-appearing nodules replace parenchyma, course calcifications, variable cystic changes in nodules	Variable	Confluent nodules in a normal or enlarged thyroid; ± abnormal thyroid function tests

Abbreviations: AIT, amiodarone-induced thyrotoxicosis; ESR, erythrocyte sedimentation rate.
* Insufficient data.

features of diffuse thyroid diseases, it is important for the radiologist to be aware of the spectrum of imaging appearances of common thyroid diseases and the distinctive imaging appearance of rare conditions affecting the thyroid gland.

THYROID ANATOMY AND ULTRASOUND SCANNING TECHNIQUE

The thyroid is a butterfly-shaped, highly vascular gland located in the anterior neck superficial to the trachea and esophagus. It is surrounded by a pencil-thin echogenic capsule on ultrasound. The thyroid plays a critical role in the regulation of many metabolic functions, such as cardiac rate and output, lipid metabolism, and skeletal growth, as well as heat production.[6] The thyroid bed is confined by strap muscles anteriorly, sternocleidomastoid muscles anterolaterally, carotid and jugular vessels laterally, and trachea, esophagus, and longus colli muscles posteriorly (**Fig. 1**). The normal thyroid parenchyma has a characteristic homogeneous, medium-level to high-level echogenicity speckle pattern created by sound waves interacting with normal follicles.[7] The gland appears darker than the surrounding hyperechoic adipose tissue and brighter than adjacent hypoechoic neck muscles.

Thyroid size can be influenced by many factors, such as alcoholic cirrhosis, renal failure,[8] smoking, parity, iodine intake, and serum thyroid-stimulating hormone (TSH) concentration, use of oral contraceptives, gender, age, body mass index (BMI, calculated as weight in kilograms divided by the square of height in meters),[9] and treatment with thyroxine or radioactive iodine. It has been reported that lean body mass and body surface area are the major determinants of thyroid size[10,11] in non–iodine-deficient areas. In most adults, the thyroid measures between 4 and 6 cm in length and between 1.3 and 1.8 cm at the thickest antero-posterior dimension. A generous estimation of normal thickness of the thyroid isthmus is up to 4 to 6 mm.[12] The thyroid gland may be considered enlarged when the anteroposterior diameter of the lobe is more than 2 cm or if the isthmus is thicker than a few millimeters.[1,13] Calculation of the thyroid volume is based on the ellipsoid model.[14] The height, width, and depth of each lobe are multiplied, the product is then multiplied by a correction factor of 0.529, and both lobe volumes are added together.[15,16] The normal thyroid volume is 18.6 $\pm$ 4.5 mL ($\pm$ standard deviation), with mildly greater volume in males (19.6 $\pm$ 4.7) compared with females (17.5 $\pm$ 4.2).[17] If available, three-dimensional ultrasound has been shown to be more accurate compared with two-dimensional ultrasound for measurement of thyroid gland volume,[18] particularly if the thyroid is large and irregular (as in patients with multinodular goiter).

The clinical history and previous relevant imaging studies should be reviewed before starting the ultrasound study. Ultrasonographic examination of the thyroid is performed in accordance with the practice guidelines published by the American Institute of Ultrasound in Medicine[19] and the American College of Radiology.[20] The patient is placed in a supine position with a rolled towel placed underneath the shoulders to hyperextend the neck and better delineate the substernal space. Scanning is performed with a high-resolution linear-array 12-MHz to 15-MHz transducer. The frequency of the transducer can be changed during the study; a tradeoff is made between selecting the highest possible frequency to optimize spatial resolution and still maintain adequate sound penetration at the necessary tissue depth. A lower-frequency (5–7 MHz) curved transducer may be used to obtain a more accurate volumetric assessment when the thyroid is markedly enlarged and extends beyond the field of view attainable on the screen.[21]

Both lobes and isthmus of the thyroid gland should be scanned in a sequential manner. Appropriate images should be documented in axial and sagittal planes. Applying slight compression with the transducer improves visualization of microcalcifications and cystic areas in thyroid nodules; compression may also improve visualization of the deep tissues in the central compartment. Saving images in cine mode maximizes anatomic coverage of the neck and allows images to be viewed close to real time for later review. Panoramic images simultaneously depict both lobes for comparison of vascularity and echogenicity and allow the entire volume to be displayed on the monitor for accurate size determination.[22] Color

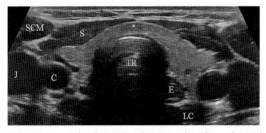

Fig. 1. Normal thyroid ultrasound. The thyroid (*asterisk*) is homogeneous and uniformly hyperechoic relative to the overlying strap muscle (S). The contour is smooth and size is normal. Note esophagus (E) posterior to the left lobe. SCM, sternocleidomastoid muscle; J, internal jugular vein; C, common carotid artery; LC, longus colli muscle; TR, trachea.

Doppler optimized for flow detection should be deliberately used to assess vascularity of the thyroid gland, any suspicious lymph nodes, and any detected focal nodules. Color Doppler may also increase the conspicuity of isoechoic thyroid nodules. Focal nodules are measured in 3 dimensions and studied for the level of echogenicity compared with normal parenchyma, presence and type of calcifications, cystic change, margins, presence of a halo, and the amount and distribution of blood flow.[13]

All patients should undergo an evaluation of the cervical lymph nodes as part of a routine thyroid ultrasound. Enlarged but morphologically normal-appearing cervical lymph nodes are common in patients with AITD (particularly Hashimoto's thyroiditis and can even be the first clue of this diagnosis. Lymph node mapping is particularly helpful when thyroid cancer has already been established[23] or when performing surveillance screening for recurrence after thyroidectomy. The likelihood that a suspicious-appearing thyroid nodule is thyroid cancer dramatically increases if malignant-appearing cervical nodes are detected.[24] In rare cases of aggressive papillary microcarcinoma, the only clue to the presence of thyroid cancer is detection of cervical adenopathy.[25] Thyroid cancer most commonly metastasizes to ipsilateral cervical lymph nodes but contralateral metastases are present up to 20% of the time; hence, both lateral nodal stations need to be examined.[26,27]

Tissues deep and inferior to the thyroid are also assessed for round or oval hypoechoic, hypervascular nodules when evaluating for enlarged parathyroid glands. Asking the patient to swallow and observing them in real time may help to elevate the lower aspect of a thyroid goiter or reveal a parathyroid gland lying deep to the clavicles.[28] It is also important to have the patients turn their head away from the side being imaged to sweep the deep cervical tissues and esophagus to the side being evaluated to improve detection of tracheoesophageal groove lesions. Occasionally, it is necessary to transiently decrease the transducer frequency (7–10 MHz) to improve sound penetration when the retrothyroid tissues are at an increased distance from the skin. Once a suspect nodule is detected, returning to higher frequencies allows better characterization.

Sonographic Technique Advances

Grayscale
The resolution of current ultrasound scanners is superb but such detailed resolution is a 2-edged sword. As smaller and smaller nodules are resolved, the clinical dilemma of how to manage this growing pool is being debated. A study performed by Guth and colleagues[29] showed that 35% more nodules were detected in a similar iodine-deficient population when imaging with a higher-resolution transducer (13 MHz) compared with 7 MHz.[30]

Several technical improvements have contributed to improved image quality. Compound imaging is a technique that averages images obtained simultaneously from different scanning angles. The images are combined into a single improved image in real time (as opposed to conventional scanning, in which images are generated from 1 angle of insonation). This technique reduces artifacts and speckle noise (the grainy appearance of the image), and improves contrast resolution. The increased contrast-to-noise ratio in thyroid images results in improved nodule conspicuity (**Fig. 2**).[31,32] Tissue harmonic imaging uses integral multiples of the transmitted frequency for image formation and results in images with improved signal-to-noise, reduced reverberation and side-lobe artifacts, and improved lateral resolution.[33,34] As with compound imaging, tissue harmonic imaging improves nodule border definition and contrast.[35,36] Although not truly a technical improvement, it is the investigators' opinion that the ability to record portions of sonographic examinations in a cine mode is indispensable. The cine mode is a series of rapidly recorded multiple images taken at sequential cycles of time. The images can be displayed in a dynamic movie format or they can be viewed as individual frames on the workstation. The thyroid (or thyroidectomy bed in patients with thyroid cancer) and the lateral compartment are captured in cine mode in the transverse, and when necessary, in the sagittal plane to improve

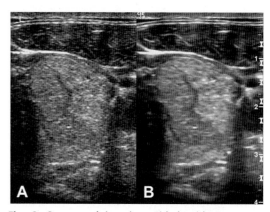

Fig. 2. Compound imaging. Side-by-side transverse views of the thyroid show a solid thyroid nodule without (*A*) and with (*B*) compound imaging. Image (*B*) is less grainy.

detection of pathologic lymph nodes and subtle thyroid nodule contour irregularity and microcalcifications. Cine virtual convex scanning may further improve anatomic coverage of the neck and thyroid. Captured cine sweeps are useful for the follow-up of a multinodular goiter when measurements of nodules are often difficult to accurately reproduce on static images alone.

Color and power Doppler

Color and power Doppler are both used to assess the degree of vascularity in the thyroid parenchyma and in nodules. Color Doppler is direction sensitive. Power Doppler may be more sensitive for detecting slow flow and it is independent of flow direction. Advanced dynamic flow (ADF) is a new technology in color flow imaging that provides superior spatial and temporal resolution, allowing more accurate measurement of blood flow. Quantitative measurement of thyroid blood flow (TBF) has been shown to be a promising method for distinguishing Graves from thyroiditis.[37]

Microbubbles

Microbubble contrast agents have been used in other organ systems. Results of studies assessing the role of microbubble contrast in the assessment of thyroid nodules have been mixed.[38] No benefit for microbubble assessment of diffuse thyroid disease has been shown.[39]

Elastography

Ultrasound elastography (USE) is a method for qualitative and quantitative estimation of tissue elasticity. It is analogous to physical palpation for evaluation of tissue stiffness of benign and malignant nodules. The rationale behind elastography is that a cancerous nodule is stiffer and that it deforms less than surrounding tissue. Elastography measures the amount of tissue deformation under applied stress. Stress can be created by external compression with a specially designed ultrasound transducer or by physiologic strain produced by a pulsating carotid artery. Depending on the method used, the data are either processed and displayed with a color map in real time in the former or postprocessed offline for the latter (**Fig. 3**). Offline postprocessing may take several hours.

Recent studies have shown the potential of USE in distinguishing between benign and malignant thyroid nodules. Rago and colleagues[40] showed a specificity and a sensitivity as high as 100% and 97%, respectively, with a positive predictive value (PPV) of 100% and negative predictive value (NPV) of 98% using external compression in 98 consecutive patients with a single thyroid nodule. USE has the potential to substantially reduce the number of fine-needle aspirations (FNAs) by 60.8%[41] because of the high specificity and NPV that can be achieved identifying benign nodules.[42] Vorlander and colleagues[43] achieved a 100% NPV in all the nodules stratified as soft using the strain index (in 96 of 309 patients, strain >0.31) in patients referred for surgery with dominant, nontoxic thyroid nodules. This technique may also play a role in selecting nodules that need to undergo biopsy in a multinodular thyroid as well as managing patients with nondiagnostic or indeterminate FNA (constituting approximately 30% of all FNAs). Promising work has recently been published by Rago and colleagues,[40] who looked at 195 nodules in 176 patients who were found to have indeterminate or nondiagnostic cytology on FNA and were able to undergo USE prior to surgical resection. The investigators reported an overall 94.9% sensitivity, 90.3% specificity, PPV of 71.1%, NPV of 98.6%, and an accuracy of 91.3% of USE in predicting malignancy. Soft nodules with high elasticity, which represent the largest proportion (73%) of nodules with indeterminate or nondiagnostic cytology, were highly associated with a benign histology. Although many patients with inconclusive biopsies currently

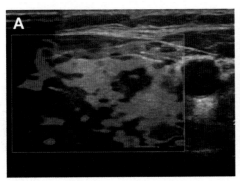
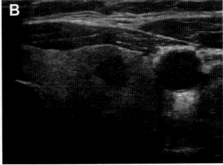

Fig. 3. Elastogram (*A*) and conventional ultrasound images (*B*) show a 7-mm left-lobe irregular solid papillary microcarcinoma, showing a homogeneously hard blue pattern.

receive surgical resection, presurgical risk stratification may reduce the number of benign thyroidectomies. A recent abstract from a meta-analysis including 8 studies with overall 639 thyroid nodules showed a mean sensitivity and specificity of 92% and 96% for the diagnosis of malignant thyroid nodules,[44] whereas mean sensitivity and specificity of FNA has been reported to be 83% and 92%, respectively.[45] Although this emerging technique is promising, it has limitations related to nodule selection. Rim or coarsely calcified nodules, those with cystic areas greater than 25% and isthmus nodules (when measuring carotid-artery–induced strain) are not amenable to USE. Because the nodule to be examined must be clearly distinguishable from other nodules, multinodular goiters with coalescent nodules are not suitable for this analysis. These encouraging feasibility studies suggest that sonoelastography may play a pivotal role in a cost-effective strategy to stratify ultrasound (and potentially FNA) indeterminate nodules in a noninvasive way. Additional validation with prospective studies is needed. There is no established role for elastography in the diagnosis of diffuse thyroid diseases.

DIFFUSE THYROID DISEASE
Hashimoto's Thyroiditis

Hashimoto's thyroiditis, synonymous with chronic lymphocytic thyroiditis (CLT), is the most common form of thyroiditis and is the most common cause of hypothyroidism in the United States.[46] As with other autoimmune diseases, women are more commonly affected than men, with an 8 to 9:1 female/male ratio.[47] Up to 2% of all women are affected.[48] The disease usually develops in young or middle-aged women who are genetically predisposed and leads to progressive thyroid failure at a rate of 4% per year in women with positive antithyroid antibodies and increased serum TSH.[49] Patients typically present with a painless, lobular, diffusely enlarged thyroid gland, often in the setting of hypothyroidism; the diagnosis is confirmed by the presence of serum autoantibodies to thyroglobulin and thyroid peroxidase.[46] The pathologic hallmark of all AITDs is thyroid infiltration by cytotoxic T cells and B-cell lymphocytes as well as plasma cells. Infiltration results in the typical histopathologic changes of Hashimoto's thyroiditis: lymphoplasmacytic aggregates with germinal centers, atrophic thyroid follicles, oxyphilic change of the epithelial cells (Hurthle cells), and variable fibrosis.[50] Because not all patients have antithyroid antibodies and many are euthyroid at the time of diagnosis, ultrasound is a useful adjunct to suggest the diagnosis when it is clinically unsuspected.[51]

Histopathologic changes of diffuse lymphocytic infiltration and severe thyroid follicle destruction lead to reduced thyroid echogenicity at ultrasound.[2] In Hashimoto's thyroiditis, diffuse thyroid hypoechogenicity is highly predictive of either current or future hypothyroidism.[52] Studies using an objective quantitative analysis of the degree of hypoechogenicity of the thyroid in patients with Hashimoto's thyroiditis compared with normal subjects showed that the degree of hypoechogenicity correlates positively with the likelihood and severity of hypothyroidism.[53,54] Although hypoechogenicity of the thyroid is a well-established parameter for detecting AITD, it has poor specificity in morbidly obese patients. Thyroid hypoechogenicity was believed to be present in 64.8% of clinically and biochemically euthyroid patients with BMI of more than 40 who underwent thyroid ultrasound.[55]

Ultrasound features of Hashimoto's thyroiditis parallel the varied clinical presentation and histopathologic changes.[56] Hence, sonographic appearances vary based on severity of follicular disruption, lymphocytic infiltration, chronicity of disease and extent of thyroid involvement. Several characteristic sonographic features have been described in patients with Hashimoto's thyroiditis. The parenchyma is heterogeneous and coarsened compared with normal thyroid. The color Doppler appearance is highly variable but either normal or increased vascularity may be shown early in the disease (Fig. 4). Deceased vascularity may be shown later in the disease course. The increase in hypervascularity seems to be associated with development of hypothyroidism, which may be caused by trophic stimulation of the thyroid by TSH.[57] The presence of innumerable hypoechoic solid micronodules ranging in size from 1 to 7 mm surrounded by an echogenic rim of fibrosis is highly specific for this disease, with an almost 95% PPV (Fig. 5).[58] At histology, these nodules correspond to parenchymal lymphocytic and plasma cell infiltrates.[50] As thyroid parenchyma is progressively destroyed, the thyroid develops echogenic linear bands of parenchymal fibrosis, which can become confluent and thicker (Fig. 6). Occasionally, involvement of the thyroid is asymmetric with preferential involvement of the anterior aspect of the gland (Fig. 7). Eventually in end-stage disease, the gland becomes atrophic and diffusely hypoechoic, similar to that of strap muscles (Fig. 8).

Several enlarged, and occasionally atypical-appearing, central compartment lymph nodes (Fig. 9) are usually found adjacent to the lower

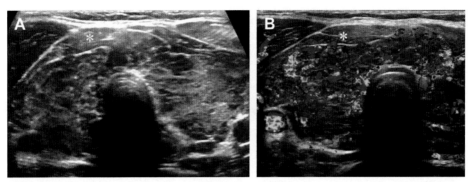

Fig. 4. Hashimoto's thyroiditis. (A) Transverse image through the midline shows a coarsened, hypoechoic, and heterogeneous gland. Thyroid parenchyma is isoechoic compared with the strap muscles (*asterisk*), and the margins appear lobular. Parenchyma is coarsened because of bright fibrous linear bands separating the hypoechoic parenchyma into patchy areas and micronodulation. Both lobes and isthmus are thickened. (B) Color Doppler of the thyroid in the same patient shows moderately to markedly increased flow. Vascular flow on color Doppler is variable in Hashimoto.

poles of both lobes.[59] These reactive lymph nodes are easily recognized and are a useful clue to the diagnosis. However, in those with Hashimoto's thyroiditis and coexisting hyperparathyroidism, detection of potential parathyroid adenomas becomes more difficult, because the grayscale appearance of a parathyroid adenoma and reactive central compartment nodes can be similar. The use of color Doppler to identify a vascular arch around a parathyroid adenoma as opposed to central hilar flow typical of a lymph node is useful, although a nuclear medicine sestamibi parathyroid scan becomes indispensible in this circumstance. Although reactive lymph nodes seen in Hashimoto's thyroiditis are mildly enlarged and hypoechoic, the presence of microcalcifications, cystic change, peripheral vascularization on color Doppler, echogenic lymph node cortex, loss of fatty hilum, and round shape are features concerning for malignant lymph node metastases, particularly from thyroid cancer.[60]

Occasionally, Hashimoto's thyroiditis can present as a focal nodule (**Fig. 10**) or nodules within a diffusely altered parenchyma or within a sonographically normal thyroid gland.[61] This form of nodular thyroiditis is found in 5% of all nodule biopsies.[62] No distinguishing sonographic features of nodular Hashimoto's thyroiditis permit a specific diagnosis. Nonetheless, one study has suggested that the most common pattern observed was that of a hyperechoic solid nodule (**Fig. 13**). The so-called "white-knight" likely represents a regenerative nodule of Hashimoto's thyroiditis.[63] However, caution should be exercised not to assume a nodule is benign simply based on hyperechogenicity, since a small subset of thyroid cancer can appear echogenic on ultrasound. Ill-defined margins, cystic changes, and intranodular calcifications were also occasionally observed.[62] It is not known whether this represents a less severe form of Hashimoto or a separate subtype.

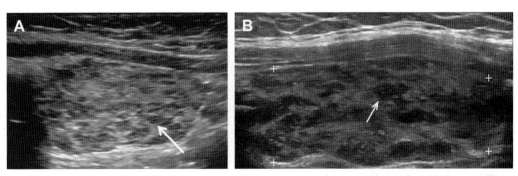

Fig. 5. Micronodular pattern in Hashimoto's thyroiditis. (A) Sagittal image of the thyroid shows diffuse, ill-marginated innumerable small hypoechoic nodules (*arrow*) surrounded by echogenic stroma termed "micronodulation," a finding specific for Hashimoto's thyroiditis. (B) Sagittal image of the thyroid in another patient with Hashimoto's thyroiditis shows Swiss-cheese appearance. Diffuse small hypoechoic lesions (*arrow*) in the thyroid create pseudocystic appearance.

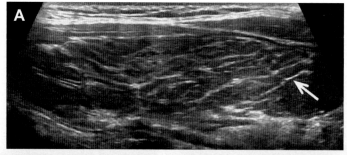

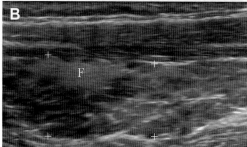

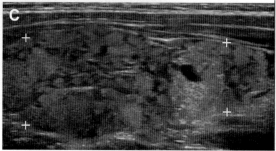

Fig. 6. Coarse septations in Hashimoto's thyroiditis. (*A*) Sagittal images of the thyroid in a patient with Hashimoto's thyroiditis show multiple course echogenic linear septations (*arrow*), representing fibrous bands. These septal lines are mostly oriented in the long axis of the gland. (*B*) Another case of Hashimoto's thyroiditis with thicker echogenic bands of fibrosis (F) separating coarse hypoechoic parenchyma. Thin septal lines are also present in the background. (*C*) "Bag of marbles" appearance; innumerable hyperechoic nodules represent areas of fibrosis.

Thyroid lymphoma is uncommon; it accounts for less than 5% of all thyroid malignancies[64] but when present it almost always develops in patients with underlying Hashimoto's thyroiditis. It has been established that Hashimoto's thyroiditis is a risk factor for development of thyroid lymphoma. One study showed that the relative risk of malignant thyroid lymphoma in these patients is 67 times increased compared with baseline.[48,65] The patient with thyroid lymphoma classically presents with a rapidly enlarging thyroid gland. Ultrasound reveals a solid, markedly hypoechoic,

ill-marginated mass in a background of chronic thyroiditis (**Fig. 11**). Lymphoma can be classified into nodular, diffuse, and mixed subtypes on ultrasound; however, the key diagnostic finding in all subtypes is enhanced through transmission posterior to the lesion (**Fig. 12**).[66] Thyroid lymphoma can be diagnosed on fine-needle aspiration biopsy (FNAB) with flow cytometry and immunohistochemistry. Core biopsy, open surgical biopsy or thyroidectomy is reserved for cases

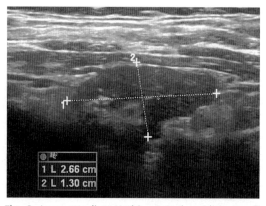

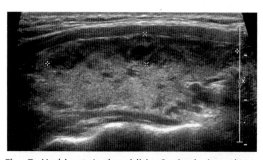

Fig. 7. Hashimoto's thyroiditis. Sagittal view shows patchy hypoechogenicity preferentially involving the anterior aspect of the thyroid (*marked by the calipers*). This area was more hypervascular on color Doppler (not shown) than the deeper aspect. Note the scattered micronodules in the remainder of the gland surrounded by normal background thyroid.

Fig. 8. Long-standing Hashimoto's thyroiditis. Small, markedly hypoechoic thyroid gland in a patient on long-term thyroid hormone replacement for hypothyroidism. Variable amount of echogenic fibrosis and lobular thyroid margins can be seen.

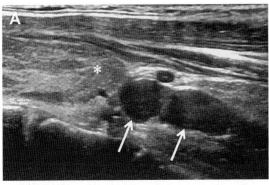
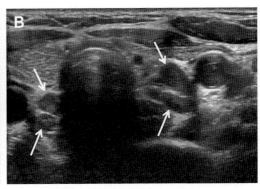

Fig. 9. Hashimoto's thyroiditis with hyperplastic adenopathy. Longitudinal (*A*) and transverse (*B*) images of the inferior thyroid in 2 different patients show enlarged, hyperplastic central compartment nodes (*arrows*) with thick, hypoechoic cortex inferior or deep to the lower pole. When present, these are often a clue to the diagnosis. Enlarged lateral compartment nodes can also be seen. Notice decreased echogenicity in the inferior aspect of the imaged thyroid gland (*asterisk*).

in which FNAB is unavailable or the diagnosis cannot be confirmed by FNA alone.[67] Surgical treatment of thyroid lymphoma is performed only if the trachea is markedly compressed by tumor; otherwise, thyroid lymphoma is the only thyroid malignancy treated nonsurgically: a combination of chemotherapy and external beam radiation is used.[68] When disease is confined to the thyroid gland, the prognosis is good.

Although still controversial, numerous studies have shown an increased frequency of papillary thyroid cancer in patients with Hashimoto.[69,70] It is unclear if this apparent increase may be

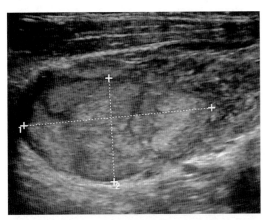

Fig. 10. Nodular Hashimoto's thyroiditis. This type of nodule has been recognized as a benign pattern seen in Hashimoto's thyroiditis. It was described by Bonavita and colleagues[63] as looking like a giraffe hide, consisting of bright blocks separated by dark bands. The background thyroid is hypoechoic and coarsened with micronodularity typical of diffuse Hashimoto's thyroiditis. FNA biopsy showed CLT. This nodule is a variation of the homogeneously echogenic nodule referred to as "white-knight" (see **Fig. 13**).

because of increased detection of cancer in this population[71] or if there is a pathologic and causative link between differentiated thyroid cancer and AITD.[72] A recent single-center prospective study in patients newly diagnosed with thyroid nodules found no significant difference between the malignancy rate of 1.0% in a cohort of 164 patients with underlying Hashimoto's thyroiditis. The incidence of thyroid cancer in the 551-person control group was 2.7%, using cytopathologic correlation.[73] The sonographic features of benign and malignant nodules within a gland affected by diffuse Hashimoto's thyroiditis are generally similar to their counterparts in the general population.[74] However, when diffuse thyroid abnormalities are present, detection of focal nodules, particularly thyroid carcinoma, is more difficult. A solid hypoechoic papillary cancer could be masked in a hypoechoic, heterogeneous thyroid gland containing pseudonodules from lymphocytic infiltrates and fibrosis. Nonetheless, a higher percentage of malignant nodules in glands with background Hashimoto have calcifications. All types of calcifications (microcalcifications, tiny nonspecific nonshadowing bright reflectors, macrocalcifications, and peripheral eggshell calcifications) (**Fig. 13**) are observed with greater frequency in this patient subset.[74] The frequency of psammoma bodies is lower, whereas the presence of dense calcifications is higher in papillary thyroid cancer in a Hashimoto's thyroid compared with papillary thyroid cancer in a normal thyroid.[75] Not only can the parenchymal heterogeneity and hypoechogenicity characteristic of Hashimoto's thyroiditis lead to false-negative studies (a malignant nodule is obscured because of surrounding parenchymal distortion) (**Fig. 14**), false-positive ultrasound examinations (a nodule is perceived

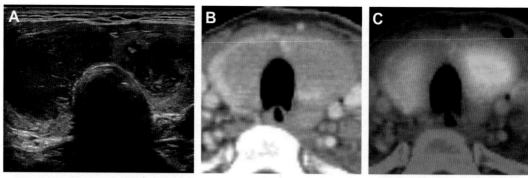

Fig. 11. Hashimoto's thyroiditis with lymphoma. (A) Profoundly hypoechoic large expansile masses were found in both lobes because of mixed type pattern of B-cell lymphoma in this patient presenting with rapidly enlarging thyroid mass. Cervical adenopathy was present (not shown). Masses were low density on computed tomography (B) and were intensely hypermetabolic on fluorodeoxyglucose-positron emission tomography scan (C).

within surrounding heterogeneous parenchyma) (Fig. 15) also occur. Careful, real-time examination, the use of cine images to differentiate true nodules from background heterogeneity, and actively searching for parenchymal calcifications is essential when evaluating for thyroid cancer. The Society of Radiologists in Ultrasound (SRU) consensus guidelines are then applied to triage each individual nodule.[71] FNA biopsy can be used in cases in which the distinction cannot be made. Rapidly enlarging and markedly hypoechoic masses in this patient subset should be evaluated with biopsy to exclude lymphoma. The use of USE may soon have a larger role to play in evaluating the gland for thyroid cancer in the difficult cases.

Graves Disease

Graves disease is a common autoimmune disorder; it occurs in 1.5–2.0% of women in the United States.[76] The disease is caused by binding of thyroid autoantibodies to the thyrotropin receptor on the follicular cells. Autoantibody binding stimulates the cells as though TSH triggered the receptor. The result is increased hormone synthesis and secretion, and growth of the thyroid gland. Diffuse hypertrophy and hyperplasia of follicular cells with colloid depletion and lymphoid infiltration are shown at histology.[76] The diagnosis is typically made in the hyperthyroid patient who presents with diffuse thyroid enlargement (diffuse toxic goiter). Secondary findings (ie, orbitopathy) may be identified in a small subset of patients with long-standing disease.

There are no specific grayscale ultrasound findings of Graves disease; findings suggestive of the

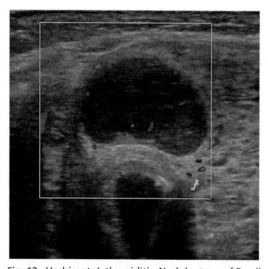

Fig. 12. Hashimoto's thyroiditis. Nodular type of B-cell lymphoma in the isthmus shows relative hypovascularity on color Doppler with typical increased through-transmission, an important finding that suggests lymphoma. Background thyroid shows micronodules. (Courtesy of Mitchell E. Tublin, MD, Pittsburgh, PA.)

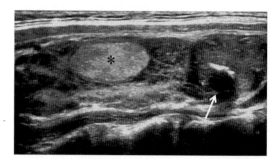

Fig. 13. Hashimoto's thyroiditis with coexistent papillary thyroid cancer and benign focal Hashimoto nodule. Lower pole focal nodule is solid and hypoechoic with course internal calcification and fine bright reflector (arrow) that proved to be a papillary thyroid cancer. The asterisk denotes an echogenic solid nodule with hypoechoic halo that has been referred to as "white-knight" and is thought to be a regenerative nodule in Hashimoto's thyroiditis.

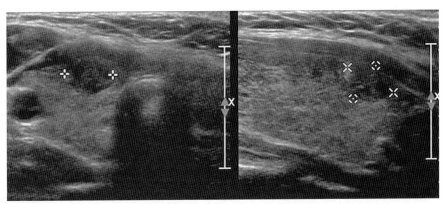

Fig. 14. Hashimoto's thyroiditis with papillary thyroid cancer. Calipers denote a subtle hypoechoic nodule in a patient with background Hashimoto that proved to be a papillary thyroid cancer. The nodule was more discrete in real time but easily blends in to the adjacent hypoechoic parenchyma on the sagittal view.

disease include diffuse enlargement, convex bowing of the anterior gland margin, and mild textural coarsening (**Fig. 16**). The echogenicity of the gland can be normal but it is often decreased to variable degrees because of increased intrathyroidal blood flow, functional changes in thyroid follicles with increased cellularity and decreased colloid content (resulting in reduction of cell/colloid interfaces), and lymphocytic infiltration. While the grayscale appearance of the thyroid in goitrous Hashimoto's thyroiditis is similar to Graves disease, the latter thyroid parenchyma typically is less heterogenous and the contour is less lobular.

Early color Doppler studies suggested that the thyroid inferno pattern[77] could be useful to differentiate between Graves and Hashimoto disease. Further work has suggested that color and spectral Doppler ultrasound might distinguish thyrotoxicosis caused by hormone overproduction from Graves disease from those with gland destruction

related to thyroiditis.[78–80] Although thyroid scintigraphy still plays a critical role in the diagnostic workup of hyperthyroidism,[81] color and spectral Doppler interrogation has been shown to differentiate Graves disease from the other causes of hyperthyroidism with high specificity. An added advantage of ultrasound is that it may also identify nodules.[82–86] Normal thyroid parenchyma shows occasional spots of flow on color Doppler; peak systolic velocities between 15 and 30 cm/s in the inferior thyroid artery and 3 to 5 cm/s in the intrathyroid arteries are considered within the range of normal.[87] Patients with untreated, active Graves disease show markedly increased vascularity at color Doppler, approximately 15-fold higher TBF measured in mL/min compared with normal,[88] and high peak systolic velocity flow on spectral Doppler in the medium-sized perithyroid and intrathyroid arteries. Saleh and colleagues[85] found that a threshold peak thyroid artery systolic velocity of more than 60 cm/s had a 100% specificity and 80% sensitivity for distinguishing Graves from other causes of diffuse toxic goiter. This increased flow is believed to be caused by thyroid stimulation from activation of the TSH receptor rather than increased levels of thyroid hormone.[89,90] Another study found that peak systolic velocity in the perithyroid artery was significantly higher in Graves disease than in Hashimoto's thyroiditis (48 ± 12.3 vs 21.7 ± 8.4 cm/s).[83] The investigators did not suggest a cutoff value for their differentiation. Advanced dynamic flow is a recently developed high-resolution power Doppler mode that can be used as a quantitative method for calculating TBF. Special software is used to calculate the percentage of flow in a region of interest. Using this technique, TBF was significantly higher in Graves disease than in patients with painless thyroiditis, subacute thyroiditis, or normal

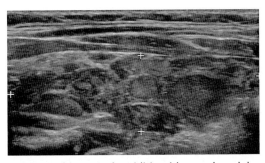

Fig. 15. Hashimoto's thyroiditis with pseudonodules. Thin and thicker fibrous septa separating the hypoechoic thyroid into lobules create the appearance of pseudonodules, causing parenchymal coarsening seen in this disease. When it is unclear if a nodule is present, FNA may be needed.

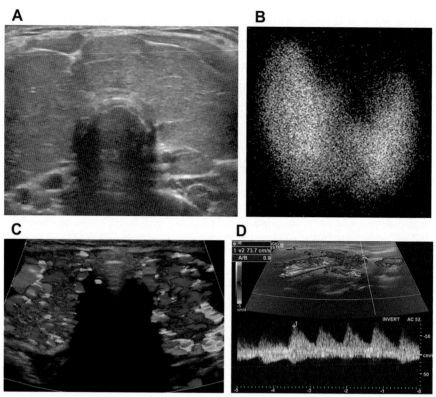

Fig. 16. Graves disease. (*A*) Diffusely enlarged, hypoechoic thyroid gland with mild heterogeneity on grayscale is not specific for Graves. (*B*) Thyroid scintigraphy shows increased tracer accumulation consistent with Graves disease. (*C*) Color Doppler reveals marked increased in hypervascularity in the parenchyma termed thyroid inferno. (*D*) Peak systolic velocity measured in the inferior thyroid artery in a different patient with long-standing untreated Graves disease measures 74 cm/s. Peak systolic velocity measurements greater than 60 cm/s are reported to be specific for Graves disease.

controls. Hence, all patients with Graves disease showed a TBF greater than 4%, whereas TBF in all other patients was less than 4%, signifying that 4% could be used as the discriminatory cutoff for distinguishing Graves disease from destruction-induced thyrotoxicosis. These findings correlated with radioactive iodine uptake scans.[37]

Thyroid vascularity and thyroid artery volumetric flow have been shown to be significantly higher when the disease was most active as determined by clinical and laboratory criteria, suggesting color Doppler imaging may be a useful marker for disease activity to monitor treatment response.[79] A significant decrease in flow velocities in the superior and inferior thyroid arteries after medical treatment has been reported. Low thyroid echogenicity and high flow in the thyroid artery and glandular parenchyma before starting medical therapy were also shown to be specific for the prediction of relapse of hyperthyroidism at the end of the treatment. Thyroid glands with low initial echogenicity showed a 93% relapse rate after treatment with methimazole was completed. The relapse rate dropped to 55% when initial thyroid echogenicity was normal.[91]

Treatment options include antithyroid medications and thyroid ablation with radioactive iodine. Radioiodine ablation should not be performed if a malignant lesion is suspected, and ultrasound-guided FNAB should precede treatment.[45] Surgical resection is reserved for patients who have contraindication to other options or when there is significant mass effect on surrounding structures.[92] Radioiodine therapy results in marked scarring and atrophy of the thyroid gland.[93] The ablated thyroid appears small and heterogeneous at ultrasound (**Fig. 17**) and is referred to as radiation thyroiditis.

De Quervain Thyroiditis

De Quervain thyroiditis also known as de Quervain's thyroiditis, subacute granulomatous thyroiditis, nonsuppurative thyroiditis or subacute thyroiditis, is an uncommon, self-limiting, inflammatory thyroid disease. It is most commonly seen in middle-aged women and often follows a viral upper respiratory tract infection. Patients with subacute granulomatous thyroiditis typically

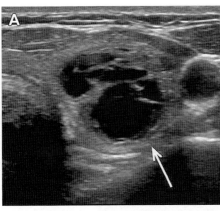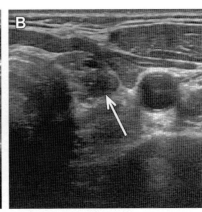

Fig. 17. Postradioablation thyroiditis. Hyperthyroid patient with Graves disease before (*A*) and after (*B*) treatment with radioiodine ablation. Both the thyroid and the incidental complex cystic colloid nodule have markedly decreased in size (*arrow*). Development of focal nodules has been described in end-stage radiation thyroiditis.

present with an enlarged, painful thyroid gland, low-grade fever, occasional dysphagia, suppressed levels of TSH, and an increased erythrocyte sedimentation rate. Pain is believed to be caused by stretching of the thyroid capsule from the underlying inflammation and edema. During the initial inflammatory phase, microabscesses form as follicles are replaced with neutrophils. Later, the macrophages and multinucleated giant cells that surround damaged follicles stimulate a granulomatous process.[76] Thyrotoxicosis occurs with follicular disruption and hormone release. A transient period of hypothyroidism often ensues. Follicles regenerate in the healing phase; hence, most patients usually recover complete thyroid function and return to a euthyroid state. If thyrotoxicosis is the presenting symptom, a radioiodine scan may be needed to confirm thyroiditis by showing diminished or absent uptake.

Ultrasound is useful to confirm the initial diagnosis and for follow-up of patients with subacute thyroiditis. The ultrasound examination is also helpful because it may identify focal nodules and help exclude other causes of neck pain. The imaging manifestations of the disease parallel the disease course: abnormalities detected by all modalities tend to resolve when the clinical symptoms abate. The characteristic ultrasound findings for this disorder are ill-defined, moderately, or markedly patchy hypoechoic areas of thyroid parenchyma that show little to no vascular flow on color Doppler interrogation (**Figs. 18** and **19**). Hypoechoic areas tend to elongate along the long axis of the thyroid; these regions can involve one area or both thyroid lobes and extend across the isthmus. Half of patients presenting with unilateral thyroid pain have bilateral hypoechoic areas of

involvement.[94] When the condition is severe, affected regions can expand the capsule. A presumptive diagnosis may be made when ill-defined hypoechoic lesions on ultrasound correspond to the patient's area of pain. Ultrasound features of malignancy (microcalcifications and taller-than-wide shape) are absent. Localized pain is also atypical in thyroid malignancy. FNAB is useful in those cases in which the hypoechoic areas cannot be distinguished from thyroid malignancy; histologic findings in thyroiditis characteristically shows multinucleated giant cells and mononuclear infiltrate. The imaging differential diagnosis includes other causes that create decreased parenchymal echogenicity although they are usually painless, such as lymphocytic thyroiditis, Graves disease, lymphoma, multinodular goiter, or occasionally thyroid malignancy. Short-term follow-up ultrasound may be useful to document regression or resolution.[95,96]

On computed tomography (CT), the involved areas of subacute thyroiditis show decreased attenuation because of follicular disruption and loss of iodine concentration (physiologic thyroid iodine concentration is responsible for thyroid attenuation between 80 and 100 HU at CT).[97] Low radioiodine uptake is shown at scintigraphy; however, uptake returns to normal when the patient returns to a euthyroid state. Magnetic resonance (MR) imaging findings reported in small series include ill-marginated areas of mild T1 signal hyperintensity with corresponding T2-weighted signal marked hyperintensity compared with the normal background thyroid signal.[98] A single case report suggested that the focal fluorodeoxyglucose uptake with subacute thyroiditis may mimic thyroid malignancy.[99] Patients are treated conservatively with antiinflammatory medications and corticosteroids.

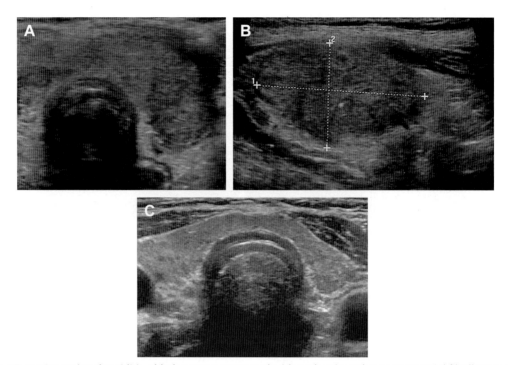

Fig. 18. De Quervain's thyroiditis. Elderly woman presented with neck pain and new-onset atrial fibrillation with transient hyperthyroidism 1 month after a viral upper respiratory tract infection. Transverse (*A*) and sagittal (*B*) ultrasound showed a poorly circumscribed, masslike enlargement of the upper left thyroid lobe extending into the isthmus with bulging of the overlying capsule. ^{123}I scan (not shown) showed markedly low iodine uptake and 2 FNA biopsies showed no malignant cells but were interpreted as lesion of undermined significance. (*C*) Repeat ultrasound approximately 5 months later showed complete sonographic resolution, supporting the diagnosed of subacute thyroiditis.

Subacute Lymphocytic Thyroiditis

Subacute lymphocytic thyroiditis is a self-limited, autoimmune disorder that comprises 29% to 50% of all cases of thyroiditis.[47] It occurs most often in women 30 to 50 years of age with increased thyroid peroxidase antibodies,[100,101] although on average the antibody levels are lower than that in Hashimoto's thyroiditis.[102] Subacute lymphocytic thyroiditis is believed to be a less severe transient, or subacute, form of Hashimoto's thyroiditis. Subacute lymphocytic thyroiditis occurring sporadically is termed painless thyroiditis or silent sporadic thyroiditis, but when it occurs within 1 year after parturition it is termed painless postpartum thyroiditis (PPT) or postpartum thyroiditis. Geographic and methodological differences probably account for a wide range of reported rates, but the mean prevalence of postpartum thyroiditis is 7.2% to and the mean incidence is 7.8% of

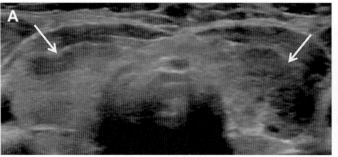
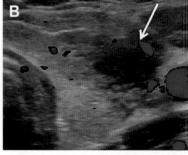

Fig. 19. De Quervain's thyroiditis. (*A*) Panoramic ultrasound of the thyroid shows bilateral broad bands of hypoechogenicity in the ventral aspect of the gland (*arrows*) in this patient who presented with tenderness of the larger left lobe lesion. (*B*) Color Doppler view of the left lobe shows typical decreased perfusion in the area of thyroiditis. (*Courtesy of* Mitchell E. Tublin, MD, Pittsburgh, PA.)

women.[103,104] The prevalence rate triples in women with type 1 diabetes.[105,106] The disease recurs in 69% of women in subsequent pregnancy.[107] Postpartum thyroiditis is believed to occur as a consequence of the immunologic flare after the immune suppression of pregnancy in genetically susceptible women.

The disease is characterized pathologically by lymphocytic infiltration of the thyroid similar to Hashimoto's thyroiditis, with the main difference being relative lack of oncocytic metaplasia, minimal to absent follicular atrophy and mild to no fibrosis.[50] Clinically, patients present with transient thyrotoxicosis followed by hypothyroidism or any combination of the two 1 to 6 months (usually 4–6 weeks) after childbirth. Symptoms usually resolve clinically and radiographically by the end of the first postpartum year.[103] There may be thyroid enlargement. Although most patients regain normal thyroid function, up to one-quarter to one-third develop permanent hypothyroidism within the next 10 years.

Although the role of ultrasound in this entity is limited, the characteristic ultrasound appearance is thyroid hypoechogenicity (**Fig. 20**), as in other forms of autoimmune thyroid disease. A prospective study showed that thyroid-antibody–positive women who developed PPT were more likely to show typical sonographic findings of thyroid hypoechogenicity compared with both antibody-positive women who did not develop PPT and a control group composed of antibody-negative women. In a subset of patients with PPT, thyroid gland hypoechogenicity preceded hypothyroidism,[107] suggesting it may be useful for identifying patients at increased risk. The usefulness of thyroid ultrasound as an independent predictor of long-term thyroid dysfunction in patients with PPT is still unclear.[108] As with De Quervain thyroiditis, when patients present with thyrotoxicosis, thyroid scintigraphy showing low radioiodine uptake is useful in distinguishing PPT from Graves disease.[107]

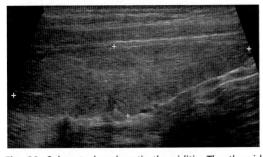

Fig. 20. Subacute lymphocytic thyroiditis. The thyroid parenchyma is mildly heterogeneous and mildly diffusely hypoechoic similar to the overlying strap muscle.

Acute Suppurative Thyroiditis

The abundant blood supply of the thyroid, its excellent lymphatic drainage, encapsulation, and high iodine content make the gland resistant to bacterial infection.[46] Acute suppurative thyroiditis is therefore an uncommon[109] but potentially life-threatening[110] infectious diseases of the thyroid. It usually affects children and young adults who have congenital fourth branchial pouch sinus tracts, especially when they present with recurrent suppurative thyroiditis.[46] These usually extend from the left (92%)[111] pyriform recess to the thyroid gland. Elderly, immunocompromised, and debilitated patients[46] can be affected by hematogenous or lymphatic seeding, or direct spread from pharyngeal or other regional infections.[112] The most common predisposing factor in adults seems to be underlying thyroid disease (ie, multinodular goiter, Hashimoto's thyroiditis, or thyroid carcinoma).[46] Infection is most often caused by a bacterial organism such as *Staphylococcus* or *Streptococcus* species, but polymicrobial infection is also common.[113] Acute suppurative thyroiditis presents with rapid onset of thyroid pain, fever, dysphagia, dysphonia, and compressive symptoms. Leukocytosis and increased erythrocyte sedimentation levels are often present.

Contrast-enhanced CT is useful in the acute setting to evaluate the extent of infection within and beyond the thyroid gland and depict the presence of an abscess. Unlike sonography, CT has the advantage of being able to evaluate the pharynx and superior mediastinum. The main role of sonography is to identify and provide guidance for percutaneous drainage of thyroid abscesses. Sonographic findings are generally nonspecific. The thyroid may appear enlarged and hypoechoic secondary to inflammation. Focal accumulation of complex fluid containing bright echoes from gas suggests an abscess. An infected sinus tract to the pyriform sinus is suspected when a left-sided, irregular tubular tract containing complex echoes extends from the thyroid gland superiorly into the neck (**Fig. 21**).[114] Patients with suspected pyriform sinus fistulae should undergo a barium esophagram when the infection is quiescent or direct inspection by endoscopic hypopharyngoscopy.[115] Fistulae are usually managed surgically, although there has been a trend toward less invasive treatment such as chemocauterization with trichloroacetic acid into the fistula opening on direct endoscopy.[115] The remaining cases are treated with aggressive antibiotics and drainage of any formed abscess.[113]

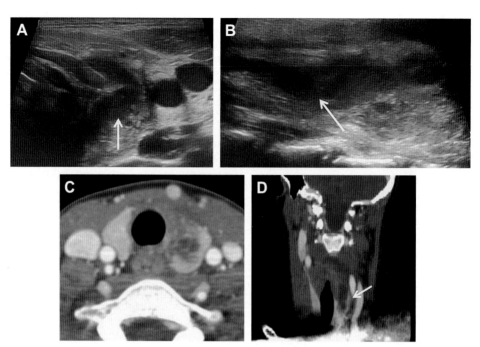

Fig. 21. Acute suppurative thyroiditis. This 17-year-old woman presented with repeated episodes of acute neck pain with fever requiring hospital admission. (*A*) Transverse and (*B*) longitudinal ultrasound images through the upper pole and axial (*C*) and coronal oblique (*D*) reconstructed contrast-enhanced neck CT images showed a tubular tract extending laterally from the hypopharynx into the left thyroid substance (*arrow*) containing complex fluid representing an infected pyriform sinus-thyroid fistula. Culture of the fine-needle aspirate fluid grew methicillin-resistant *Staphylococcus aureus*. Because of recurrent symptoms after antibiotic therapy, the patient required left thyroid lobectomy. (*Courtesy of* Ka-Kai Ngan, MD, Pittsburgh, PA.)

Simple/multinodular Goiter

Goiter refers to generalized enlargement of the thyroid. It can be seen with most diffuse (or nodular) thyroid diseases. Simple diffuse nontoxic goiter refers to diffuse, nonnodular thyroid enlargement in a euthyroid patient (**Fig. 22**), which may eventually progress to multinodular goiter in the absence of underlying thyroid disease. The cause of simple goiter is multifactorial and involves complex interactions between environmental (iodine intake), genetic, and endogenous (female gender) factors.[116] The most common cause of goiter outside the United States is dietary iodine deficiency. To compensate for inadequate thyroid hormone output, follicular epithelium undergoes compensatory hypertrophy to achieve a euthyroid state.[97] Pathologically, the nodularity observed in multinodular goiter consists of ordinary, polyclonal follicles that expand in a nodular fashion because they replicate within a mold made out of a poorly distensible network of connective tissue resulting from scarring caused by hemorrhagic necrosis over the course of goiter growth.[117] It is reminiscent to the development of round regenerative nodules in a cirrhotic liver.

On ultrasound, multinodular goiter, also known as adenomatous (although nodules are not true adenomas) or colloid goiter, is characterized by focal or diffuse replacement of the thyroid parenchyma by closely opposed, isoechoic solid nodules containing variable amount of cystic change, without normal intervening parenchyma and background heterogeneity (**Fig. 23**).

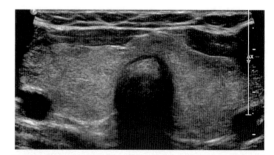

Fig. 22. Simple diffuse goiter. A transverse ultrasound image through the isthmus of a euthyroid patient shows a moderately to markedly enlarged thyroid gland with normal homogenous thyroid echogenicity. Notice that both thyroid lobes extend lateral to the carotid artery.

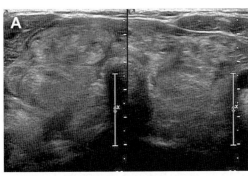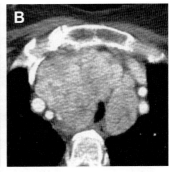

Fig. 23. Multinodular goiter. Transverse ultrasound (*A*) and contrast-enhanced CT (*B*) of the thyroid at the level of the superior mediastinum show massive thyroid enlargement. The parenchyma is entirely replaced by similar-appearing innumerable confluent solid nodules abutting one another with variable cystic degeneration. Course, shadowing parenchymal calcification is often present. It is important to evaluate all nodules for suspicious features.

Parenchymal nodularity and inability to reproduce the borders of individual nodules in 3 dimensions is often accentuated during real-time examination. In other cases, multiple discrete nodules can be seen throughout an otherwise normal-appearing gland.[118] When involvement is asymmetric, the lower lobes are often preferentially affected. Similar-appearing nodules with borders that blend together can be difficult to distinguish from one another. Over time, the nodules undergo a varying degree of cystic or complex cystic changes because of necrosis, colloid accumulation, or hemorrhage; this accounts for the varying size and composition of the nodules in multinodular goiter. Dystrophic calcifications are common; the calcifications are typically coarse and cause posterior acoustic shadowing. The internal matrix of the nodules may be obscured by shadowing from rim calcifications. When all nodules appear similar, representative nodules, or nodule clusters when involvement is focal, can be selected for measurement with emphasis on the ones that are most reproducible for follow-up purposes. Nodules that appear dominant, enlarging,[119] different, or those that have malignant sonographic features (microcalcifications, hypoechogenicity, tall configuration) are targeted for ultrasound-guided FNA.

CT and MR imaging can also reveal multiple variably sized nodules containing complex cystic change, but they are better suited than ultrasound to assess the intrathoracic extension of a substernal goiter, compression of adjacent trachea and esophagus, and mass effect on surrounding vessels. Although ultrasound is the modality of choice for evaluating patients with mild to moderate thyroid enlargement, its inability to penetrate through lung and bone limit the usefulness of ultrasound for evaluating the mediastinal

extension of goiter. T2-weighted MR images show heterogeneous signal, and T1-weighted images show high signal foci, representing colloid-containing or hemorrhage-containing cysts.[97] Parenchymal calcifications are better shown on ultrasound or CT. Treatment is focused on maintaining or restoring normal thyroid function and reducing gland volume in patients whose main symptoms are related to mass effect. Reduction of thyroid volume may be achieved by levothyroxine suppression, surgical resection, or ^{131}I radioiodine ablation.[116]

Multiple studies have shown that the risk of thyroid cancer in each patient is the same, and independent of the number of thyroid nodules present.[120,121] Therefore, the risk of malignancy in each individual nodule within a multinodular gland decreases by a rate proportional to the number of nodules.[122] In a prospective study by Deandrea and colleagues[120] in a cohort of 402 patients with nonpalpable or single palpable nodules, it was shown that 22% of malignant thyroid nodules evaluated by FNA were found in multinodular thyroids, whereas 33% were found in a uninodular goiter. Not only should the presence of multiple nodules not be dismissed as a sign of benignity but each nodule should be scrutinized for the presence of suspicious features. Both the SRU[122] and American Thyroid Association[123] recommend analyzing the sonographic features of individual nodules in a multinodular gland to triage the nodules rather than using nodule size as the primary criteria for biopsy in patients with multiple nodules.[120,124–126] A study by Frates and colleagues[127] found that among 120 patients with multiple nodules, the nodule harboring the thyroid cancer was in the largest nodule only 72% of the time. The likelihood that the largest nodule was malignant decreased as the number of nodules increased. Many laboratories consider nodules that are sonographically similar to be histologically similar. When nodules with different sonographic features are present, each nodule should be evaluated individually by applying the criteria established for solitary nodules, discussed in the subsequent article. The nodules with more suspicious features should be selected for biopsy first, followed by other nodules that are representative of the remaining nodules.[120,123–126] Nodules that are not biopsied and do not seem suspicious can be followed to evaluate for rapid growth or other features that cause concern.[71]

Riedel Thyroiditis

Riedel thyroiditis, or Riedel's thyroiditis, is a rare, local manifestation of a systemic form of systemic fibrosclerosis. Its cause is obscure but it is characterized at histology by a fibroinflammatory process that destroys all or portions of the thyroid gland. Fibrosis and inflammation may extend beyond the capsule into the surrounding tissues[128,129]; the adjacent carotid artery and jugular vein may be encased by fibrosis. Riedel thyroiditis may occur in isolation, or as part of a systemic fibrosclerosing process that may include retroperitoneal fibrosis, mediastinal fibrosis, orbital pseudotumor, and sclerosing cholangitis.

Most patients are between 30 and 50 years old at the time of diagnosis. Riedel thyroiditis is rare: the estimated incidence of Riedel thyroiditis among thyroidectomy specimens has been reported to be between 0.04% and 0.30%.[130,131] The patients typically present with an enlarged, fixed, rock-hard, painless goiter. Tracheal and esophageal compression by periglandular fibrosis may cause dysphagia and dyspnea.[46] Most patient are euthyroid at the time of diagnosis, but in 30–40% hypothyroidism eventually develops when the thyroid becomes nearly completely replaced by fibrosis.[132] Forty-five percent of patients have increased thyroglobulin and thyroid peroxidase antibodies,[132] although it is unclear if this is a cause or the effect of fibrotic destruction. Riedel thyroiditis should be distinguished from the fibrotic form of Hashimoto. The fibrotic form of Hashimoto's thyroiditis seen in up to 13% of patients with Hashimoto's thyroiditis,[133] and also results in a rock-hard thyroid gland on palpation, was previously believed to represent a variation of Riedel thyroiditis but they are now considered separate entities but in earlier correction it was as is. In contrast to the fibrous form of Hashimoto, Riedel shows extrathyroid extension and loss of normal thyroid lobulation.[128]

The rarity of Riedel thyroiditis accounts for the paucity of literature describing its imaging appearance. The radiographic findings reflect the fibrotic and locally aggressive nature of the process. Sonographic findings include an enlarged, hypoechoic gland or coarsened echotexture with fibrous septations resulting in pseudonodular morphology.[132,134,135] Involvement of the neck and thyroid gland can be focal or diffuse. CT shows an enlarged, hypodense to normal attenuation gland, which slightly enhances after the administration of intravenous contrast.[131] MR may be more useful than CT in that fibrous tissue shortens T2 relaxation times and results in characteristic low T1-weighted and T2-weighted signal intensity (**Fig. 24**).[135,136] Both minimal and marked enhancement after contrast administration have been described.[136,137] CT and MR imaging are better suited than ultrasound to determine the extent of tracheal and esophageal compression, and extrathyroidal soft-tissue involvement but either modality may show encasement of jugular vessels.

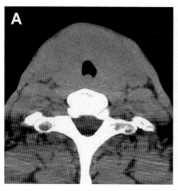 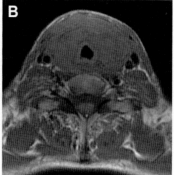 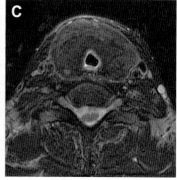

Fig. 24. Riedel thyroiditis. The thyroid is diffusely enlarged and hypodense on CT (*A*) and low signal on T1-weighted and T2-weighted MR imaging (*B* and *C*) consistent with fibrosis. The thyroid is encircling the trachea and esophagus posteriorly.

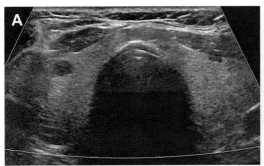
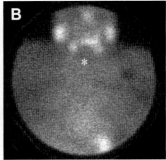

Fig. 25. AIT type 2. (*A*) Color Doppler of the thyroid shows normal grayscale appearance with striking absence of thyroid perfusion consistent with type 2 AIT. (*B*) Thyroid scan shows complete absence of tracer uptake in the thyroid gland (*). Activity in the salivary glands is normal.

Extracapsular extension is neither a sensitive nor specific finding of Riedel thyroiditis. Periglandular fibrosis may be absent in early stages of Riedel disease and when present the differential diagnosis expands to include thyroid lymphoma and anaplastic thyroid carcinoma. Anaplastic thyroid cancer is expected to show more heterogeneous echogenicity on ultrasound and higher T2 signal intensity on MR imaging because of tumor necrosis.[138] FNAB is typically inconclusive; the ultimate diagnosis of Riedel thyroiditis is usually made by surgical wedge resection. The treatment may involve surgical resection for compressive symptoms if medical therapy fails.

Amiodarone-associated Thyroid Disease

Amiodarone is an iodine-rich antiarrhythmic cardiac drug used to treat certain arrhythmias refractory to standard therapy. Although most patients remain euthyroid, 15% to 20% develop either amiodarone-induced thyrotoxicosis (AIT) or amiodarone-induced hypothyroidism. There is no role of imaging for the latter because these patients are all generally treated with thyroid hormone replacement. There are 2 main types of AIT. Type 1 is a form of iodine-induced hyperthyroidism that develops in abnormal glands (multinodular goiter or latent Graves disease). The thyrotoxicosis in type 1 AIT is caused by excessive thyroid hormone synthesis and is treated with antithyroid drugs. The more common type 2 AIT occurs in patients without underlying thyroid disease. Thyrotoxicosis in these patients is caused by amiodarone-induced destructive thyroiditis; the disease is treated with steroids.[139,140]

Although there are mixed forms, classifying patients with AIT into the correct subtype is vital for determining appropriate therapy. Ultrasound with color Doppler has an important role to play in this regard.[139,141] Ultrasound in patients with type 1 AIT reveals a diffuse or nodular goiter. On the other hand, a normal thyroid or small diffuse goiter is shown in patients with type 2 AIT. Color Doppler is particularly useful in distinguishing between the 2 types of AIT. Mildly to markedly increased flow is shown within the thyroid in patients with type 1 AIT, whereas flow within the thyroid is markedly diminished or absent in patients with type 2 AIT (**Fig. 25**).[142,143] Therefore, the presence of vascular flow on color Doppler suggests type 1 AIT. Color Doppler flow evaluation should be directed at the thyroid parenchyma and not discrete nodules, if present. Thyroid radioactive iodine uptake values are likewise usually low to absent in type 2 AIT and are normal or increased in type 1 AIT.[144] Preliminary work by Piga and colleagues[145] has found that thyroid technetium 99m methoxyisobutylisonitrile scintigraphy may also be a useful tool in differentiating the different forms of AIT and potentially identifying the mixed form. In this study, diffuse retention of the radioactive tracer was present in all patients with type 1 AIT, which indicates hyperfunctioning tissue, whereas no significant uptake was found in type 2 AIT, suggestive of a destructive process. Other

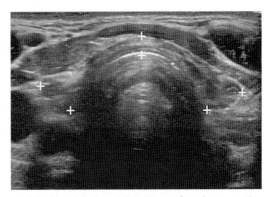

Fig. 26. Atrophic thyroiditis. Young female presenting with hypothyroidism. The thyroid gland is small to normal in size and diffusely hypoechoic with micronodulation.

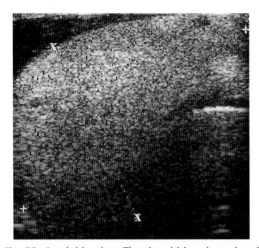

Fig. 27. Amyloid goiter. The thyroid is enlarged and shows increased ground glass echogenicity with acoustic impedance of sound to the deep aspect of the thyroid. (*From* Sbaï A, Wechsler B, Leenhardt L, et al. Amyloid goiter as the initial manifestation of systemic amyloidosis due to familial Mediterranean fever with homozygous MEFV mutation. Thyroid 2001;11(4):398; with permission.)

drugs that are associated with thyroid abnormalities include lithium, interferon alfa, and interleukin 2.

Atrophic Thyroiditis

Atrophic thyroiditis is an AITD characterized by a small (atrophic) thyroid gland with lymphocytic infiltration, fibrosis, and parenchymal destruction, leading to clinical hypothyroidism. Serum autoantibodies to thyroid peroxidase and thyroglobulin are present, similar to Hashimoto's thyroiditis. The main distinction from Hashimoto's thyroiditis is the absence of a palpable goiter. A higher percentage of patients with atrophic thyroiditis

have also been found to have antibodies blocking the TSH receptor compared with classic goiterous Hashimoto.[146] TSH receptor blockade (as opposed to the TSH stimulation of Graves disease) is believed to cause thyroid atrophy and hypothyroidism.[147] The typical sonographic appearance of atrophic thyroiditis is a small, hypoechoic thyroid (**Fig. 26**). Whether atrophic thyroiditis represents a separate disease entity from Hashimoto, end stage of Hashimoto, or is simply an extreme within a normal distribution of thyroid volume has been a topic of continued debate.[148,149]

Thyroid Amyloid

Systemic amyloidosis can affect any organ of the body including the thyroid. Although this condition is rarely encountered in clinical practice, specific sonographic appearances have been described. In 1 small series, in which histopathologic examination of the thyroid was performed, distinctive sonographic findings included enlargement of 1 or both lobes of the thyroid, high echogenicity approaching that of the connective tissue of the neck, decreased ultrasound penetration, and a very fine homogenous echotexture (**Fig. 27**) suggestive of ground glass appearance. Tiny cystic cavities within the thyroid believed to be dilated follicles were occasionally observed.[150]

Metastatic Disease

Most thyroid metastases are clinically silent and most nodules in patients with known malignancy are still benign. Although detection of clinically apparent palpable metastatic disease to the thyroid is uncommon (5% of 188 in 1 autopsy series),[151] when meticulous autopsy is performed, the incidence is as high as 24%.[152] Lymphoma, melanoma, renal cell carcinoma, lung, colorectal carcinoma, and breast cancer metastases to the

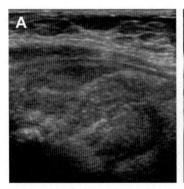
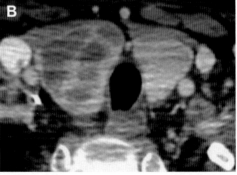

Fig. 28. Thyroid metastasis. Unilateral patchy infiltrative areas of hypoechogenicity on ultrasound (*A*) and low attenuation on contrast-enhanced CT (*B*). CT also showed malignant cervical and mediastinal adenopathy and spiculated lung nodule. Biopsy of a right cervical lymph node showed high-grade small-cell and non–small-cell cancer, believed to represent lung cancer metastasis.

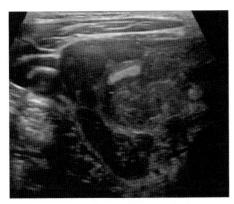

Fig. 29. Diffuse thyroid lymphoma. Transverse ultrasound through the right lobe shows a markedly enlarged gland diffusely replaced by a profoundly hypoechoic and heterogeneous mass in a 63-year-old man. Deep aspect of the right lobe has a pseudocystic appearance. Biopsy confirmed B-cell lymphoma.

thyroid have been described, seen in association with diffuse metastatic disease elsewhere. Although thyroid metastases have highly variable imaging appearances, sonographic findings in a series of 11 patients showed all metastasis to be either hypoechoic or markedly hypoechoic, most with well-defined margins and lack of a halo and calcifications (**Figs. 28** and **29**). It is not unexpected that most metastases were hypodense compared with the usually hyperdense, iodine-rich, thyroid gland on CT. Signal characteristics on MR imaging were variable.[153] Multiple, similar appearing solid nodules are the most common presentation; but a single nodule or a heterogenous pattern can also occur when the thyroid is diffusely involved. Multiple markedly hypoechoic thyroid nodules with concurrent cervical adenopathy may suggest lymphoma.[152] Tissue sampling with FNA is used to establish the diagnosis.

SUMMARY

Optimized technique, improved scanner platforms, and color Doppler have made it possible to quickly evaluate thyroid anatomy and perfusion. Thyroid hypoechogenicity and parenchymal heterogeneity are easily appreciated and are the hallmark of AITD. A wide range of diffuse thyroid diseases are often first evaluated with ultrasound; although the imaging features of these diseases often overlap, a reasonable differential diagnosis can often be made when clinical and laboratory values are considered. Color Doppler may play an ancillary role in assessing disease activity

in several causes of thyrotoxicosis. The potential role of recent ultrasound advancements (elastography, microbubbles) in the assessment of thyroid disease is under investigation.

REFERENCES

1. Solbiati L, Charboneau JW. The thyroid gland. In: Rumack CM, editor. Diagnostic ultrasound. St Louis (MO): Mosby; 2004. p. 703–29.
2. Hayashi N, Tamaki N, Konishi J, et al. Sonography of Hashimoto's thyroiditis. J Clin Ultrasound 1986; 14:123–6.
3. Pedersen OM, Aardal NP, Larssen TB, et al. The value of ultrasonography in predicting autoimmune thyroid disease. Thyroid 2000;10:251–9.
4. Slatosky J, Shipton B, Wahba H. Thyroiditis: differential diagnosis and management. Am Fam Physician 2000;61:1047–52, 1054.
5. Rapoport B. Pathophysiology of Hashimoto's thyroiditis and hypothyroidism. Annu Rev Med 1991;42:91–6.
6. Fadel BM, Ellahham S, Ringel MD, et al. Hyperthyroid heart disease. Clin Cardiol 2000;23:402–8.
7. Muller HW, Schroder S, Schneider C, et al. Sonographic tissue characterisation in thyroid gland diagnosis. A correlation between sonography and histology. Klin Wochenschr 1985;63:706–10.
8. Hegedus L. Thyroid size determined by ultrasound. Influence of physiological factors and nonthyroidal disease. Dan Med Bull 1990;37:249–63.
9. Knudsen N, Laurberg P, Perrild H, et al. Risk factors for goiter and thyroid nodules. Thyroid 2002;12:879–88.
10. Gomez JM, Maravall FJ, Gomez N, et al. Determinants of thyroid volume as measured by ultrasonography in healthy adults randomly selected. Clin Endocrinol (Oxf) 2000;53:629–34.
11. Wesche MF, Wiersinga WM, Smits NJ. Lean body mass as a determinant of thyroid size. Clin Endocrinol (Oxf) 1998;48:701–6.
12. Middleton WD, Kurtz AB. Ultrasound: the requisites. Philadelphia (PA): Mosby; 2004.
13. Solbiati L, Osti V, Cova L, et al. Ultrasound of thyroid, parathyroid glands and neck lymph nodes. Eur Radiol 2001;11:2411–24.
14. Brown MC, Spencer R. Thyroid gland volume estimated by use of ultrasound in addition to scintigraphy. Acta Radiol Oncol Radiat Phys Biol 1978; 17:337–41.
15. Knudsen N, Bols B, Bulow I, et al. Validation of ultrasonography of the thyroid gland for epidemiological purposes. Thyroid 1999;9:1069–74.
16. Shabana W, Peeters E, De Maeseneer M. Measuring thyroid gland volume: should we change the correction factor? AJR Am J Roentgenol 2006; 186:234–6.

17. Hegedus L, Perrild H, Poulsen LR, et al. The determination of thyroid volume by ultrasound and its relationship to body weight, age, and sex in normal subjects. J Clin Endocrinol Metab 1983;56:260–3.

18. Schlogl S, Werner E, Lassmann M, et al. The use of three-dimensional ultrasound for thyroid volumetry. Thyroid 2001;11:569–74.

19. AIUM, editor. American Institute of Ultrasound in Medicine Practice guideline for the performance of a thyroid and parathyroid ultrasound examination 2007. Leurel (MD): AIUM; 2007.

20. ACR, editor. American College of Radiology-American Institute of Ultrasound in Medicine Practice guideline for the performance of a thyroid and parathyroid ultrasound examinations. ACR; 2007.

21. Peeters EY, Shabana WM, Verbeek PA, et al. Use of a curved-array transducer to reduce interobserver variation in sonographic measurement of thyroid volume in healthy adults. J Clin Ultrasound 2003; 31:189–93.

22. Shapiro RS. Panoramic ultrasound of the thyroid. Thyroid 2003;13:177–81.

23. Langer JE, Mandel SJ. Sonographic imaging of cervical lymph nodes in patients with thyroid cancer. Neuroimaging Clin N Am 2008;18:479–89, vii–viii.

24. Koike E, Noguchi S, Yamashita H, et al. Ultrasonographic characteristics of thyroid nodules: prediction of malignancy. Arch Surg 2001;136:334–7.

25. Chow SM, Law SC, Chan JK, et al. Papillary microcarcinoma of the thyroid–prognostic significance of lymph node metastasis and multifocality. Cancer 2003;98:31–40.

26. Kouvaraki MA, Shapiro SE, Fornage BD, et al. Role of preoperative ultrasonography in the surgical management of patients with thyroid cancer. Surgery 2003;134:946–54 [discussion: 54–5].

27. Shimamoto K, Satake H, Sawaki A, et al. Preoperative staging of thyroid papillary carcinoma with ultrasonography. Eur J Radiol 1998;29:4–10.

28. Johnson NA, Tublin ME, Ogilvie JB. Parathyroid imaging: technique and role in the preoperative evaluation of primary hyperparathyroidism. AJR Am J Roentgenol 2007;188:1706–15.

29. Guth S, Theune U, Aberle J, et al. Very high prevalence of thyroid nodules detected by high frequency (13 MHz) ultrasound examination. Eur J Clin Invest 2009;39:699–706.

30. Reiners C, Wegscheider K, Schicha H, et al. Prevalence of thyroid disorders in the working population of Germany: ultrasonography screening in 96,278 unselected employees. Thyroid 2004;14:926–32.

31. Dahl JJ, Soo MS, Trahey GE. Spatial and temporal aberrator stability for real-time adaptive imaging. IEEE Trans Ultrason Ferroelectr Freq Control 2005;52:1504–17.

32. Shapiro RS, Simpson WL, Rausch DL, et al. Compound spatial sonography of the thyroid gland: evaluation of freedom from artifacts and of nodule conspicuity. AJR Am J Roentgenol 2001; 177:1195–8.

33. Tranquart F, Grenier N, Eder V, et al. Clinical use of ultrasound tissue harmonic imaging. Ultrasound Med Biol 1999;25:889–94.

34. Whittingham TA. Tissue harmonic imaging. Eur Radiol 1999;9(Suppl 3):S323–6.

35. Saleh A, Cupisti K, Cohnen M, et al. Early postoperative tissue harmonic sonography of the thyroid gland. Acta Radiol 2002;43:147–50.

36. Szopinski K, Slapa RZ. Harmonic imaging in ultrasonography: basic concepts and applications. Pol Merkur Lekarski 2003;14:139–41 [in Polish].

37. Ota H, Amino N, Morita S, et al. Quantitative measurement of thyroid blood flow for differentiation of painless thyroiditis from Graves' disease. Clin Endocrinol (Oxf) 2007;67:41–5.

38. Bartolotta TV, Midiri M, Galia M, et al. Qualitative and quantitative evaluation of solitary thyroid nodules with contrast-enhanced ultrasound: initial results. Eur Radiol 2006;16:2234–41.

39. Claudon M, Cosgrove D, Albrecht T, et al. Guidelines and good clinical practice recommendations for contrast enhanced ultrasound (CEUS)–update 2008. Ultraschall Med 2008;29:28–44.

40. Rago T, Scutari M, Santini F, et al. Real-time elastosonography: useful tool for refining the presurgical diagnosis in thyroid nodules with indeterminate or nondiagnostic cytology. J Clin Endocrinol Metab 2010;95(12):5274–80.

41. Dighe M, Kim J, Luo S, et al. Utility of the ultrasound elastographic systolic thyroid stiffness index in reducing fine-needle aspirations. J Ultrasound Med 2010;29:565–74.

42. Kagoya R, Monobe H, Tojima H. Utility of elastography for differential diagnosis of benign and malignant thyroid nodules. Otolaryngol Head Neck Surg 2010;143:230–4.

43. Vorlander C, Wolff J, Saalabian S, et al. Real-time ultrasound elastography–a noninvasive diagnostic procedure for evaluating dominant thyroid nodules. Langenbecks Arch Surg 2010;395:865–71.

44. Bojunga JX, Herrmann E, Meyer G, et al. Real-time elastography for the differentiation of benign and malignant thyroid nodules: a meta-analysis. Thyroid 2010;20:1145–50.

45. Gharib H, Papini E, Valcavi R, et al. American Association of Clinical Endocrinologists and Associazione Medici Endocrinologi medical guidelines for clinical practice for the diagnosis and management of thyroid nodules. Endocr Pract 2006;12:63–102.

46. Pearce EN, Farwell AP, Braverman LE. Thyroiditis. N Engl J Med 2003;348:2646–55.

47. Farwell AP, Braverman LE. Inflammatory thyroid disorders. Otolaryngol Clin North Am 1996;29: 541–56.

48. Holm LE, Blomgren H, Lowhagen T. Cancer risks in patients with chronic lymphocytic thyroiditis. N Engl J Med 1985;312:601–4.

49. Vanderpump MP, Tunbridge WM. Epidemiology and prevention of clinical and subclinical hypothyroidism. Thyroid 2002;12:839–47.

50. LiVolsi VA. The pathology of autoimmune thyroid disease: a review. Thyroid 1994;4:333–9.

51. Poropatich C, Marcus D, Oertel YC. Hashimoto's thyroiditis: fine-needle aspirations of 50 asymptomatic cases. Diagn Cytopathol 1994;11:141–5.

52. Marcocci C, Vitti P, Cetani F, et al. Thyroid ultrasonography helps to identify patients with diffuse lymphocytic thyroiditis who are prone to develop hypothyroidism. J Clin Endocrinol Metab 1991;72: 209–13.

53. Loy M, Cianchetti ME, Cardia F, et al. Correlation of computerized gray-scale sonographic findings with thyroid function and thyroid autoimmune activity in patients with Hashimoto's thyroiditis. J Clin Ultrasound 2004;32:136–40.

54. Mazziotti G, Sorvillo F, Iorio S, et al. Grey-scale analysis allows a quantitative evaluation of thyroid echogenicity in the patients with Hashimoto's thyroiditis. Clin Endocrinol (Oxf) 2003;59:223–9.

55. Rotondi M, Cappelli C, Leporati P, et al. A hypoechoic pattern of the thyroid at ultrasound does not indicate autoimmune thyroid diseases in patients with morbid obesity. Eur J Endocrinol 2010;163:105–9.

56. Mizukami Y, Michigishi T, Kawato M, et al. Chronic thyroiditis: thyroid function and histologic correlations in 601 cases. Hum Pathol 1992;23:980–8.

57. Kerr L. High resolution ultrasound: value of color Doppler. Ultrasound Q 1994;12:21–43.

58. Yeh HC, Futterweit W, Gilbert P. Micronodulation: ultrasonographic sign of Hashimoto thyroiditis. J Ultrasound Med 1996;15:813–9.

59. Serres-Creixams X, Castells-Fuste I, Pruna-Comella X, et al. Paratracheal lymph nodes: a new sonographic finding in autoimmune thyroiditis. J Clin Ultrasound 2008;36:418–21.

60. Leboulleux S, Girard E, Rose M, et al. Ultrasound criteria of malignancy for cervical lymph nodes in patients followed up for differentiated thyroid cancer. J Clin Endocrinol Metab 2007; 92:3590–4.

61. Anderson L, Middleton WD, Teefey SA, et al. Hashimoto thyroiditis: part 1, sonographic analysis of the nodular form of Hashimoto thyroiditis. AJR Am J Roentgenol 2010;195:208–15.

62. Langer JE, Khan A, Nisenbaum HL, et al. Sonographic appearance of focal thyroiditis. AJR Am J Roentgenol 2001;176:751–4.

63. Bonavita JA, Mayo J, Babb J, et al. Pattern recognition of benign nodules at ultrasound of the thyroid: which nodules can be left alone? AJR Am J Roentgenol 2009;193:207–13.

64. Pasieka JL. Hashimoto's disease and thyroid lymphoma: role of the surgeon. World J Surg 2000;24:966–70.

65. Takashima S, Matsuzuka F, Nagareda T, et al. Thyroid nodules associated with Hashimoto thyroiditis: assessment with US. Radiology 1992; 185:125–30.

66. Ito Y, Amino N, Miyauchi A. Thyroid ultrasonography. World J Surg 2010;34:1171–80.

67. Wirtzfeld DA, Winston JS, Hicks WL Jr, et al. Clinical presentation and treatment of non-Hodgkin's lymphoma of the thyroid gland. Ann Surg Oncol 2001;8:338–41.

68. McDougall IR. Metastatic struma ovarii: the burden of truth. Clin Nucl Med 2006;31:321–4.

69. Gul K, Dirikoc A, Kiyak G, et al. The association between thyroid carcinoma and Hashimoto's thyroiditis: the ultrasonographic and histopathologic characteristics of malignant nodules. Thyroid 2010;20:873–8.

70. Matsubayashi S, Kawai K, Matsumoto Y, et al. The correlation between papillary thyroid carcinoma and lymphocytic infiltration in the thyroid gland. J Clin Endocrinol Metab 1995;80:3421–4.

71. Langer JE. Invited Commentary: US features of thyroid malignancy: pearls and pitfalls. Radiographics 2007;27:861–5.

72. Feldt-Rasmussen U, Rasmussen AK. Autoimmunity in differentiated thyroid cancer: significance and related clinical problems. Hormones (Athens) 2010;9:109–17.

73. Anil C, Goksel S, Gursoy A. Hashimoto's thyroiditis is not associated with increased risk of thyroid cancer in patients with thyroid nodules: a single-center prospective study. Thyroid 2010;20:601–6.

74. Anderson L, Middleton WD, Teefey SA, et al. Hashimoto thyroiditis: part 2, sonographic analysis of benign and malignant nodules in patients with diffuse Hashimoto thyroiditis. AJR Am J Roentgenol 2010;195:216–22.

75. Ohmori N, Miyakawa M, Ohmori K, et al. Ultrasonographic findings of papillary thyroid carcinoma with Hashimoto's thyroiditis. Intern Med 2007;46:547–50.

76. Maitra A. The endocrine system. In: Kumar V, Abbas AK, Fausto N, et al, editors. Robbins & Cotran pathologic basis of disease. 8th edition. Philadelphia: WB Saunders; 2009.

77. Ralls PW, Mayekawa DS, Lee KP, et al. Color-flow Doppler sonography in Graves disease: "thyroid inferno". AJR Am J Roentgenol 1988;150:781–4.

78. Arslan H, Unal O, Algun E, et al. Power Doppler sonography in the diagnosis of Graves' disease. Eur J Ultrasound 2000;11:117–22.

79. Castagnone D, Rivolta R, Rescalli S, et al. Color Doppler sonography in Graves' disease: value in assessing activity of disease and predicting outcome. AJR Am J Roentgenol 1996;166:203–7.

80. Vitti P. Grey scale thyroid ultrasonography in the evaluation of patients with Graves' disease. Eur J Endocrinol 2000;142:22–4.

81. Singer PA, Cooper DS, Levy EG, et al. Treatment guidelines for patients with hyperthyroidism and hypothyroidism. Standards of Care Committee, American Thyroid Association. JAMA 1995;273:808–12.

82. Boi F, Loy M, Piga M, et al. The usefulness of conventional and echo colour Doppler sonography in the differential diagnosis of toxic multinodular goitres. Eur J Endocrinol 2000;143:339–46.

83. Erdogan MF, Anil C, Cesur M, et al. Color flow Doppler sonography for the etiologic diagnosis of hyperthyroidism. Thyroid 2007;17:223–8.

84. Kurita S, Sakurai M, Kita Y, et al. Measurement of thyroid blood flow area is useful for diagnosing the cause of thyrotoxicosis. Thyroid 2005;15:1249–52.

85. Saleh A, Cohnen M, Furst G, et al. Differential diagnosis of hyperthyroidism: Doppler sonographic quantification of thyroid blood flow distinguishes between Graves' disease and diffuse toxic goiter. Exp Clin Endocrinol Diabetes 2002;110:32–6.

86. Vitti P, Rago T, Mazzeo S, et al. Thyroid blood flow evaluation by color-flow Doppler sonography distinguishes Graves' disease from Hashimoto's thyroiditis. J Endocrinol Invest 1995;18:857–61.

87. Bogazzi F. Color flow Doppler sonography of the thyroid. In: Baskin HJ, editor. Thyroid ultrasound and ultrasound-guided FNA Biopsy. Boston: Kluwer Academic Publishers; 2000. p. 215–38.

88. Baldini M, Castagnone D, Rivolta R, et al. Thyroid vascularization by color Doppler ultrasonography in Graves' disease. Changes related to different phases and to the long-term outcome of the disease. Thyroid 1997;7:823–8.

89. Bogazzi F, Bartalena L, Brogioni S, et al. Thyroid vascularity and blood flow are not dependent on serum thyroid hormone levels: studies in vivo by color flow Doppler sonography. Eur J Endocrinol 1999;140:452–6.

90. Baldini M, Orsatti A, Bonfanti MT, et al. Relationship between the sonographic appearance of the thyroid and the clinical course and autoimmune activity of Graves' disease. J Clin Ultrasound 2005;33:381–5.

91. Vitti P, Rago T, Mancusi F, et al. Thyroid hypoechogenic pattern at ultrasonography as a tool for predicting recurrence of hyperthyroidism after medical treatment in patients with Graves' disease. Acta Endocrinol (Copenh) 1992;126:128–31.

92. Streetman DD, Khanderia U. Diagnosis and treatment of Graves disease. Ann Pharmacother 2003;37:1100–9.

93. Shih WJ, Mitchell B, Schott JC. Scarred atrophic thyroid after I-131 therapy for Graves' disease documented at autopsy. J Natl Med Assoc 2002;94:915–9.

94. Nishihara E, Ohye H, Amino N, et al. Clinical characteristics of 852 patients with subacute thyroiditis before treatment. Intern Med 2008;47:725–9.

95. Tokuda Y, Kasagi K, Iida Y, et al. Sonography of subacute thyroiditis: changes in the findings during the course of the disease. J Clin Ultrasound 1990;18:21–6.

96. Park SY, Kim EK, Kim MJ, et al. Ultrasonographic characteristics of subacute granulomatous thyroiditis. Korean J Radiol 2006;7:229–34.

97. Loevner LA, Kaplan SL, Cunnane ME, et al. Cross-sectional imaging of the thyroid gland. Neuroimaging Clin N Am 2008;18:445–61, vii.

98. Otsuka N, Nagai K, Morita K, et al. Magnetic resonance imaging of subacute thyroiditis. Radiat Med 1994;12:273–6.

99. Yeo SH, Lee SK, Hwang I, et al. Subacute thyroiditis presenting as a focal lesion on [18F] Fluorodeoxyglucose whole-body positron-emission tomography and CT. AJNR Am J Neuroradiol 2010. [Epub ahead of print].

100. Schubert MF, Kountz DS. Thyroiditis. A disease with many faces. Postgrad Med 1995;98:101–3 107–8, 112.

101. Singer PA. Thyroiditis. Acute, subacute, and chronic. Med Clin North Am 1991;75:61–77.

102. Woolf PD. Transient painless thyroiditis with hyperthyroidism: a variant of lymphocytic thyroiditis? Endocr Rev 1980;1:411–20.

103. Stagnaro-Green A. Postpartum thyroiditis. Best Pract Res Clin Endocrinol Metab 2004;18:303–16.

104. Lucas A, Pizarro E, Granada ML, et al. Postpartum thyroiditis: epidemiology and clinical evolution in a nonselected population. Thyroid 2000;10:71–7.

105. Alvarez-Marfany M, Roman SH, Drexler AJ, et al. Long-term prospective study of postpartum thyroid dysfunction in women with insulin dependent diabetes mellitus. J Clin Endocrinol Metab 1994;79:10–6.

106. Gerstein HC. Incidence of postpartum thyroid dysfunction in patients with type I diabetes mellitus. Ann Intern Med 1993;118:419–23.

107. Roti E, Uberti E. Post-partum thyroiditis–a clinical update. Eur J Endocrinol 2002;146:275–9.

108. Premawardhana LD, Parkes AB, Ammari F, et al. Postpartum thyroiditis and long-term thyroid status: prognostic influence of thyroid peroxidase antibodies and ultrasound echogenicity. J Clin Endocrinol Metab 2000;85:71–5.

109. Cases JA, Wenig BM, Silver CE, et al. Recurrent acute suppurative thyroiditis in an adult due to

a fourth branchial pouch fistula. J Clin Endocrinol Metab 2000;85:953–6.

110. Pereira O, Prasad DS, Bal AM, et al. Fatal descending necrotizing mediastinitis secondary to acute suppurative thyroiditis developing in an apparently healthy woman. Thyroid 2010;20:571–2.

111. Chen HL, Chen PL. Recurrent acute suppurative thyroiditis in a patient without pyriform sinus fistula: a case report. J Intern Med Taiwan 2007;18:134–9.

112. Farwell AP. Subacute thyroiditis and acute infectious thyroiditis. In: Braverman LE, Utiger RD, editors. Werner and Ingbar's the thyroid: a fundamental and clinical text. 9th edition. Philadelphia (PA): Lippincott Williams & Wilkins; 2005. p. 536–47.

113. Paes JE, Burman KD, Cohen J, et al. Acute bacterial suppurative thyroiditis: a clinical review and expert opinion. Thyroid 2010;20:247–55.

114. Brant WE. The core curriculum: ultrasound. 1st edition. Philadelphia (PA): Lippincott Williams & Wilkins; 2001.

115. Kim KH, Sung MW, Koh TY, et al. Pyriform sinus fistula: management with chemocauterization of the internal opening. Ann Otol Rhinol Laryngol 2000;109:452–6.

116. Hegedus L, Bonnema SJ, Bennedbaek FN. Management of simple nodular goiter: current status and future perspectives. Endocr Rev 2003; 24:102–32.

117. Ramelli F, Studer H, Bruggisser D. Pathogenesis of thyroid nodules in multinodular goiter. Am J Pathol 1982;109:215–23.

118. Simeone JF, Daniels GH, Mueller PR, et al. High-resolution real-time sonography of the thyroid. Radiology 1982;145:431–5.

119. Shulkin BL, Shapiro B. The role of imaging tests in the diagnosis of thyroid carcinoma. Endocrinol Metab Clin North Am 1990;19:523–43.

120. Deandrea M, Mormile A, Veglio M, et al. Fine-needle aspiration biopsy of the thyroid: comparison between thyroid palpation and ultrasonography. Endocr Pract 2002;8:282–6.

121. McCall A, Jarosz H, Lawrence AM, et al. The incidence of thyroid carcinoma in solitary cold nodules and in multinodular goiters. Surgery 1986;100: 1128–32.

122. Frates MC, Benson CB, Charboneau JW, et al. Management of thyroid nodules detected at US: Society of Radiologists in Ultrasound consensus conference statement. Radiology 2005;237: 794–800.

123. Cooper DS, Doherty GM, Haugen BR, et al. Revised American Thyroid Association management guidelines for patients with thyroid nodules and differentiated thyroid cancer. Thyroid 2009; 19:1167–214.

124. Cooper DS, Doherty GM, Haugen BR, et al. Management guidelines for patients with thyroid nodules and differentiated thyroid cancer. Thyroid 2006;16:109–42.

125. Leenhardt L, Hejblum G, Franc B, et al. Indications and limits of ultrasound-guided cytology in the management of nonpalpable thyroid nodules. J Clin Endocrinol Metab 1999;84:24–8.

126. Wienke JR, Chong WK, Fielding JR, et al. Sonographic features of benign thyroid nodules: interobserver reliability and overlap with malignancy. J Ultrasound Med 2003;22:1027–31.

127. Frates MC, Benson CB, Doubilet PM, et al. Prevalence and distribution of carcinoma in patients with solitary and multiple thyroid nodules on sonography. J Clin Endocrinol Metab 2006;91:3411–7.

128. Comings DE, Skubi KB, Van Eyes J, et al. Familial multifocal fibrosclerosis. Findings suggesting that retroperitoneal fibrosis, mediastinal fibrosis, sclerosing cholangitis, Riedel's thyroiditis, and pseudotumor of the orbit may be different manifestations of a single disease. Ann Intern Med 1967;66:884–92.

129. Schwaegerle SM, Bauer TW, Esselstyn CB Jr. Riedel's thyroiditis. Am J Clin Pathol 1988;90:715–22.

130. Hay ID. Thyroiditis: a clinical update. Mayo Clin Proc 1985;60:836–43.

131. Malotte MJ, Chonkich GD, Zuppan CW. Riedel's thyroiditis. Arch Otolaryngol Head Neck Surg 1991;117:214–7.

132. Papi G, LiVolsi VA. Current concepts on Riedel thyroiditis. Am J Clin Pathol 2004;121(Suppl):S50–63.

133. Katz SM, Vickery AL Jr. The fibrous variant of Hashimoto's thyroiditis. Hum Pathol 1974;5:161–70.

134. Ozbayrak M, Kantarci F, Olgun DC, et al. Riedel thyroiditis associated with massive neck fibrosis. J Ultrasound Med 2009;28:267–71.

135. Perez Fontan FJ, Cordido Carballido F, Pombo Felipe F, et al. Riedel thyroiditis: US, CT, and MR evaluation. J Comput Assist Tomogr 1993;17:324–5.

136. Lo JC, Loh KC, Rubin AL, et al. Riedel's thyroiditis presenting with hypothyroidism and hypoparathyroidism: dramatic response to glucocorticoid and thyroxine therapy. Clin Endocrinol (Oxf) 1998;48: 815–8.

137. Ozgen A, Cila A. Riedel's thyroiditis in multifocal fibrosclerosis: CT and MR imaging findings. AJNR Am J Neuroradiol 2000;21:320–1.

138. Takashima S, Morimoto S, Ikezoe J, et al. CT evaluation of anaplastic thyroid carcinoma. AJNR Am J Neuroradiol 1990;11:361–7.

139. Bogazzi F, Bartalena L, Dell'Unto E, et al. Proportion of type 1 and type 2 amiodarone-induced thyrotoxicosis has changed over a 27-year period in Italy. Clin Endocrinol (Oxf) 2007;67:533–7.

140. Martino E, Bartalena L, Bogazzi F, et al. The effects of amiodarone on the thyroid. Endocr Rev 2001;22: 240–54.

141. Eaton SE, Euinton HA, Newman CM, et al. Clinical experience of amiodarone-induced thyrotoxicosis

over a 3-year period: role of colour-flow Doppler sonography. Clin Endocrinol (Oxf) 2002;56:33–8.

142. Bogazzi F, Bartalena L, Brogioni S, et al. Color flow Doppler sonography rapidly differentiates type I and type II amiodarone-induced thyrotoxicosis. Thyroid 1997;7:541–5.

143. Loy M, Perra E, Melis A, et al. Color-flow Doppler sonography in the differential diagnosis and management of amiodarone-induced thyrotoxicosis. Acta Radiol 2007;48:628–34.

144. Martino E, Aghini-Lombardi F, Lippi F, et al. Twenty-four hour radioactive iodine uptake in 35 patients with amiodarone associated thyrotoxicosis. J Nucl Med 1985;26:1402–7.

145. Piga M, Cocco MC, Serra A, et al. The usefulness of 99mTc-sestaMIBI thyroid scan in the differential diagnosis and management of amiodarone-induced thyrotoxicosis. Eur J Endocrinol 2008; 159:423–9.

146. Orgiazzi J. Anti-TSH receptor antibodies in clinical practice. Endocrinol Metab Clin North Am 2000;29: 339–55, vii.

147. Takasu N, Yoshimura Noh J. Hashimoto's thyroiditis: TGAb, TPOAb, TRAb and recovery from hypothyroidism. Expert Rev Clin Immunol 2008;4:221–37.

148. Carle A, Pedersen IB, Knudsen N, et al. Thyroid volume in hypothyroidism due to autoimmune disease follows a unimodal distribution: evidence against primary thyroid atrophy and autoimmune thyroiditis being distinct diseases. J Clin Endocrinol Metab 2009;94:833–9.

149. Davies TF, Amino N. A new classification for human autoimmune thyroid disease. Thyroid 1993;3:331–3.

150. el-Reshaid K, al-Tamami M, Johny KV, et al. Amyloidosis of the thyroid gland: role of ultrasonography. J Clin Ultrasound 1994;22:239–44.

151. Shimaoka K, Sokal JE, Pickren JW. Metastatic neoplasms in the thyroid gland. Pathological and clinical findings. Cancer 1962;15:557–65.

152. Silverberg SG, Vidone VA. Metastatic tumors in the thyroid. Pacif Med Surg 1966;74:175–80.

153. Takashima S, Takayama F, Wang JC, et al. Radiologic assessment of metastases to the thyroid gland. J Comput Assist Tomogr 2000;24:539–45.

Thyroid Ultrasonography. Part 2: Nodules

Tara L. Henrichsen, MD*, Carl C. Reading, MD

KEYWORDS
- Thyroid • Thyroid ultrasonography • Thyroid nodules
- Thyroid cancer

THYROID NODULE FORMATION AND INCIDENCE

Thyroid nodules are sonographically discrete lesions that may be identified in normal or abnormal background thyroid parenchyma. Nodules imaged by ultrasonography may have been detected on physical examination or imaging examinations such as MR imaging, positron emission tomography, computed tomography, ultrasonography of the neck performed for other reasons, and nuclear medicine studies. Multiple physical examination studies, ultrasonographic studies, and pathologic postmortem studies have shown the incidence of thyroid nodules, which ranges from 6.5% on physical examination studies to at least 50% on pathologic studies.[1,2] Ultrasonography demonstrates nodules in approximately 41% of the population; among patients referred for ultrasonography of a palpable solitary nodule, up to 48% had additional nodules.[3] The incidence of nodular thyroid disease is also known to increase with age. The causes of thyroid nodules are varied. Nodules commonly occur in patients with iodine deficiency, thyroiditis, and multiple endocrine neoplasia (MEN) syndromes. Most nodules occur secondary to benign hyperplasia. Previous radiation exposure is known to increase the risk of malignant thyroid nodules.

The term nodule when used to describe a pathologic condition of the thyroid includes both cystic and solid masses. Some thyroid nodules are completely cystic and may represent simple cysts, even though these are rare. Most cystic-appearing nodules are colloid filled and termed as colloid cysts. Alternatively, some cystic nodules may be hemorrhagic. Benign solid, and partially cystic nodules are most commonly hyperplastic and may also be called colloid or adenomatoid nodules. Solid nodules are often found in Hashimoto thyroiditis, most of which are nodular Hashimoto thyroiditis and nodular hyperplasia.[4] Solid neoplasms include benign follicular adenomas, follicular carcinomas, Hürthle cell adenomas, Hürthle cell carcinomas, papillary carcinomas, medullary carcinomas, anaplastic carcinomas, primary thyroid lymphomas, and metastatic disease. Although solid nodules may be benign or malignant, it should be remembered that the overwhelming majority of thyroid nodules are benign.[5]

THYROID CANCER

The American Cancer Society estimated 37,200 new cases of thyroid cancer in the United States in 2009. This estimate corresponds to 2.5% of the total cancer diagnoses. The estimated number of deaths attributed to thyroid cancer were 1630 or 0.2% of cancer deaths.[6] The incidence of thyroid carcinoma has increased over the last several decades.[7-10] In fact, there has been a 2.4-fold increase between the years 1973 and 2002.[7] The greatest increase has been in papillary carcinomas, which was found throughout all racial/ethnic groups. The incidence of follicular carcinoma has also increased slightly. An increase in the incidence of medullary carcinomas was seen

The authors have nothing to disclose.
Department of Radiology, Mayo Clinic, 200 1st Street, SW Rochester, MN 55905, USA
* Corresponding author.
E-mail address: Henrichsen.tara@may.edu

radiologic.theclinics.com

only in Hispanic males, and the data set for anaplastic carcinomas was too small to determine a trend.[8,10] Some have speculated that this increase is secondary to increased imaging use and the detection of nonpalpable subcentimeter nodules. However, using data from the Surveillance, Epidemiology and End Results (SEER) program of the National Cancer Institute, Enewold and colleagues[8] found that between the years 1992 to 1995 and 2003 to 2005, only half of the increase in papillary carcinomas was attributable to cancers less than 1 cm. About 30% of the incidence increase was due to cancers 1.1 to 2.0 cm, and 20% of the incidence increase was secondary to cancers greater than 2 cm. Therefore, the increased incidence of thyroid carcinoma cannot be solely linked to imaging detection.

The overall incidence of thyroid carcinoma still remains low, and when present, the disease is typically indolent. Additional data analysis from the SEER project and National Vital Statistics program has shown that the 20-year survival rate is 99% for patients with newly diagnosed papillary thyroid cancer, who undergo immediate (within 1 year) definitive treatment. Those who did not undergo immediate treatment had a 20-year survival rate of 97%. According to Davies and Welch,[11] these outcomes are still considered satisfactory. This observation leads to a discussion of whether or not nodules can and should be watched. Many professional societies have addressed the dilemma of the thyroid nodule and have published recommendations. A comparison of these guidelines is summarized later, and nodule characterization at ultrasonography is a primary determinant in all recent guidelines.

APPROACH TO NODULE CHARACTERIZATION

Once a thyroid nodule has been identified, there are 2 main considerations to categorizing and determining whether the nodule should undergo fine-needle aspiration (FNA): nodule appearance and size. There is extensive overlap of many reported individual nodule descriptors, which may be seen in both benign and malignant nodules. The only single sonographic feature that is considered safely benign is a purely cystic nodule. There are no other single characteristics that are sensitive and specific[12]; however, combining features into a pattern may be helpful when triaging thyroid nodules.[13,14] There are five patterns that have been shown to have high specificity for benignity.[14] This pattern approach is an initial step in dividing the nodules into those for which FNA should be considered and those that are likely benign, for which FNA is not recommended.

LIKELY BENIGN PATTERNS, FNA NOT NECESSARY

Cystic Nodules With or Without Internal Echogenic Foci

Nodules that are small, less than 10 mm, fluid filled, and solitary or multiple are benign and nonneoplastic. These nodules are thought to be caused by thyroid nodular hyperplasia leaving colloid-filled cysts.[13] Often, these colloid cysts contain tiny echogenic foci that may demonstrate a posterior reverberation also known as comet-tail or ring-down artifact (Fig. 1). This artifact may be secondary to condensed or inspissated colloid, which has been shown to be benign.[15] Bonavita and colleagues[14] described a pattern of larger cystic nodules with retracted-appearing nonvascular debris, dubbed as a colloid clot or colloid plug. In this appearance, the colloid clot has the benign honeycomb or spongiform pattern. This pattern was reported to have 100% specificity for a benign lesion.

Honeycomb or Spongiform Pattern

This pattern appears as innumerable tiny cystic spaces separated by thin bands or septations (Fig. 2).[13] The honeycomb pattern of fluid separated by attenuated strands of thyroid tissue or septations is benign and nonneoplastic. Although a honeycomb nodule is usually avascular, vascularity may be identified in the tissue strands.[14] Echogenic foci are often encountered when high-frequency probes are used. Careful examination shows that these echogenic foci are linear and associated with the back wall of the tiny cysts. This feature is an important contradistinction to the microcalcifications identified in solid malignant nodules. Ginat and colleagues[16] found that the honeycomb morphology was 100% specific

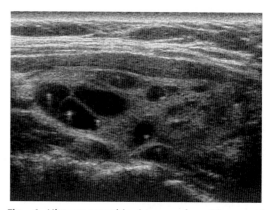

Fig. 1. Ultrasonographic image of a 50-year-old woman with benign colloid cysts demonstrating the ring-down artifact in several cysts.

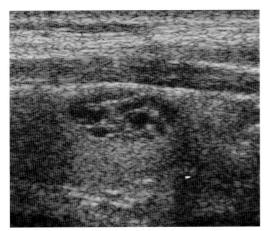

Fig. 2. Ultrasonographic image of a 33-year-old woman with a benign thyroid nodule demonstrating the classic spongiform or honeycomb pattern.

for benign nodular hyperplasia. In the study by Bonavita and colleagues,[14] all the 210 nodules with this appearance were benign and the vast majority were read pathologically as benign colloid nodules (196 of 210), the remainder were nodular Hashimoto thyroiditis or hyperplasia.

Large Predominately Cystic Nodules

A nodule with a predominately cystic pattern is considered highly likely to be benign (**Fig. 3**).[13] The large amount of fluid may be secondary to degeneration, colloid, or sequela of previous hemorrhage. It has been repeatedly demonstrated that benign nodules commonly demonstrate cystic change.[12,17,18] Although a small percentage (6%) of thyroid carcinoma may also be partially cystic,[19]

it is rare to find cystic change occupying more than 50% of the nodule.[20] In the extremely rare case of a malignant nodule with a more than 50% cystic change, other worrisome features such as microcalcifications, vascular mural nodules, increased vascularity, or thick irregular walls are typically present.[20,21] A caveat is that this pattern can only be applied to a nodule within the thyroid because it is commonly known that nodal metastases from papillary thyroid carcinoma are often cystic.

Innumerable Tiny Nodules

Another classic benign pattern is that of innumerable tiny hypoechoic nodules throughout both thyroid lobes, which are separated by coarse echogenic bands.[13] The histologic correlate is multiple lymphoid follicles and surrounding fibrosis. This pattern has a 95% positive predictive value for Hashimoto thyroiditis.[22] In addition, more discrete larger nodules may form in Hashimoto thyroiditis (**Fig. 4**). Most of these nodules are benign and typically caused by focal or nodular Hashimoto thyroiditis, nodular hyperplasia, and follicular adenomas. However, up to 16% of these larger nodules are malignant (usually papillary carcinoma and rarely lymphoma). This incidence is higher than that in the general population and that in those who undergo thyroid FNA.[4] Therefore, it is important to carefully evaluate any discrete nodule larger than the background nodularity.

Markedly Hyperechoic

Another pattern described as 100% specific for benignity is a markedly hyperechoic nodule.[14]

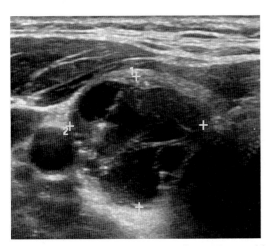

Fig. 3. Ultrasonographic image of a 36-year-old woman with a benign nodule demonstrating marked cystic change.

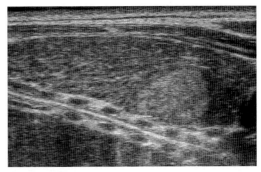

Fig. 4. Ultrasonographic image of a 16-year-old boy with a pattern of multiple tiny hypoechoic nodules consistent with his known diagnosis of chronic lymphocytic thyroiditis (Hashimoto thyroiditis) as well as a well-defined echogenic nodule that was surgically removed and demonstrated nodular Hashimoto thyroiditis).

This can be a colloid-type nodule or focal nodular Hashimoto thyroiditis. In the authors' experience, the markedly hyperechoic nodule is a benign nodule, although rare hyperechoic malignancies can be seen.

WORRISOME PATTERNS THAT SHOULD PROMPT FNA
Solid Hypoechoic Nodules With Discrete Echogenic Foci

A hypoechoic nodule with discrete punctate echogenic foci indicates a high probability of papillary thyroid carcinoma.[13] It is widely known that most (86%–90%) papillary carcinomas are hypoechoic compared with the background thyroid parenchyma.[19,23] This knowledge holds true for even tiny tumors from 8 to 15 mm. Papini and colleagues[24] demonstrated that 87% of these small tumors were hypoechoic. However, hypoechogenicity, in and of itself, is not specific because a large number of benign nodules may have a similar appearance. On the other hand, the combination of hypoechogenicity with another characteristic that has high specificity creates a useful pattern for triaging nodules to FNA. The specificity of microcalcifications for malignancy is 93% to 97%.[16,24,25] The sensitivity is lower, only 42% of papillary carcinomas contain microcalcifications,[19] but the positive predictive value for microcalcifications has been shown to be 70% to 71%.[26,27] These microcalcifications are likely secondary to psammoma bodies, which are lamellated spheres formed from necrotic cells.

During sonography, individual microcalcifications do not shadow (**Fig. 5**A), but if they cluster and form aggregates, posterior shadowing may be seen (see **Fig. 5**B). With careful sonographic interrogation, these microcalcifications can often be distinguished from the echogenic back walls of tiny cysts.

Solid Hypoechoic Nodules With Coarse Echogenic Foci

Another pattern that should prompt FNA is a hypoechoic nodule with coarse central calcification. This pattern can be seen with either papillary or medullary carcinoma.[13] Medullary carcinomas are even more likely to be hypoechoic than papillary carcinomas. Nonetheless, because medullary carcinomas are relatively rare (3%–5% of all thyroid carcinomas), the vast majority of nodules with this pattern are papillary carcinomas. In patients with the MEN syndrome, this pattern is worrisome for medullary carcinoma; the recognition of a hypoechoic nodule with coarse echogenic foci should prompt a thorough evaluation of both thyroid lobes because cancer in these patients may be multicentric. As with microcalcifications, the cause of the coarse calcifications may be psammoma bodies; however, in medullary cancer, the calcifications may be secondary to amyloid deposits that have fibrosed and become calcified.[28] Coarse calcification is also commonly seen in benign nodules, which has been observed in nodules followed over time. These calcifications are usually dystrophic. Although coarse calcification has not been shown to be specific for either

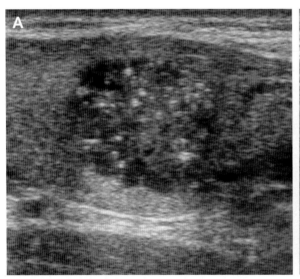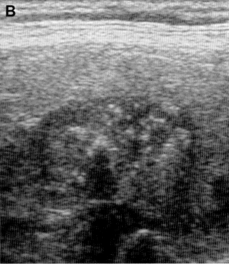

Fig. 5. Ultrasonographic images of (*A*) a 33-year-old man with papillary thyroid cancer demonstrating the classic pattern of a hypoechoic nodule with microcalcifications and (*B*) a 54-year-old woman with papillary carcinoma and coalesced microcalcifications appearing coarse.

benign or malignant nodules, it is the combination of coarse central calcification and nodule hypoechogenicity (**Fig. 6**) that is worrisome and should prompt FNA.

Solid Homogeneous Egg-Shaped Nodules With a Thin Capsule

Follicular lesions are usually solid and homogeneous in echotexture, are oval, and have a thin capsule (**Fig. 7**). These lesions may be isoechoic, hyperechoic, or hypoechoic. Mixed echogenicity, cystic change, and calcifications are less-common features.[13] Both benign and malignant neoplasms have this appearance. Sillery and colleagues[29] found that hypoechogenicity, a lack of cystic change or halo, and a larger size favor malignant follicular carcinoma. In addition, a meta-analysis by Iared and colleagues[30] showed that intranodular vascularity favored malignancy; absent intranodular flow or a predominantly peripheral flow had a lower probability of malignancy. However, these features still lack specificity; therefore, FNA of the lesion is usually performed to establish a follicular neoplastic process. Cytologic diagnosis of a follicular lesion typically prompts diagnostic lobectomy or thyroidectomy. FNA and even core biopsy specimens are insufficient to exclude vascular or capsular invasion, which is the differentiating factor between follicular adenomas and malignant follicular lesions (follicular carcinoma, follicular variant of papillary carcinoma). Most follicular lesions are ultimately confirmed to be follicular adenomas.

Refractive Shadow from the Edge of a Solid Lesion

A refractive shadow at the border of a nodule increases the likelihood that a nodule is

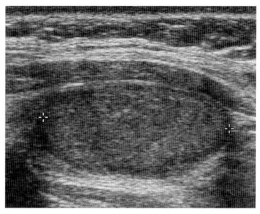

Fig. 7. Ultrasonographic image of a 56-year-old woman with a benign follicular adenoma demonstrating the classic pattern of a homogeneous oval nodule with a thin capsule.

malignant.[13] The refractive shadow occurs at the juncture of 2 tissues with differing sound propagation velocities at an oblique angle to the sound wave. This oblique angle results in diminished transmission, which is manifested as shadowing posterior to the juncture (**Fig. 8**). On gross pathologic examination, most papillary carcinomas contain dense fibrous tissue at the periphery of the nodule. This fibrous reaction likely results in characteristic refractive shadows. Refractive shadow may also be identified posterior to the border of predominately cystic nodules, but the other benign features of these nodules should still allow for correct characterization.

Several other individual descriptors have been described that lack specificity; diffusely increased

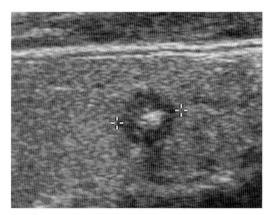

Fig. 6. Ultrasonographic image of a 69-year-old woman with medullary thyroid carcinoma showing the classic pattern of a hypoechoic nodule with coarse central calcification.

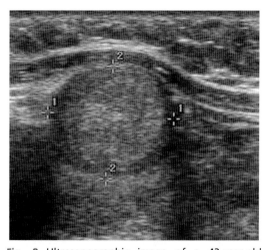

Fig. 8. Ultrasonographic image of a 43-year-old woman with papillary carcinoma demonstrating the pattern of a solid nodule with refractive shadow off the margins.

vascularity, peripheral vascularity, irregular margins, and a halo (or lack of a halo) may be seen with both benign and malignant nodules.[14]

NODULE SIZE

Size is used as a criterion in the decision tree for thyroid nodule biopsy. Size does not aid in upfront diagnosis, but the size of the nodule clearly affects the likelihood of a diagnostic FNA specimen. Moreover, Alexander and colleagues[31] have demonstrated that a significant portion of benign thyroid nodules grow over time.

CLINICAL HISTORY

Pertinent aspects of a patient's clinical history that increase the risk of thyroid malignancy may trump other classification schemes. For example, a small hypoechoic nodule in a patient with a history of head and neck radiation (a significant risk factor for thyroid carcinoma) should prompt FNA even if other worrisome features are absent. The threshold for biopsy in patients with a personal or strong family history of thyroid malignancy is similarly decreased. Finally, nodules in patients with genetic syndromes associated with thyroid cancer, such as MEN, should be viewed with concern.

SOCIETY RECOMMENDATIONS

Many professional societies have published guidelines for thyroid nodule biopsy. As with all consensus documents, these recommendations are based on a combination of scientific research of varying strength and expert opinion.[32,33] These guidelines are based on a combination of nodule characteristics, and nodule size. The recommendations of the Society of Radiologists in Ultrasound (SRU) and the American Thyroid Association (ATA) are summarized in Table 1. This simplified table provides guidelines for the vast majority of nodules encountered in clinical practice, although several unique scenarios are not accounted for. For example, the table does not describe the increasingly accepted observation approach for thyroid glands that are replaced by innumerable similar-appearing nodules. The thyroid-stimulating hormone (TSH) values can also be incorporated into the decision tree. The ATA recommends obtaining serum TSH levels before nodule biopsy: FNA should be performed if the TSH level is elevated or normal and other criteria for biopsy are present. On the other hand, a low TSH level should prompt radionuclide imaging: FNA is not recommended if the nodule is hot (ie, hyperfunctioning) and there are no other worrisome ultrasonographic features. The ATA recommendations listed in Table 1 are for those nodules that are either isofunctioning or hypofunctioning in patients with a low TSH level or for nodules in patients with normal or elevated TSH levels. Both the ATA and SRU guidelines suggest biopsy of any abnormal lymph node discovered during the neck ultrasonographic examination.

Several studies have attempted to validate the effectiveness of published guidelines.[34,35] The results have been variable, and no single set of guideline criteria is more reliable than others. McCartney and Stukenborg,[34] for example, found that the SRU guidelines were particularly useful for triaging nodules that measured between 10 and 14 mm. These results were likely skewed by a selection bias; however, differing size thresholds for biopsy resulted in fewer FNA procedures being performed when the SRU guidelines were applied.

Table 1
Criteria for biopsy

Size of Nodule (mm)	ATA	SRU
5–10	FNA if clinical risk factors and suspicious ultrasonographic features	No recommendation
10–15	FNA if nodule contains microcalcifications or is solid	Strongly consider FNA if nodule contains microcalcifications
15–20	FNA if nodule contains microcalcifications, is solid, or is both solid and cystic with suspicious features	Strongly consider FNA if nodules contain microcalcifications, or is solid with coarse calcifications
>20	FNA for all nodules except the purely cystic ones	Strongly consider FNA if nodule contains microcalcifications, is solid with coarse calcifications, is both solid and cystic, or is cystic with mural nodules or substantial growth

In another study, Ahn and colleagues[35] found that the Kim criteria and the American Association of Clinical Endocrinologists criteria were more accurate. This increased accuracy, however, was a direct result of the decreased emphasis of nodule size in these classifications schemes. The Kim criteria for biopsy include marked hypoechogenicity, irregular or microlobulated margins, microcalcifications, and height greater than width, whereas the American Association of Clinical Endocrinologists criteria for FNA include hypoechogenicity with at least 1 additional worrisome feature such as irregular margins, microcalcifications, and longer-than-wide shape. Both decision trees advocate biopsy of nodules with worrisome features, regardless of size. Such an approach may not take into account the clinical effect of biopsy on the so-called papillary microcarcinomas (<10 mm papillary thyroid carcinomas). This controversy is clearly beyond the scope of this review, but controversy still remains regarding the outcome of the typical patient with small-volume differentiated thyroid cancer.

SUMMARY

The current epidemic of thyroid nodules makes it imperative that practitioners effectively divide nodules into those that should be left alone and those that should be biopsied. This article has reviewed a reliable pattern approach to categorizing thyroid nodules into likely benign patterns for which FNA is not necessary and worrisome patterns that require FNA. Nodules that are cystic and may contain echogenic foci, spongiform nodules, large predominately cystic nodules, and innumerable tiny nodules are all likely benign patterns that do not require FNA. Conversely, solid hypoechoic nodules with discrete tiny echogenic foci, solid hypoechoic nodules with coarse echogenic foci, solid homogeneous nodules with thin capsules, and solid nodules with refractive edge shadows are worrisome findings that should prompt FNA. In addition, the SRU and ATA recommendations for nodule triage are also summarized; both the guidelines heavily incorporate nodule size into the decision tree. Although size alone does not indicate the biological behavior, the likelihood of ultimate successful characterization, by FNA, improves with larger-size nodules.

REFERENCES

1. Brander A, Viikinkoski P, Nickels J, et al. Thyroid gland: US screening in a random adult population. Radiology 1991;181(3):683–7.

2. Mortensen JD, Woolner LB, Bennett WA. Gross and microscopic findings in clinically normal thyroid glands. J Clin Endocrinol Metab 1955;15(10):1270–80.

3. Tan GH, Gharib H. Thyroid incidentalomas: management approaches to nonpalpable nodules discovered incidentally on thyroid imaging. Ann Intern Med 1997;126(3):226–31.

4. Anderson L, Middleton WD, Teefey SA, et al. Hashimoto thyroiditis: part 2, sonographic analysis of benign and malignant nodules in patients with diffuse Hashimoto thyroiditis. AJR Am J Roentgenol 2010;195(1):216–22.

5. Brander AE, Viikinkoski VP, Nickels JI, et al. Importance of thyroid abnormalities detected at US screening: a 5-year follow-up. Radiology 2000;215(3):801–6.

6. Jemal A, Siegel R, Ward E, et al. Cancer statistics, 2009. CA Cancer J Clin 2009;59(4):225–49.

7. Davies L, Welch HG. Increasing incidence of thyroid cancer in the United States, 1973–2002. JAMA 2006;295(18):2164–7.

8. Enewold L, Zhu K, Ron E, et al. Rising thyroid cancer incidence in the United States by demographic and tumor characteristics, 1980–2005. Cancer Epidemiol Biomarkers Prev 2009;18(3):784–91.

9. Burke JP, Hay ID, Dignan F, et al. Long-term trends in thyroid carcinoma: a population-based study in Olmsted County, Minnesota, 1935–1999. Mayo Clin Proc 2005;80(6):753–8.

10. Yu GP, Li JC-L, Branovan D, et al. Thyroid cancer incidence and survival in the National Cancer Institute Surveillance, Epidemiology, and End Results race/ethnicity groups. Thyroid 2010;20(5):465–73.

11. Davies L, Welch HG. Thyroid cancer survival in the United States: observational data from 1973 to 2005. Arch Otolaryngol Head Neck Surg 2010;136(5):440–4.

12. Wienke JR, Chong WK, Fielding JR, et al. Sonographic features of benign thyroid nodules: interobserver reliability and overlap with malignancy. J Ultrasound Med 2003;22(10):1027–31.

13. Reading CC, Charboneau JW, Hay ID, et al. Sonography of thyroid nodules: a "classic pattern" diagnostic approach. Ultrasound Q 2005;21(3):157–65.

14. Bonavita JA, Mayo J, Babb J, et al. Pattern recognition of benign nodules at ultrasound of the thyroid: which nodules can be left alone? AJR Am J Roentgenol 2009;193(1):207–13.

15. Ahuja A, Chick W, King W, et al. Clinical significance of the comet-tail artifact in thyroid ultrasound. J Clin Ultrasound 1996;24(3):129–33.

16. Ginat DT, Butani D, Giampoli EJ, et al. Pearls and pitfalls of thyroid nodule sonography and fine-needle aspiration. Ultrasound Q 2010;26(3):171–8.

17. Frates MC, Benson CB, Doubilet PM, et al. Can color Doppler sonography aid in the prediction of

malignancy of thyroid nodules? J Ultrasound Med 2003;22(2):127–31 [quiz: 132–4].

18. Grant CS, Goellner JR. Cystic thyroid nodules. The dilemma of malignant lesions. Arch Intern Med 1990;150(7):1376–7.

19. Chan BK, Desser TS, McDougall IR, et al. Common and uncommon sonographic features of papillary thyroid carcinoma. J Ultrasound Med 2003;22(10): 1083–90.

20. Henrichsen TL, Reading CC, Charboneau JW, et al. Cystic change in thyroid carcinoma: prevalence and estimated volume in 360 carcinomas. J Clin Ultrasound 2010;38(7):361–6.

21. Hatabu H, Kasagi K, Yamamoto K, et al. Cystic papillary carcinoma of the thyroid gland: a new sonographic sign. Clin Radiol 1991;43(2):121–4.

22. Yeh HC, Futterweit W, Gilbert P. Micronodulation: ultrasonographic sign of Hashimoto thyroiditis. J Ultrasound Med 1996;15(12):813–9.

23. Jun P, Chow LC, Jeffrey RB. The sonographic features of papillary thyroid carcinomas: pictorial essay. Ultrasound Q 2005;21(1):39–45.

24. Papini E, Guglielmi R, Bianchini A, et al. Risk of malignancy in nonpalpable thyroid nodules: predictive value of ultrasound and color-Doppler features. J Clin Endocrinol Metab 2002;87(5):1941–6.

25. Takashima S, Fukuda H, Nomura N, et al. Thyroid nodules: re-evaluation with ultrasound. J Clin Ultrasound 1995;23(3):179–84.

26. Kakkos SK, Scopa CD, Chalmoukis AK, et al. Relative risk of cancer in sonographically detected thyroid nodules with calcifications. J Clin Ultrasound 2000;28(7):347–52.

27. Kim EK, Park CS, Chung WY, et al. New sonographic criteria for recommending fine-needle aspiration biopsy of nonpalpable solid nodules of the thyroid. AJR Am J Roentgenol 2002;178(3):687–91.

28. Gorman B, Charboneau JW, James EM, et al. Medullary thyroid carcinoma: role of high-resolution US. Radiology 1987;162(1 Pt 1):147–50.

29. Sillery JC, Reading CC, Charboneau JW, et al. Thyroid follicular carcinoma: sonographic features of 50 cases. AJR Am J Roentgenol 2010;194(1):44–54.

30. Iared W, Shigueoka DC, Cristofoli JC, et al. Use of color Doppler ultrasonography for the prediction of malignancy in follicular thyroid neoplasms: systematic review and meta-analysis. J Ultrasound Med 2010;29(3):419–25.

31. Alexander EK, Hurwitz S, Heering JP, et al. Natural history of benign solid and cystic thyroid nodules. [summary for patients in Ann Intern Med 2003; 138(4):I60; PMID: 12585849]. Ann Intern Med 2003; 138(4):315–8.

32. Frates MC, Benson CB, Charboneau JW, et al. Management of thyroid nodules detected at US: Society of Radiologists in Ultrasound consensus conference statement. Radiology 2005;237(3): 794–800.

33. American Thyroid Association Guidelines Taskforce on Thyroid Nodules and Differentiated Thyroid Cancer, Cooper DS, Doherty GM, et al. Revised American Thyroid Association management guidelines for patients with thyroid nodules and differentiated thyroid cancer. Thyroid 2009;19(11):1167–214.

34. McCartney CR, Stukenborg GJ. Decision analysis of discordant thyroid nodule biopsy guideline criteria. J Clin Endocrinol Metab 2008;93(8):3037–44.

35. Ahn SS, Kim EK, Kang DR, et al. Biopsy of thyroid nodules: comparison of three sets of guidelines. AJR Am J Roentgenol 2010;194(1):31–7.

Thyroid: Nuclear Medicine Update

Judith M. Joyce, MD*, Andrew Swihart, MD

KEYWORDS

- Nuclear medicine • Iodine 131 • Iodine 123
- Tc 99m pertechnetate • FDG PET/CT • SPECT/CT

Nuclear medicine has played a vital role in the evaluation and treatment of thyroid disease since it was first introduced in the 1930s. The unique ability of radiotracers to evaluate and, when used in sufficient doses, treat thyroid disease (by ablating benign overactive or malignant thyroid tissue) has not been replicated by any other imaging modality or medication. Some of the radionuclides initially developed, such as iodine 131 (^{131}I), are still widely used. Other radiotracers, such as Tc 99m pertechnetate, iodine 123 (^{123}I), and fluorodeoxyglucose (FDG), have assumed a larger role in the nuclear medicine armamentarium for the diagnosis of thyroid disease. In addition, imaging techniques have gradually advanced from the basic gamma camera to highly specialized hybrid imaging equipment, single-photon emission computed tomography (SPECT)/computed tomography (CT) and positron emission tomography (PET)/CT. The preparation for thyroid imaging and treatment of thyroid cancer has also evolved. Traditional thyroid hormone withdrawal still is used, but patient preparation with recombinant *thyroid-stimulating hormone* (rTSH) is now routinely used at many centers. An increased number of radiotracers, improved imaging capabilities, and better patient preparation have reinforced the special role of nuclear medicine in the evaluation and treatment of thyroid disease. Despite rapid improvements in cross-sectional imaging, the ability of nuclear medicine to assess physiology and function and treat makes it an indispensable tool in the management of the patient with thyroid disease.

HISTORY

One day in the spring of 1938, Joe Hamilton ran into Glenn Seaborg on the steps of the physics building at Berkeley University and complained about the short half-life of iodine 128 (28 minutes). Joe asked Glenn if he could produce an iodine with a longer half-life, like "about a week." A few months later, after working with Jack Livingood on tellurium targets and chemical separation, they identified a new isotope, ^{131}I.[1] The birth of this new agent, ^{131}I, revolutionized the evaluation and treatment of thyroid disease and may be one of the most important factors in the origin and growth of nuclear medicine.

RADIONUCLIDES
Iodine 131

Despite being more than 70 years old, ^{131}I remains a major agent of choice for the treatment of benign and malignant thyroid disease. It is still used to image thyroid cancer and quantify thyroid uptake measurements. Iodine 131 has unique gamma and beta emitting properties; the gamma radiation allows for imaging, and the beta radiation is used for therapy. Initially, ^{131}I was also an important tracer for the imaging of benign thyroid disease, but its high radiation dose (^{131}I emits approximately 1 rad/μCi to the thyroid gland) and unfavorable imaging characteristics (its principal photon has a high energy of 364 keV) are less than optimal. The introduction of newer radiotracers with lower radiation doses, such as ^{123}I and Tc

The authors have nothing to disclose.
Division of Nuclear Medicine, Department of Radiology, University of Pittsburgh Medical Center, 200 Lothrop Street, Pittsburgh, PA 15213, USA
* Corresponding author.
E-mail address: joycejm@upmc.edu

Radiol Clin N Am 49 (2011) 425–434
doi:10.1016/j.rcl.2011.02.004

99m pertechnetate, has resulted in a decreasing role of ^{131}I in the imaging and uptake evaluation of benign thyroid disease. However, ^{131}I continues to play a major role in the imaging of patients with thyroid cancer after thyroidectomy and the treatment of hyperthyroidism and thyroid cancer.[2]

Iodine 123

Iodine 123 has become the imaging and uptake agent of choice for routine benign thyroid imaging because of its more ideal properties (a half-life of 13 hours and energy of 159 keV). Like ^{131}I, ^{123}I is trapped and organified by the thyroid gland and is administered orally. With ^{123}I, a low dose (0.3–0.5 mCi) is given for both imaging and uptake evaluation. Imaging and uptake values are acquired 4 to 24 hours after ingestion; this timing is based on a long half-life and retention of the tracer in the gland after organification. The approach is convenient because uptake values can be determined using the same dose of ^{123}I administered for imaging.[2]

Tc 99m Pertechnetate

Tc 99m pertechnetate also has ideal imaging properties and a low radiation dose (half-life of 6 hours and 140 keV). An additional benefit is that it is usually readily available for clinical use. Because Tc 99m pertechnetate is trapped but not organified by the thyroid gland and has a shorter half-life, imaging is performed 15 to 20 minutes after intravenous injection. A higher dose (5–10 mCi) of tracer is also administered. Tc 99m pertechnetate is not typically used to obtain uptake values because it is not organified by the thyroid gland and requires special valid and reproducible acquisition methods. A very low dose of [131]I (3–5 μCi) may be given concurrently with Tc 99m pertechnetate if both uptake values and imaging are needed.

[18]F Fluorodeoxyglucose

[18]F FDG is a glucose analogue labeled with the positron emitter, fluorine 18 (^{18}F). It is now routinely used to image tumors that are highly metabolically active. Because of its half-life of almost 2 hours, ^{18}F can be labeled to deoxyglucose and distributed by regional radiopharmacies to multiple clinical sites on a daily basis with reasonable cost and dependability. The typical dose of FDG injected is 12 to 20 mCi; imaging is performed approximately 45 to 90 minutes postinjection.

After injection, FDG is taken up by normal-glucose-using sites throughout the body and metabolically active tumor cells. FDG undergoes phosphorylation to FDG 6-PO_4 and accumulates within malignant cells. Increased FDG uptake within tumor cells is selectively detected by PET.[3] FDG PET is now commonly used for multiple approved oncological indications, including thyroid cancer.

INSTRUMENTATION/EQUIPMENT
Gamma Camera

The gamma camera was a major breakthrough in nuclear medicine because it vastly improved the capability of imaging gamma-emitting radionuclides, such as technetium and iodine agents. A collimator attached to the gamma camera acts as a grid; the collimator improves resolution and decreases undesired scatter, which can degrade the image. For routine Tc 99m and ^{123}I agents, a low-energy collimator is used. The high energy of ^{131}I requires a high-energy collimator with thicker lead septa. A more optimal collimator for imaging the thyroid gland is the pinhole collimator, a cone-shaped device attached to the gamma camera, with the small aperture placed closest to the patient. This special collimator magnifies small structures and permits high-resolution scans. Typically, this is the collimator used when imaging patients with their native thyroid glands with Tc 99m pertechnetate or [123]I.[2]

Uptake Probe

A basic measurement of the overall function of the thyroid can be obtained by using a thyroid uptake probe, a single-crystal counting device. This simple procedure starts with the measuring of the standard by the uptake probe before its administration to the patient on day 1. The patient returns for subsequent evaluation, typically at 4 and 24 hours after ingestion, for measurements of the uptake in the neck, thigh (patient background), and room background. The mathematical calculation of the thyroid uptake is performed by using the decay-corrected standard measurement in the neck (thyroid uptake) and subtracting the patient background activity (thigh activity), which is then divided by the amount of activity in the decay-corrected standard (given to the patient on day 1) subtracting the room background activity.[4] Previously, these calculations were performed by hand, but modern computer-integrated probes quickly and automatically calculate the percentage uptake.

SPECT, PET, and Hybrid Imaging

SPECT has been available for many years on state-of-the-art gamma camera/computer. Specialized acquisition protocols and processing generate tomographic slices. Although traditional planar imaging provides 2-dimensional pictures of 3-dimensional (3D) objects, SPECT allows the user to more accurately view the radiotracer distribution and localization within the body using a 3D representation.[5]

FDG PET imaging has also been available for many years. However, its use was limited to research applications until the US Centers for Medicare and Medicaid Services approved reimbursement for clinical usage in the 1990s. The subsequent development of multiple sites for manufacturing and delivering FDG in the late 1990s facilitated the rapid expansion of this modality. PET scanners are composed of multiple highly specialized thick detectors that have a stopping power to accept high-energy 511-keV coincident positron emissions and are capable of resolving the time of this detection in nanoseconds. The coincidence detection of these positrons by the PET scanner results in a 100-fold increase in photon sensitivity for PET compared with SPECT for the same spatial resolution. This sensitivity results in excellent image quality as well as reliable quantitative assessment.[5]

SPECT and PET cameras have been further improved by the introduction of hybrid imaging equipment that can perform both nuclear medicine and CT imaging. These scanners can not only produce images from each of these modalities separately but can also combine the emission data from the nuclear medicine images with the CT data to produce images with improved attenuation correction and anatomic localization. Both SPECT/CT and PET/CT imaging have improved the accuracy of benign and malignant disease detection.[6–9]

IMAGING PROTOCOLS
Thyroid Nodules

Routine thyroid scanning for the evaluation of thyroid nodules is performed with Tc 99m pertechnetate or [123]I. A pinhole collimator attached to the gamma camera magnifies the gland and improves resolution. Although this approach provides relatively good images of the intrinsic uptake within the thyroid gland, nuclear medicine thyroid imaging cannot achieve the anatomic detail obtained with ultrasonography. However, the unique benefit of nuclear medicine scanning is its ability to determine function within the thyroid gland, a valuable capability not paralleled by any other imaging modality. Neither ultrasonography nor CT (or MR imaging) can determine if a hyperfunctioning nodule appears "hot" or a hypofunctioning nodule appears "cold."[4]

Hyperthyroidism

The workup of hyperthyroidism entails obtaining anatomic images of the thyroid gland and uptake values of its overall function. Images of the gland are obtained with ^{123}I or Tc 99m pertechnetate. The pattern of uptake in the gland may help determine the cause of the hyperthyroidism. In addition, the overall function of the thyroid gland is quantitatively determined with a thyroid uptake probe. The most commonly used uptake measurement for hyperthyroidism is obtained at 24 hours following ingestion of ^{123}I or [131]I. It is also helpful to obtain a 4- to 6-hour measurement to avoid missing the occasional occurrence of a rapid turnover, which can occur when the gland quickly organifies the radiotracer and releases radiolabeled thyroid hormone into the system before 24 hours.[4]

Hypothyroidism

Evaluation of the thyroid gland is an essential step in the workup of pediatric hypothyroidism. A thyroid scan can readily be performed for this purpose; Tc 99m pertechnetate is usually given intravenously. Iodine 123 may also be given orally, although it may be difficult to administer effectively to an infant. Pinhole images are obtained to magnify the small structures in the neck, and imaging from the base of the tongue to the base of the neck is performed to evaluate for the presence and location of normal or ectopic thyroid tissue.[5]

Thyroid Cancer

Nuclear medicine imaging protocols for evaluation of thyroid cancer have rapidly evolved over the past few years. Improved approaches have been recommended in recently published guidelines.[10] For many years, patients have undergone thyroidectomy and then thyroid hormone withdrawal to cause hypothyroidism. Such an approach maximizes the uptake of the radiotracer into residual thyroid tissue or functioning thyroid tumor. The traditional imaging radiotracer has been ^{131}I, which is a high-energy radionuclide with poor imaging characteristics.

This traditional approach requires the patient to be taken off thyroxine (T_4) for 4 to 6 weeks. The patient is often placed on triiodothyronine (T_3) for the next 2 to 4 weeks, and then all thyroid hormone replacement is withdrawn for approximately 2 weeks.[11] This preparation requires that the patient become hypothyroid with an elevated TSH level, which is often difficult for the patient to endure. In addition, the patient should follow a low-iodine diet during the 1 to 2 weeks before the initial ingestion of the ^{131}I for diagnostic imaging. A low-iodine diet has been shown to improve the detection of tissue and/or tumor.[12]

rTSH is now routinely used in lieu of thyroid hormone withdrawal before thyroid cancer diagnostic imaging and therapy. rTSH was first approved by the US Food and Drug Administration (FDA) in 1998 as an alternate method for preparation for radioiodine imaging in the follow-up of patients with well-differentiated thyroid cancer. In 2007, the FDA granted supplemental approval of rTSH for preparation for radioiodine ablation of thyroid tissue remnants in patients who have undergone a near-total or total thyroidectomy for well-differentiated thyroid cancer without evidence of metastatic thyroid cancer. This new method of preparation for thyroid cancer imaging and therapy has not only allowed many patients to avoid the inconvenience of hypothyroidism but also has minimized the likelihood of other side effects, such as salivary gland symptoms.[13]

For imaging of patients with thyroid cancer with ^{131}I, usually 1 to 4 mCi is given orally and the patient returns 48 to 72 hours later for whole-body imaging. Iodine 131 imaging requires a high-energy collimator with thick parallel "holes" (created by lead septa) caused by the strength of the gamma energy of this radionuclide. The pictures include whole-body images from the head to toes, along with a dedicated separate planar image of the neck. More recently, ^{123}I has been introduced for imaging of thyroid cancer. A low-energy high-resolution parallel-hole collimator is used for this radiotracer. The ^{123}I is given in similar doses of 1 to 4 mCi. The lower and more optimal imaging energy results in better resolution imaging than when ^{131}I is used; earlier imaging at 24 hours is also possible because of its shorter half-life (**Fig. 1**). Nonetheless, ^{123}I is more expensive, and its use may not significantly change the overall clinical results.[14]

A valuable complement to the imaging examination is a quantitative determination of the thyroid bed uptake on ^{123}I or ^{131}I static images of the neck. To perform this measurement, a standard must be placed in the field of view and the counts from the thyroid bed, standard, patient, and image background are entered into a formula that calculates the percentage uptake in the thyroid bed. This uptake value is very helpful in determining the appropriate management of patients with thyroid cancer because it permits a more individualized ^{131}I doses for the patient.

The introduction of rTSH for imaging and therapy preparation and the better logistics of ^{123}I whole-body imaging at 24 hours have prompted a more streamlined imaging and treatment

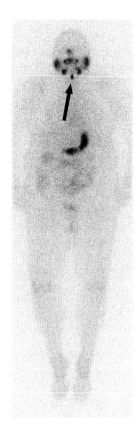

Fig. 1. Iodine 123 whole-body scan on a 69-year-old woman after thyroidectomy for papillary thyroid carcinoma, follicular variant, which demonstrates a small amount of midline residual thyroid tissue present (*arrow*); thyroid bed uptake was calculated at 0.24%.

protocol based on a single 2 course of rTSH. The rTSH is given on the first and second days (typically at the same time each morning), followed by ^{123}I on the afternoon of the second day. Imaging and therapy are then performed on the third day. This approach has been found to be helpful, particularly for first timers with low-risk disease.

Several institutions have developed more sophisticated dosimetric methods to determine the optimal ^{131}I dose to administer to each patient with thyroid cancer.[15,16] These more demanding protocols may not be feasible at all institutions, but the tailored dose may especially be helpful when treating patients with advanced disease. When the authors perform dosimetry, the patient ingests the ^{131}I and returns for 4 days for whole-body imaging and after a week for blood sampling. These results are then used to determine the highest dose the patient can receive, keeping the exposure less than 200 rads to the blood and less than 80 mCi to the lungs. This more complicated procedure is primarily performed in patients with significantly advanced metastatic thyroid cancer, so that the maximum dose can be administered. This approach is also useful to evaluate an appropriate dose in patients with renal dysfunction and poor iodine clearance.

INTERPRETATION
Normal

Images of the normal thyroid gland typically demonstrate homogeneous uptake of radiotracer in both lobes with the characteristic butterfly pattern, along with uptake in the isthmus if present. With pertechnetate imaging, physiologic uptake is also seen in the salivary glands, which normally show slightly less-intense uptake than the normal thyroid gland. This relative uptake can be used as a visual qualitative assessment of thyroid function. Uptake is then quantitatively confirmed by the calculated uptake measurement. A range of normal values has been used, including 5% to 15% at 4 to 6 hours and 10% to 30% at 24 hours.

Nodules

Nodules in the thyroid gland can show varying levels of uptake based on their function in relation to the surrounding thyroid gland. Most thyroid nodules are hypofunctioning in relation to the

normally functioning thyroid gland and are detected as cold on the images (**Fig. 2**). Cold nodules have an approximate 5% to 35% chance of malignancy and should be further worked up with ultrasonography and possible biopsy. Occasionally, thyroid nodules are hyperfunctioning in relation to the adjacent gland and are considered hot. If this is first evaluated with a pertechnetate scan, reimaging with an ^{123}I scan is necessary to exclude the rare occurrence of a discordant nodule, which might be hot on the pertechnetate scan but is actually cold on the ^{123}I scan. If the uptake in the lesion is similar to that in the adjacent gland, the nodule would be considered a "warm" nodule, which is essentially managed as a cold nodule because it is not truly hyperfunctioning.[4]

The utility of thyroid scintigraphy to characterize thyroid nodules has significantly decreased over the past decade because of the increasing use of thyroid ultrasonography and *fine needle aspiration* (FNA) biopsy. Nonetheless, nuclear medicine thyroid scanning can still play a role in specific situations. The recently revised American Thyroid Association (ATA) guidelines recommend the use of thyroid scintigraphy in the initial workup of patients who present with a nodule and a low TSH value.[10] If the nodule is hyperfunctioning, then the patient is further evaluated and treated for hyperthyroidism and no cytologic evaluation

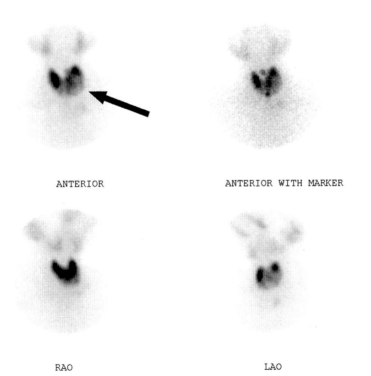

ANTERIOR

ANTERIOR WITH MARKER

RAO

LAO

Fig. 2. Tc 99m pertechnetate scan on a 37-year-old woman with a large cold nodule (*arrow*) in the left thyroid lobe. LAO, left anterior oblique; RAO, right anterior oblique.

is necessary. These guidelines also recommend a thyroid scan in the evaluation of an FNA biopsy, suggesting a follicular neoplasm, because a hyperfunctioning (hot) nodule indicates a benign cause. The limited resolution of thyroid scintigraphy, even with pinhole imaging, should be kept in mind when contemplating its use, particularly for nodules smaller than 1 to 1.5 cm.

Hyperthyroidism

The thyroid uptake and scan has proved to be useful in the diagnosis and treatment of hyperthyroidism. The uptake plays a primary role in distinguishing between the major causes of hyperthyroidism. A very low thyroid uptake indicates causes such as subacute thyroiditis, postpartum thyroiditis, or amiodarone toxicity, whereas uptake is usually normal to high in toxic nodular disease (20%–40%) and high (often >50%) in Grave disease.[17] The last 2 causes can be further evaluated by analyzing the pattern of uptake on the images from the scan: a homogeneous uptake may indicate Grave disease (**Fig. 3**), whereas a heterogeneous pattern suggests nodular disease. After the diagnostic evaluation, the quantitative uptake value can be used to determine the dose of ^{131}I appropriate for treatment of hyperthyroidism due to Grave disease or toxic nodular glands.

Hypothyroidism

Recognition of the severe effects of hypothyroidism has lead to the mandatory screening of

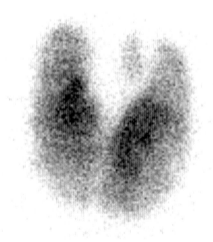

Fig. 3. Iodine 123 scan with a pinhole collimator in a 26-year-old woman with Grave disease demonstrating an enlarged thyroid gland with diffusely increased uptake throughout both the right and left lobes and in the pyramidal lobe, with an elevated uptake measurement of 55%.

neonatal hypothyroidism in the United States. The workup includes thyroid ultrasonography and a thyroid scan to visualize the presence and location of normal or ectopic thyroid tissue in the neck. Ectopic tissue can be located from the base of the tongue to the base of the neck, based on its embryologic migration (**Fig. 4**). If the thyroid gland is not visualized on nuclear medicine imaging but is identified on ultrasonography, TSH receptor blocking antibodies may be present. Thyroid agenesis is likely if the thyroid is not be identified by either method.[17]

Thyroid Cancer

The use of radioiodine whole-body scanning for thyroid cancer evaluation before ^{131}I therapy has been controversial. Prior reports have suggested the potential of the low dose of ^{131}I used for pretreatment imaging to stun the remaining thyroid tissue/tumor and diminish the effectiveness of ablation.[18] Some sites, such as the authors' institution, routinely use the pretreatment scan and thyroid bed uptake to help determine the treatment dose based on the degree of uptake as well as the extent of distant metastases. Other institutions do not always perform a pretherapy scan but may routinely obtain a neck ultrasonogram instead.[11]

Most sites do perform posttherapy scans. Current ATA guidelines recommend that the posttherapy scan be performed 2 to 10 days after treatment.[10] The rationale for these posttreatment scans is the ability to potentially detect additional sites of metastatic disease not visualized on the pretreatment scan. Additional sites of tumor have been reported in 10% to 26% of patients following high radioactive iodine treatment compared with the diagnostic scan. Recognition of more sites of disease than initially appreciated might affect subsequent management.[19]

THYROID DISEASE TREATMENTS
Hyperthyroidism

Hyperthyroidism is a benign thyroid disease that requires a proper workup to determine its cause to assure appropriate treatment. When hyperthyroidism due to a toxic nodular gland or Grave disease is confirmed, antithyroid medication may be initially used as a temporary treatment, but more permanent therapy with radioactive iodine or surgery is usually necessary. Treatment with ^{131}I has proved to be a valuable noninvasive approach with minimal side effects. Because of the beta radiation properties of ^{131}I, effective radiation is delivered locally to the thyroid; radiation gradually ablates the thyroid cells over several

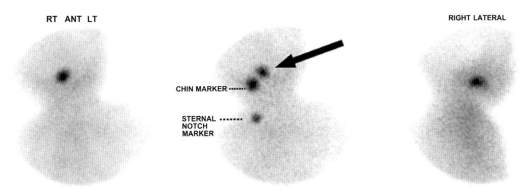

RT ANT LT

RIGHT LATERAL

CHIN MARKER ·······

STERNAL ········
NOTCH
MARKER

Fig. 4. Tc 99m pertechnetate scan in a 12-month-old child with hypothyroidism with an ectopic lingual thyroid (*arrow*).

months. The gamma properties of ^{131}I mandate several short-term radiation precautions, including keeping a distance away from others and preventing exposure to others of bodily fluids.[17]

The methods for determining ^{131}I treatment doses for hyperthyroidism due to Grave disease or a toxic nodular goiter vary among practitioners. Initially, multiple smaller doses were used, with the rationale being that such an approach might ultimately result in euthyroidism. In practice, if euthyroidism is achieved, it is usually only temporary. Multiple small doses eventually lead to hypothyroidism or even recurrent hyperthyroidism. For Grave disease, high cure rates usually occur with doses of at least 15 mCi. These doses result in retained activity in the thyroid of at least 8 mCi, 150 to 200 μCi/g, and an absorbed thyroid radiation dose of 25,000 rads (250 Gy). Toxic multinodular goiters typically required higher doses of up to 25 to 30 mCi or greater.[17] Recent reports of the use of rTSH to increase the ^{131}I uptake describe improved results with a greater reduction in thyroid volume.[20]

Thyroid Cancer

Thyroid cancer therapy with ^{131}I is still considered an important part of the treatment regimen for differentiated thyroid cancer. The preparation for this therapy requires that the patient undergo initial total thyroidectomy, become endogenously hypothyroid by thyroid hormone withdrawal, or receive exogenous rTSH and follow a low-iodine diet in order that the residual thyroid tissue or tumor effectively localizes the radioiodine internally.[11] Depending on the institution, the patient may undergo a pretreatment whole-body ^{123}I or ^{131}I scan to evaluate the amount of residual thyroid tissue and the extent of metastatic tumor. Whole-body scans may also be supplemented by neck ultrasonography. These measures can then be followed by ^{131}I therapy if indicated.

A key issue that has undergone recent scrutiny is the categorization of patients with low-risk differentiated thyroid cancer to undergo surgery, ^{131}I therapy, and routine ^{131}I imaging surveillance. Treatment strategies weigh the need and risks of surgery and radiation versus the long-term prognosis for patients with low-risk disease. The newly revised ATA guidelines outline possible algorithms to use based on the nodule size, the patient's pathology from lobectomy or thyroidectomy, imaging results, and thyroglobulin (Tg) levels. This risk stratification has become paramount not only in the initial decision making of whether the patient needs surgery and radioiodine therapy but also in the determination of the follow-up after initial treatment. For example, a patient with a single well-differentiated thyroid cancer less than 1 cm may only need lobectomy, and not thyroidectomy with subsequent ^{131}I therapy. A patient with a thyroid cancer greater than 1 cm but less than 4 cm and no nodal involvement may need only 50 mCi ^{131}I, which is less than the usual 100 mCi or more that previously was commonly prescribed. Furthermore, the guidelines recommend that after the initial ^{131}I treatment (remnant ablation), low-risk patients with undetectable Tg levels and negative results on ultrasonography do not need to undergo routine follow-up with ^{131}I whole-body scans, which previously were performed annually as a part of routine surveillance.[10]

In contrast, most experts agree that patients with moderate- to high-risk disease should undergo ^{131}I treatment with higher ^{131}I doses and that these patients should have routine follow-up radioiodine scans and determination of Tg levels. These patients include those with suspected residual disease, extrathyroidal extension, more aggressive histology, or metastatic disease. Such patients require special management because the intensity of follow-up depends on multiple factors, such as age, initial pathology, genetic markers, subsequent surgical findings, location and extent of disease, radioactive iodine avidity, and Tg levels. Multimodal imaging with ultrasound, CT, as well as PET/CT and SPECT/CT, may be appropriate.[7]

In patients with moderate- to high-risk disease, increasing the dose to 100 to 200 mCi or even higher may be indicated, but dosing should be determined on a case-by-case basis. However, empiric doses of more than 200 mCi are not recommended for patients older than 70 years.[10] At our institution, when a dose greater than 200 mCi is considered, dosimetric evaluation as previously described is performed to limit the blood and lung exposure to acceptable levels (with the caveat that, the superiority of dosimetry-determined doses vs empiric dosing has not been proven).[8]

Iodine 131 therapy for patients with differentiated thyroid cancer is not risk-free. Despite the valuable role of ^{131}I therapy in destroying residual thyroid tissue and/or tumor, the short- and long-term risks of this therapy need to be considered before dosing. The transient nausea that many patients experience can usually be controlled with antinausea medications. However, the salivary gland injury that can occur may lead to bothersome long-term symptoms, such as a dry mouth (one of the additional benefits of lower-dose regimens advocated in the new guidelines is a decreased incidence of this long-term complication). Even more concerning is the occurrence of secondary malignancies following treatment.[21]

USE OF NEW IMAGING TECHNIQUES IN THYROID DISEASE MANAGEMENT

FDG PET/CT has become an important imaging modality for the diagnosis and evaluation of treatment response in patients with cancer. Although most patients with differentiated thyroid cancer have low-risk disease, an unfortunate few have more aggressive tumors that spread, especially to the lymph nodes, lung, and bone. To evaluate these patients, numerous studies have investigated the role of FDG PET imaging to detect thyroid cancer metastases. The overall sensitivity and specificity were found to range from 45% to 100% and 42% to 90%, respectively.[3]

An important subset of these patients with thyroid cancer is those with elevated Tg levels and dedifferentiated tumor that is not radioiodine avid (and not detectable on ^{131}I scans) (Fig. 5). In this setting of Tg-positive but iodine-negative disease, the sensitivity of FDG PET scanning has been reported to increase from 75% for all patients with thyroid cancer up to 85% in patients with negative radioiodine scans.[22] Consequently, FDG

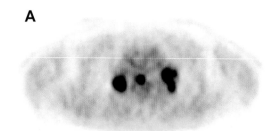

A

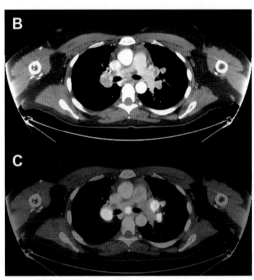

B

C

Fig. 5. (A–C) PET/CT imaging in a 44-year-old woman with papillary thyroid carcinoma who had an elevated Tg level of 716 and negative ^{131}I whole-body scan. Intensely FDG-avid metastatic mediastinal and bilateral hilar lymphadenopathy is demonstrated on the transaxial FDG PET image (A), corresponding CT slice (B), and PET/CT fusion image (C).

PET imaging has proved helpful in determining if there is disease present in these patients, if the disease is resectable, and if further treatment with high-dose ^{131}I might be successful (see Fig. 5).[7,23] Newer chemotherapy agents are also being developed, which may add further treatment options in these difficult situations.[24]

A pitfall of interpreting FDG PET images has been the difficulty in distinguishing areas of uptake under normal physiologic versus pathologic conditions. PET/CT has significantly improved localization, because it improves attenuation correction and fuses FDG uptake (function) with CT (anatomy). One study reported an increase of 78% to 93% in accuracy between PET and PET/CT imaging.[25] As this dual imaging technology improves, it will likely have an increasing impact on patient management because of its ability to accurately detect even smaller foci of disease.[3]

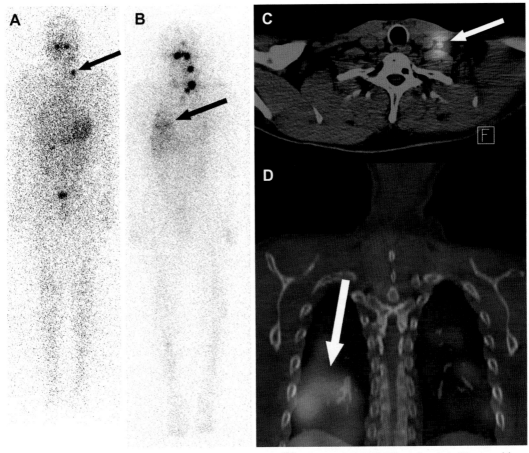

Fig. 6. (A–D) Pretreatment and posttreatment whole-body ^{131}I scans and SPECT/CT imaging in a 57-year-old man with a remote history of papillary thyroid cancer treated with radioactive iodine 35 years prior and recent development of increasing Tg levels. (A) Pretreatment whole-body radioiodine scan revealed a single focus of ^{131}I uptake in the left neck (arrow). (B) After treatment with 153 mCi of ^{131}I, the posttreatment scan showed multiple left neck foci and uptake in the lungs (arrow). (C) Transaxial SPECT/CT imaging demonstrated that the neck uptake corresponded to left level III cervical and a left supraclavicular (arrow) lymph node, not residual thyroid bed tissue. (D) Coronal SPECT/CT imaging showed diffuse lung uptake, greater on the right (arrow), compatible with iodine-avid pulmonary metastatic disease.

SPECT/CT is another important new modality that can help localize the presence and extent of disease.[26] By fusing the [131]Inuclear medicine imaging information with the anatomic CT data, detection and localization of the radioiodine-avid disease can be enhanced (Fig. 6). A recent study reported that SPECT/CT performed in patients with differentiated thyroid cancer after treatment with ^{131}I enabled more accurate localization of ^{131}I uptake in 20% of patients. The investigators also noted that adding SPECT/CT imaging to traditional planar imaging changed patient management in 6.4% of patients.[8]

SUMMARY

The essential role of nuclear medicine in the evaluation and treatment of benign and malignant thyroid disease remains strong and continues to evolve. Radiotracer and imaging methodology has been significantly enhanced with advancements such as FDG, SPECT/CT, and PET/CT. Treatment guidelines with ^{131}I continue to evolve, with the ultimate goal being appropriate risk stratification and individualized therapy. Further improvements in nuclear medicine imaging and treatments for thyroid are anticipated in the near future.

REFERENCES

1. Brucer MA. Chronology of nuclear medicine, 1600–1989. St Louis (MO): Heritage Publications, Inc; 1990. p. 228.
2. Freeman L. Freeman and Johnson's clinical radionuclide imaging. New York: Grune & Stratton, Inc; 1984. p. 1275–317.

3. Fanti S, Alavi A. Positron emission tomography and thyroid cancer. PET imaging in endocrine disorders. PET Clin 2007;2:295–304.

4. Palmer E, Scott J, Strauss H. Practical nuclear medicine. Philadelphia: WB Saunders Company; 1992. p. 311–41.

5. Treves S. Pediatric nuclear medicine/PET. 3rd edition. New York: Springer; 2007. p. 57–86, 437–504.

6. Grunwald F, Menzel C, Bender H, et al. Comparison of 18FDG-PET with 131-iodine and 99m Tc-sestamibi scintigraphy in differentiated thyroid cancer. Thyroid 1997;7:327–35.

7. Lind P, Kohlfurst S. Respective roles of thyroglobulin, radioiodine imaging, and positron emission tomography in the assessment of thyroid cancer. Semin Nucl Med 2006;36:194–205.

8. Grewal R, Tuttle R, Fox J, et al. The effect of posttherapy I-131 SPECT/CT on risk classification and management of patients with differentiated thyroid cancer. J Nucl Med 2010;51:1361–7.

9. Wong K, Zarshevsky N, Cahill J, et al. Incremental value of diagnostic I-131 SPECT/CT fusion imaging in the evaluation of differentiated thyroid carcinoma. AJR Am J Roentgenol 2008;191:1785–94.

10. Cooper D, Doherty G, Haugen B, et al. Revised American Thyroid Association management guidelines for patients with thyroid nodules and differentiated thyroid cancer. Thyroid 2009;19:1–47.

11. Amdur R, Mazzaferri E. Essentials of thyroid cancer management. New York: Springer; 2005. p. 229–46.

12. Pluijmen M, Eustatia-Rutten C, Goslings B, et al. Effects of low-iodide diet on postsurgical radioiodide ablation therapy in patients with differentiated thyroid carcinoma. Clin Endocrinol 2003;58:428–35.

13. Pacini F, Ladenson P, Schlumberger M, et al. Radioiodine ablation of thyroid remnants after preparation with recombinant human thyrotropin in differentiated thyroid carcinoma: results of international, randomized, controlled study. J Clin Endocrinol Metab 2006;91:926–32.

14. Silberstein E. Comparison of outcomes after I-123 versus I-131 pre-ablation imaging before radioiodine ablation in differentiated thyroid cancer. J Nucl Med 2007;48:1043–6.

15. Sgouros G, Kolbert K, Sheikh A, et al. Patient-specific dosimetry for I-131 thyroid cancer therapy using I-124 PET and 3-dimentional internal dosimetry (3D-ID) software. J Nucl Med 2004;45:1366–72.

16. Van Nostrand D, Atkins F, Yeganeh F, et al. Dosimetrically determined doses of radioiodine for the treatment of metastatic thyroid carcinoma. Thyroid 2002;12:121–34.

17. Sarkar S. Benign thyroid disease: what is the role of nuclear medicine? Semin Nucl Med 2006;36:185–93.

18. Park H, Perkins O, Edmondson R, et al. Influence of diagnostic radioiodines on the uptake of ablative dose of I-131. Thyroid 1994;88(4):49–54.

19. Sherman S, Tielens E, Sostre S, et al. Clinical utility of posttreatment radioiodine scans in the management of patients with thyroid carcinoma. J Clin Endocrinol Metab 1994;78:629–34.

20. Albino C, Junior M, Olandoski M, et al. Recombinant human thyrotropin as adjuvant in the treatment of multinodular goiters with radioiodine. J Clin Endocrinol Metab 2005;990:2775–80.

21. Subramanian S, Goldstein D, Parlea L, et al. Second primary malignancy risk in thyroid cancer survivors: a systematic review and meta-analysis. Thyroid 2007;17:1277–88.

22. Grunwald F, Kalicki T, Feine U, et al. Fluorine 18 fluorodeoxyglucose positron emission tomography in thyroid cancer: results of multicentre study. Eur J Nucl Med 1999;26:1547–52.

23. Schluter B, Bohuslavizk K, Beyer W, et al. Impact of FDG-PET on patients with differentiated thyroid cancer who present with elevated thyroglobulin and negative I-131 scan. J Nucl Med 2001;42:71–6.

24. Middendorp M, Grunwald F. Update on recent developments in the therapy of differentiated thyroid cancer. Semin Nucl Med 2010;40:145–52.

25. Palmedo H, Bucerius J, Joe A, et al. Integrated PET/CT in differentiated thyroid cancer: diagnostic accuracy and impact on patient management. J Nucl Med 2006;47:616–24.

26. Chen L, Luo Q, Shen Y, et al. Incremental value of I-131 SPECT/CT in the management of patients with differentiated thyroid carcinoma. J Nucl Med 2008;49:1952–7.

Thyroid Cytology: Challenges in the Pursuit of Low-Grade Malignancies

N. Paul Ohori, MD*, Karen E. Schoedel, MD

KEYWORDS

• Thyroid • Fine needle aspiration • Bethesda classification

Thyroid nodules are common and are found in approximately 5% of the general population,[1,2] translating to 15 million people in the United States. Each year, approximately 5% of these people seek medical attention and are evaluated. Among these, thyroid cancer is found in only a few percent and represents approximately 37,000 cases in the United States each year.[3] Thyroid cancer accounts for 2.5% of all cancers, but only 0.28% of all cancer deaths.[4] After clinical and radiologic examination of the thyroid gland, fine needle aspiration (FNA) biopsies are often performed for concerning nodules. Although other factors have been implicated, the increased sensitivity of imaging for detecting thyroid nodules has largely accounted for the increased incidence of thyroid cancer over the past several decades.

FNA of thyroid has become an important tool in evaluating nodules, and the definitively positive and negative diagnoses have high sensitivity and specificity.[5] However, sensitivity and specificity calculations do not take into account the 30% to 40% of indeterminate and unsatisfactory cases. From the cytopathologic perspective, most thyroid cancers are low grade and have pathologic features that overlap with other benign hyperplastic or neoplastic nodules. These characteristics combined with the technical challenges associated with procuring an adequate thyroid FNA sample highlight the main difficulties associated with diagnostic thyroid cytology. This article primarily focuses on the issues surrounding the diagnosis of differentiated follicular patterned lesions and neoplasms. The pathogenesis of thyroid nodules, factors related to obtaining and processing thyroid FNA samples, interpretation and reporting of cytologic diagnoses, and application of ancillary studies for the diagnostic refinement are described (**Table 1**).

PATHOGENESIS OF NODULAR GROWTH

Thyroid nodules grow by one or a combination of mechanisms. Most commonly, nodules form because of distention of the follicles that are filled with colloid (goiter, colloid nodule). Nodules also form through cellular hyperplasia (adenomatous hyperplasia) or neoplasia, in which cells densely proliferate in an encapsulated or otherwise roughly demarcated area. Infiltration by nonthyroid follicular-type cells, such as inflammatory cells (eg, thyroiditis), may result in localized enlargement. Finally, nodules are encountered when extracellular material (eg, fibrosis, amyloid) occupies a localized area. For each mechanism, the pathologic features of some entities are distinct, allowing a definitive diagnosis with cytologic sampling. However, in other situations, the features may be shared by a variety of entities.

Multinodular goiter (MNG) represents a general enlargement of the thyroid gland. As the name implies, most of these show multiple nodules, and the growth and size of the more conspicuous nodules raise clinical concern. Nodules in

The authors have nothing to disclose.
Department of Pathology, A610, University of Pittsburgh Medical Center-Presbyterian, 200 Lothrop Street, Pittsburgh, PA 15213, USA
* Corresponding author.
E-mail address: ohorinp@upmc.edu

Radiol Clin N Am 49 (2011) 435–451
doi:10.1016/j.rcl.2011.02.005
0033-8389/11/$ – see front matter

Table 1
Components of thyroid FNA cytology

Component	Description	Optimization
Pathology	Follicular derived lesions and neoplasms have overlapping features. Certain neoplasms (eg, classic papillary carcinoma) have characteristic features.	Development of tests distinguishing pathobiologic nature of lesions
FNA operator	Aspiration technique Capillary (nonaspiration) technique	Cellular specimen reflecting architectural pattern of cell proliferation
Specimen processing	Direct smears Liquid-based slides Cell block Collection in molecular preservative	Slides: monolayer of well-preserved and well-stained cells without artifacts Ancillary studies: preservation of nucleic acid and protein molecules
Interpretation and reporting	Bethesda classification (six-tiered)	Standardization and application of criteria for uniform diagnostic practice
Ancillary studies	Molecular markers: *BRAF, RAS, RET/PTC, PAX8/PPARgamma* Immunohistochemical markers: HBME-1, Galectin-3, CITED-1 Others under development	High sensitivity and specificity for malignant neoplasms

multinodular goiter are often colloid nodules or cellular adenomatous (hyperplastic) nodules. The origin of multinodular goiter seems to be multifactorial and involves dietary, hereditary, and environmental factors. The contributions of iodine deficiency and ingestion of goitrogenic foods are well-known. Smoking also seems to be associated with the risk for nodular hyperplasia, especially in iodine deficient areas.[6] Medications that interfere with thyroid hormone synthesis or release are also associated with nodular hyperplasia. Common examples include lithium, perchlorate, iodine, amiodarone, and other iodine-containing drugs.

Although these entities represent known associations, most multinodular goiters are caused by intrinsic characteristics of the follicular epithelial cells combined with environmental and hereditary factors. The molecular basis for the hyperplastic process has been a topic of many investigations. Candidate genes speculated to be associated with hyperplastic processes include genes involved in the synthesis of thyroglobulin, thyroperoxidase, sodium iodide symporter, and thyroid-stimulating hormone (TSH) receptor.[7] Linkage analysis has identified a locus on chromosome 14q named *MNG1*, which may be involved in thyroid growth and hormone synthesis.[8]

Whether through TSH stimulation or autonomous growth, the hyperplastic process is manifested by an increase in the number of follicular cells, number of follicles, or size of selected follicles. In the overall process of hyperplasia, the follicular epithelial cells do not respond to stimuli uniformly. Therefore, the cellular populations grow at different rates, creating subpopulations of nodules of different sizes. The rapid growth of certain nodules leads to focal hemorrhage and necrosis. With subsequent repair, fibrosis and accentuation of certain nodular foci result. Macrofollicles that are filled with thin watery colloid are a result of the high production of thyroglobulin and colloid and low rate of endocytosis and hormone release (**Fig. 1**). For some patients, the massively enlarged thyroid gland may reach 1000 g or greater.

Whether multinodular goiter should be considered a neoplastic process is a matter of debate, because monoclonality has been shown in discrete nodules by some investigators. However, the clonality of the nodules may be explained by the relatively large patch size of the embryonal thyroid gland. Therefore, hyperplastic growth in thyroid nodules may appear monoclonal but may represent normal thyroid growth.[9]

Diffuse hyperplasia (Graves disease) is an autoimmune condition resulting in diffuse enlargement of the thyroid gland. The origin of diffuse hyperplasia is unknown. However, the pathogenesis

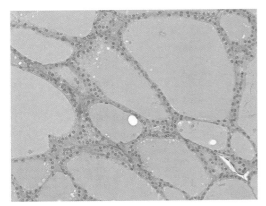

Fig. 1. Macrofollicles from a multinodular goiter are filled with watery colloid and lined by low cuboidal epithelium (hematoxylin and eosin, original magnification ×200).

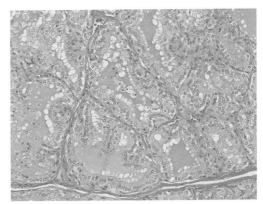

Fig. 2. In Graves disease (diffuse hyperplasia), the follicular epithelial cells are columnar and the hyperplastic process produces papillary infoldings into the lumen. Also, the hyperfunctioning nature of the follicular cells produces vacuoles at the periphery of the follicular lumen (hematoxylin and eosin, original magnification ×200).

involves an autoimmune mechanism possibly related to hereditary and environmental factors. Women are more commonly affected than men, and the overall process seems to involve dysregulation of the immune system. The hyperthyroid manifestation in Graves disease is thought to be from the production of autoantibodies directed to TSH receptor (TSHR) on follicular epithelial cells.[10] In general, antibodies involved in autoimmune thyroid disease may be grouped in three categories: stimulatory, blocking, or neutral. In Graves disease, the autoantibodies have a different stimulatory effect than lymphocytic (Hashimoto) thyroiditis, which commonly involves blocking autoantibodies. However, in some cases of diffuse hyperplasia, both stimulatory and blocking antibodies are identified.

The autoantibodies of Graves disease activate TSHR, resulting in thyroid hormone synthesis and secretion, and diffuse proliferation of the follicular epithelial cells with papillary configuration. Cytologically, the follicular cells acquire columnar morphology from the original low cuboidal state. With the increased proliferation, the follicle size decreases and the follicular lumens contain less colloid. Furthermore, as a reflection of the hyperplastic process, "scalloping" of the colloid material at the periphery of the follicular lumen is identified (**Fig. 2**). For the most part, the hyperplasia is diffusely and evenly distributed throughout the thyroid gland. However, in certain instances, nodularity may develop, and these nodules may raise clinical concern. Malignancy found in the context of diffuse hyperplasia is rare.

Chronic lymphocytic thyroiditis is another autoimmune process that most likely involves complex interactions of a variety of hereditary and environmental factors. Like Graves disease, the presence of circulating autoantibodies is involved in lymphocytic thyroiditis. However, the antibodies of lymphocytic thyroiditis are more commonly of the blocking type.

Lymphocytic thyroiditis has several clinical and pathologic manifestations, depending on the individual patient and stage of disease. Most commonly, lymphocytic thyroiditis involves infiltration predominantly by T lymphocytes (CD4-positive majority and CD8-positive minority).[11] In addition, germinal center formation (with B lymphocytes) may be found (**Fig. 3**). These lymphoid cells often are accompanied by macrophages and natural killer cells. The resulting enlargement may be twice to four times that of

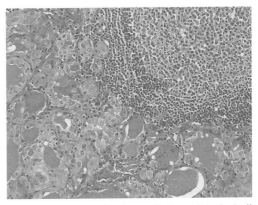

Fig. 3. Lymphocytic (Hashimoto) thyroiditis typically shows proliferation of oncocytic (Hürthle) cells (*left*) and reactive lymphoid cells with germinal center formation (*right*) (hematoxylin and eosin, original magnification ×200).

normal thyroid glands and is often diffuse, although lobular accentuation and nodular growth may be seen. Nodules are composed of areas rich in lymphocytic infiltrates, hyperplastic or metaplastic (especially oncocytic) epithelial cells, colloid (colloid nodules), or fibrosis and may raise clinical concern. With progression of the disease and increasing numbers of lymphocytes infiltrating the thyroid gland, further follicular epithelial cell damage results.

The pathogenesis of follicular epithelial cell injury seems to involve cytokines, such as interferon gamma, autoantibodies, perforin, and other cytotoxic agents. The fate of some epithelial cells is apoptosis (cell death), whereas other injured cells undergo metaplasia to the oncocytic (Hürthle cell) phenotype. Squamous metaplasia also may be seen as a result of epithelial cell injury. Damage to the thyroid epithelial cells leads to parenchymal fibrosis, often surrounding atrophic follicular epithelial cells. Lymphoepithelial lesions, follicular atrophy, and fibrosis are histologic manifestations of the regressive phase of the process. Although lymphocytic infiltrates are characteristic of lymphocytic thyroiditis, they are not specific for this entity, because they are commonly observed in other thyroid diseases. Therefore, the diagnosis of lymphocytic (Hashimoto) thyroiditis, defined as an autoimmune disease, requires clinical and pathologic correlation.

Follicular adenoma is the most common benign neoplasm of the thyroid gland. It accounts for approximately two-thirds to three-quarters of solitary thyroid nodules. As with any neoplasm, the pathogenesis involves monoclonal proliferation of genetically altered cells through one or more pathways. Although certain syndromes (eg, Cowden disease and Carney complex) are associated with the development of follicular adenomas, most follicular adenomas are sporadic.[12,13] Etiologic associations include radiation, iodine deficiency, and medications such as the cholesterol-lowering agent HMG-CoA reductase inhibitor, Simvastatin.[14]

In follicular adenoma, the neoplastic cells typically proliferate as crowded cell clusters, often with very little or no intraluminal colloid. However, the appearance may be heterogeneous; areas with large follicles filled with watery colloid may be identified. By definition, follicular adenoma is surrounded by a dense fibrotic capsule with small vessels within the capsule. The architectural patterns of the neoplastic cells include solid, trabecular, microfollicular, normal follicular, macrofollicular, and, rarely, papillary patterns. Cytologically, most cells are cuboidal to polygonal with round nuclei showing mild variation in size.

Occasionally, large nuclei may be identified. Most nuclei are hyperchromatic with coarse nuclear chromatin and occasional nucleoli. Nuclear membranes are smooth and regular (**Fig. 4**).

The diagnosis of follicular adenoma requires the absence of capsular invasion. Because this feature cannot be shown through cytologic sampling, the final diagnosis of follicular adenoma depends on the thorough histologic examination of the entire capsule. The oncocytic variant of follicular adenoma is composed predominantly (at least 75%) of oncocytic cells. These cells show cytoplasmic granularity because of the abundance of abnormal mitochondria.

Most clonality studies show that follicular adenomas are of monoclonal origin. Cytogenetic changes have shown relatively frequent gains in chromosomes 7, 12, and 5. Furthermore, translocation involving chromosome 19q13 and 2p21 have been shown.[15–17] Other genetic abnormalities of follicular adenomas include loss of heterozygosity, which involves on average 6% per chromosome arm (in contrast to 20% for follicular carcinoma).[18] Somatic mutations associated with follicular adenoma involve the RAS family of genes (NRAS, KRAS, and HRAS). These mutations are found in approximately 30% of follicular adenomas.[19] In a smaller minority (5%–10%) of follicular adenomas, PAX8/PPARgamma rearrangement is found.[20] However, many of these neoplasms may represent follicular carcinomas that were underdiagnosed because of insufficient sampling of the capsule.

Follicular carcinomas share many pathologic features with follicular adenomas, including the architectural patterns and cytologic features of

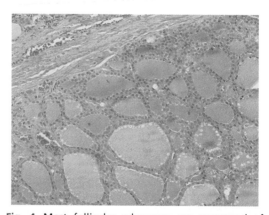

Fig. 4. Most follicular adenomas are composed of follicles of smaller size in an encapsulated area. The upper left area of the image shows the dense fibrous capsule (hematoxylin and eosin, original magnification ×200).

the neoplastic cells. The two are distinguished primarily through the identification of capsular or vascular invasion (**Fig. 5**). Somatic mutations, such as those of the *RAS* family of genes, are shared by follicular adenomas and follicular carcinomas.[19] However, the frequency of mutation is higher in carcinomas. Therefore, some investigators believe that follicular carcinomas develop after additional genetic alterations in follicular adenomas. However, some evidence suggests that follicular carcinomas and follicular adenomas develop in separate pathways. For example, *PAX8/PPARgamma* rearrangement is found in a significant number of follicular carcinomas but is rare in follicular adenomas.[20] Translocations involving chromosome loci on 19q13 and 2p21 are common in follicular adenomas but rare in carcinomas.[21] This evidence suggests that adenomas with these translocations may have a low probability of progression to carcinoma.

Most papillary carcinomas are sporadic, and the etiology is often unclear. Some associations include iodine-rich diets and ionizing radiation. Regions of the world that have higher dietary intake of iodine have been reported to have higher incidences of papillary carcinoma. Similarly, a history of radiation therapy (latency period ranging from 4–40 years) is known to be associated with papillary carcinoma.

In a minority of cases (approximately 5%), papillary carcinomas arise in the setting of hereditary disorders.[22] These disorders are grouped into two categories. The first category involves hereditary multicancer syndromes, such as familial adenomatous polyposis (FAP) syndrome, Carney complex, and Werner syndrome. In the second category, familial cases without multicancer syndromes characteristically show an autosomal dominant inheritance pattern.

The pathogenesis of papillary carcinoma involves clonal expansion of the neoplastic cell population and, in some cases, multiple foci are present. In approximately half of the cases, these represent intrathyroidal spread of the primary papillary carcinoma. However, in other cases, the multiple foci represent independent clones that show distinct genetic alterations (eg, *BRAF, RAS, RET/PTC*). Cytogenetic abnormalities are found in 20% to 40% of papillary carcinomas.[23–25] Using comparative genomic hybridization, most common chromosomal losses are found on 22q and 9q and chromosomal gains are found at 17q, 1q, and 9q. The chromosomal imbalances for follicular variant papillary carcinoma are more similar to those of follicular adenoma and follicular carcinoma than to those of classic papillary carcinoma.

Papillary carcinomas have a relatively low rate of loss of heterozygosity (LOH). LOH studies have shown a 2.5% rate of LOH per chromosomal arm compared with 20% for follicular carcinoma.[18] Loci on 3p, 4p, and 10q are more frequently deleted in papillary carcinoma.[26,27] Somatic mutations, in particular those involving the mitogen-activated protein kinase (MAPK) pathway, are important in the pathogenesis of papillary carcinoma.[28] Common alterations include point mutations of the *BRAF* and *RAS* genes and *RET/PTC* gene rearrangements, which are mutually exclusive. These alterations influence tumor growth, differentiation, and survival, and are involved in most papillary carcinoma cases. However, approximately 30% of papillary carcinomas do not show alterations using current methodologies.[29] The known genetic alterations result in neoplastic growth and the characteristic pathologic features of papillary carcinoma.

No one particular feature is pathognomonic of papillary carcinoma, and the cytologic diagnosis relies on the combination of architectural and cytologic features, with most emphasis placed on the nuclear characteristics. The typical architectural pattern of papillary carcinoma is the papillary growth pattern. However, papillary growth may be seen in benign processes such as papillary hyperplasia and even in follicular adenoma, and not all papillary carcinomas exhibit a papillary pattern. Therefore, the architecture must be viewed in conjunction with the cytologic features.

The cytologic features that are important in making the diagnosis of papillary carcinoma include nuclear enlargement, crowding and overlapping, chromatin clearing, irregular nuclear membranes, intranuclear pseudoinclusions, and

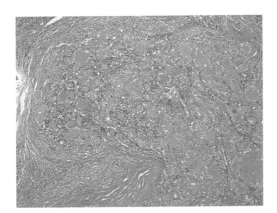

Fig. 5. The diagnosis of a well differentiated follicular carcinoma is based often on capsular invasion. The invasive front of the follicular carcinoma protrudes through the capsule (*lower left*) (hematoxylin and eosin, original magnification ×200).

nuclear groove formation (**Fig. 6**). In most cases of papillary carcinoma, the nuclear features are readily identified and widely recognized. However, in a minority of cases, the changes are subtle and interobserver variability is noted. The cases that involve the highest degree of interobserver variability include the follicular variant of papillary carcinoma and oncocytic papillary carcinoma.

The nodular growths described earlier are collectively classified as "follicular-derived lesions" and constitute most thyroid nodules.[30] In some instances (eg, classic papillary carcinoma), the cytologic features of the epithelial cells are distinct. Other lesions show cytologic features that overlap with other entities (eg, encapsulated follicular variant papillary carcinoma, follicular carcinoma, hyperplastic adenomatous nodule in goiter). For some low-grade, well-differentiated papillary or follicular carcinomas, the malignant features are so subtle that the diagnosis remains challenging at histologic examination of the resected neoplasm. Given the nature of these lesions, cytologic examination has inherent limitations, and even under the best circumstances the diagnostic end point may be a differential diagnostic category, such as follicular neoplasm, which implies a set of differential diagnoses (see later discussion).

FNA PROCEDURE OPERATOR FACTORS

Thyroid FNA is deceptively simple, and a common misconception is that placing the needle inside the lesion will automatically yield an adequate specimen. Although the localization of the needle is challenging, the ability to extract lesional material is an important aspect of the FNA procedure. After

the needle is placed in the lesion, one may ask the question "Is the lesion in the needle?" For the practices involved in thyroid FNA, procurement of high-quality samples perhaps could be better emphasized. Furthermore, the quantitative aspect of the adequacy criteria ("six groups of well-preserved, well-stained follicular cell groups with ten cells each") is misunderstood at times, especially in the setting of immediate on-site evaluations.[31]

The expected cellularity of the specimen is related to the diagnostic category of its cytology (**Table 2**). For example, although six groups of follicular cells is adequate for the negative/benign diagnosis, initial aspirates that are "quantitatively minimally adequate" and show some degree of architectural (eg, microfollicles) or cytologic atypia (eg, occasional nuclear grooves) probably do not represent the entire lesion well. In these cases, obtaining additional passes in an attempt to clarify the lesional characteristics probably would be beneficial. With the use of proper techniques, most neoplasms yield cellular specimens. For these reasons, the value of good sampling and proficiency in specimen processing cannot be overemphasized because the overall specimen quality influences the diagnostic accuracy.

FNA sampling of thyroid nodules has been performed in North America since the 1980s.[32] Several variables regarding the specific aspects of FNA have evolved during this time. Some of these variables include the type of specialist involved in performing the FNA, choice of needle (eg, gauge, length), apparatus, and the efficacy

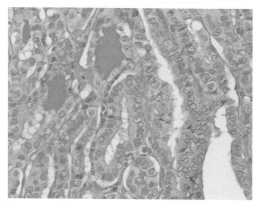

Fig. 6. Papillary carcinomas often show nuclear enlargement, crowding and overlapping, chromatin clearing, irregular nuclear membranes, intranuclear pseudoinclusions, and nuclear groove formation (hematoxylin and eosin, original magnification ×200).

Table 2	
Expected cellularity of diagnostic categories in the Bethesda system for thyroid cytology	
Diagnostic Category	**Cellularity**
Unsatisfactory/ nondiagnostic	Markedly hypocellular or severely comprised by artifact
Negative/benign	Low to moderate in cellularity
Follicular lesion/ atypia of undetermined significance	Variable – some are low in cellularity
Follicular neoplasm	Highly cellular
Suspicious for malignancy	Variable
Positive/malignant	Moderate to highly cellular

of aspiration or capillary (nonaspiration) techniques. In general, the FNA sampling technique involves the use of fine staccato vibratory oscillations of 3 to 5 per second in the targeted lesion.[31]

The ideal FNA specimen has the thick consistency of potato soup. However, this result may not be achieved with thyroid FNAs because of the vascular nature of thyroid lesions (in particular follicular neoplasms). To avoid bloody specimens, some operators advocate the capillary (nonaspiration) technique.[33] However, depending on the operator, excellent cellular material may be obtained using either the capillary or aspiration technique. Therefore, the choice may be based on the skill, experience, and preference of the individual operator. Operator performance may be monitored through tracking the rate of unsatisfactory specimens.

During the procedure, the patient is placed in the supine position with the neck extended. The lesion is localized through palpation or with the assistance of an ultrasonographic device. Local anesthesia (eg, 1% lidocaine hydrochloride) may be used to anesthetize the surrounding skin and soft tissue. Ice may be substituted as a local anesthetic,[34] and some operators advocate its use because of its vasoconstrictive effect and because it decreases bleeding during the FNA procedure.

Most FNAs are performed using 22- to 27-gauge needles. If the aspiration technique is used, the needle is attached to a 2 to 20 cm^3 syringe. For solid lesions, thinner-gauge needles (eg, 25- or 27-gauge) tend to yield less bloody specimens. In general, bloody specimens should be avoided because excessive hemorrhage dilutes the cellular content and contributes to a higher probability of a nondiagnostic specimen. However, if the lesion is cystic, a larger-gauge needle (eg, 22-gauge) is needed to successfully drain the cystic contents. Multiple passes are usually necessary to ensure adequacy of the specimen. Some operators suggest starting the FNA procedure with the capillary (nonaspiration) technique and switching to the aspiration technique if the specimen does not appear adequate.

Core biopsies, alone or in conjunction with FNA, have been used by some operators.[35,36] The procurement of a greater amount of lesional tissue correlates with greater diagnostic sensitivity and specificity. However, some reports have indicated an increased incidence of complications as a result of core needle biopsy. Therefore, the risks and benefits should be carefully considered when adopting this technique. On-site evaluation increases the yield of the FNA procedure because immediate feedback is provided to the operator.

However, the process may be time-consuming, and for busy practices performing a large volume of FNA cases, the added time may not be beneficial to the overall practice, especially if the adequacy and diagnostic rate is high.[37] For these practices, on-site evaluation may be used judiciously, at the discretion of the operator, when a lesion is deemed challenging.

SPECIMEN PROCESSING

The goal of specimen processing depends on the type of evaluation. For cytomorphologic evaluation, the goal is to produce cytology slides with a monolayer of well-preserved diagnostic cells without artifactual distortion, and is achieved by making direct smears or liquid-based slides. For best results, the needle removed after the aspiration procedure should be handled immediately for slide preparation and other specimen processing procedures. Efficiency is important in avoiding clot formation and artifactual distortion of cells. Direct smears are performed using standard smear preparation techniques.[31]

Because thyroid specimens tend to be more dilute than other FNA samples, the operator should be careful to place only a small amount of lesional material near the top of the glass slide for smearing. Another glass slide is used to smear the material on the diagnostic slide and produce a monolayer of cellular material. Once the smear is made, slides may be fixed in alcohol for Papanicolaou staining or air dried for Diff-Quik or other types of Romanowsky staining. The air-dried slides stained with Diff-Quik often are used for immediate evaluation.

Many cytopathologists believe that the cytomorphologic presentation is best with direct smears because these show good nuclear detail with demonstration of nuclear grooves and intranuclear inclusions. Direct smears also show the presence of colloid, both in thin watery and thick forms. The disadvantages of direct smears include the high degree of technical skill required for smear preparation. Also, the thyroid cytology practices using direct smears are often confronted with a large volume of slides per case. The increased volume of slides is associated with higher use of cytotechnology resources and slower throughput.

Alternatively, the aspirated material may be placed without delay in a specific preparatory solution (eg, Cytolyt) to produce liquid-based slides, or in formalin for cell block preparation. The slides produced using liquid-based techniques cover a round area and are alcohol-fixed and stained using the Papanicolaou method.

The use of ThinPrep and other liquid-based techniques has some advantages. Manual skills for smear-making are not required because the material is placed directly in a vial of solution and the processing instrument produces slides with an even monolayer of cells. Colloid on liquid-based slides has a distinct appearance (orangeophilic and "glassy") and can be separated from serum material. This distinction may be difficult on direct smear slides. For hypocellular specimens, follicular epithelial cells are better identified on liquid-based slides than on direct smears. In practices that primarily use liquid-based cytology, only one slide is produced. Because of the low slide volume, the screening time for the cytotechnologist is minimized and the throughput is faster.

The disadvantages of liquid-based cytology for thyroid FNA cytology are the strengths of direct smears. Immediate evaluation cannot be performed because the FNA material is placed directly in the liquid-based solution. Liquid-based cytology produces follicular epithelial cells that are relatively small in cluster size. Some cytopathologists believe that the cytomorphologic appearance (eg, nuclear detail) of the diagnostic cells is inferior to that of direct smears.

Liquid-based cytology was originally designed for gynecologic Papanicolaou smear processing and has a mucolytic and hemolytic quality that removes mucus and blood. The same process removes colloid material, which is often diminished in quantity or possibly lost. Analyses of these methodologies have shown that a higher percentage of definitive diagnoses is made based on direct smears of cancer cases than on liquid-based cytology.[38]

Clotted or other solid aspirated material from the FNA procedure may be submitted in formalin for cell block preparation and processed similarly to biopsied tissue material. The slides produced are similar to histologic sections and stained with hematoxylin and eosin. Because residual material often is present in the paraffin block, additional special and immunohistochemical stains may be performed. Cell blocks and special stains are particularly helpful in confirming medullary carcinoma and lymphoproliferative conditions, and evaluating the origin of metastatic disease.

In addition to slide preparations, the aspirated material may be placed in other media for specific studies (eg, microbiology if infection is suspected; molecular studies to evaluate the malignant potential of the follicular epithelial cell population). Molecular testing may be performed from previously stained smears; however, the test slide is sacrificed and the process may be problematic if diagnostic cellular material is limited and present on only the test slide. Molecular tests may be performed on cell block material also, if sufficient. However, RNA is not well preserved on previously stained smears or cell block material. Regarding the quality of nucleic acid for DNA and RNA tests, samples separately collected in nuclear acid preservative solution are optimal, although visualization of the cellular lesional material is not possible and sampling variability may be an issue. However, if the test addresses a specific and focused issue (eg, evaluation of epithelial cells), molecular markers (eg, keratin) may be included in the test panel as a molecular control to ensure the presence of particular cells. Overall, the processing methods described earlier may be used alone or in combination with the other methods.

CYTOLOGIC INTERPRETATION AND REPORTING SYSTEM

Over the past few decades, the widespread use of thyroid FNA resulted in a large volume of knowledge regarding the cytologic characteristics of thyroid lesions. Specific features of benign conditions, such as nodular hyperplasia (goiter), and malignant neoplasms, such as papillary carcinoma, have become well-known. Based on these experiences, the evaluation of thyroid FNA evolved into a systematic review of basic cytologic elements that are categorized into background, epithelial cell, and inflammatory cell components (Table 3).

The background information is crucial and should not be overlooked. Thyroid nodules arise for several reasons, including an increase in the number of cells, distention of the follicles from increased amount of intraluminal colloid, hemorrhage into the nodule, other extracellular material (eg, amyloid), or any combination of the these. Distinction of colloid from serum may be difficult and in this regard, and having a liquid-based slide (eg, ThinPrep) may be beneficial. The sources of

Table 3	
Key components of thyroid FNA specimens	
Component	**Elements**
Background	Colloid, serum, amyloid
Epithelial cells	Follicular cells, oncocytic cells, papillary carcinoma cells
Inflammatory cells	Lymphocytes, macrophages, neutrophils

epithelial cells are follicular-type epithelial cells (including oncocytic cells), neuroendocrine C-cells, and metastatic cells. The follicular-type epithelial cells are most commonly encountered, and the cytologic features and architectural organization are important to appreciate because the pattern reflects the arrangement of these cells in tissue. The number of inflammatory cells range from rare (eg, classic benign colloid nodule) to numerous (eg, lymphocytic thyroiditis).

The lymphocytes that are characteristic of lymphocytic thyroiditis are mostly small and round, with a moderate degree of polymorphism. Tingible body macrophages are often identified. The presence of hemosiderin-laden macrophages alone indicates degenerative or cystic change, and may be seen in conjunction with benign or malignant lesions. The ability of cytologic evaluation to specify the type of nodular lesion depends on the presence or absence of distinctive features. Therefore, some nodules, such as classic papillary carcinoma, may be specified precisely by cytologic evaluation, whereas others such as follicular carcinoma cannot be diagnosed using cytology (**Table 4**).

A benign/negative diagnosis is based on certain premises. Benign hyperplastic nodules are usually colloid-rich nodules, nodules representing lymphocytic thyroiditis (Hashimoto thyroiditis), or nodules in Graves disease (diffuse hyperplasia). In colloid nodules, the distension of the colloid-filled follicles results in flattening of the follicular epithelial cells. When these follicular epithelial cells are aspirated and smeared onto a glass slide, they appear as two-dimensional sheets with a regular honeycomb configuration in the background of

Table 4
Typical cytologic diagnosis for thyroid nodules with or without distinctive cytologic features

Type of Thyroid Nodule at Resection	Distinctive Cytologic Features Usually Present	Distinctive Cytologic Features Usually Absent
Colloid nodule (MNG)	Negative/benign	
Cellular adenomatous nodule (MNG)		Follicular Neoplasm
Diffuse hyperplasia	Negative/benign	
Lymphocytic thyroiditis	Negative/benign	
Follicular adenoma		Follicular neoplasm
Follicular carcinoma		Follicular neoplasm
Follicular variant, PTC		Follicular neoplasm or suspicious for malignancy
Classic PTC	Positive/malignant - PTC	
Tall cell variant, PTC	Positive/malignant - PTC	
Medullary carcinoma	Positive/malignant – medullary carcinoma	
Poorly differentiated carcinoma		Follicular neoplasm or suspicious for malignancy (some cases may be called positive/malignant)
Anaplastic carcinoma	Positive/malignant (need to exclude metastasis)	
Lymphoma (high-grade)	Positive/malignant (perform flow cytometry and specify if possible)	
Lymphoma (low-grade)		Atypia of undetermined significance (may be called positive/malignant if flow cytometry is diagnostic)
Metastasis	Positive/malignant (search for specific features)	

Abbreviations: MNG, multinodular goiter; PTC, papillary carcinoma.

watery colloid (**Fig. 7**). Lymphocytic thyroiditis presents with a cellular population of polymorphous lymphocytes and epithelial cells (follicular or oncocytic).

The pitfalls for this diagnosis are low-grade lymphoma and a well-differentiated papillary carcinoma arising in the background of lymphocytic thyroiditis. FNA specimens from Graves disease show large sheets of hyperplastic cells with abundant cytoplasm. Oncocytes and lymphocytes may be seen in the background. To provide a negative/benign diagnosis for these entities, the features are found in the absence of a significant microfollicular component and significant nuclear atypia. Unfortunately, the patterns associated with the benign/negative diagnoses are not entirely specific and occasionally may be seen in neoplasms, such as follicular adenoma, follicular carcinoma, and follicular variant papillary carcinoma. Therefore, a false-negative diagnosis in approximately 3% of cases cannot be avoided in thyroid cytology.

The basis for a malignant primary thyroid diagnosis usually refers to papillary carcinoma, because follicular carcinoma and oncocytic (Hürthle cell) carcinoma cannot be diagnosed using cytologic methods. Other malignancies that are less frequently diagnosed with FNA include medullary carcinoma, anaplastic carcinoma, lymphoma, metastasis, and other rare neoplasms. The key features of papillary carcinoma are nuclear enlargement, elongation, crowding, nuclear groove formation, and intranuclear pseudoinclusion formation. The chromatin pattern tends to be powdery and nucleoli are small and eccentrically located (**Fig. 8**). Pitfalls and sources

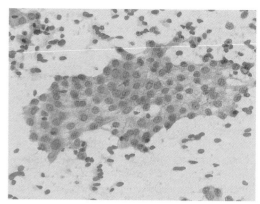

Fig. 8. Fine needle aspiration specimens of papillary carcinoma show nuclear characteristics found in histologic specimens. The key diagnostic features include nuclear enlargement, elongation, crowding, groove formation, and intranuclear pseudoinclusion formation (Diff-Quik, original magnification ×400).

of false-positive results often are caused by atypia induced by extremely reactive conditions or oncocytic (Hürthle) cell change with features mimicking papillary carcinoma. However, some malignancies (eg, follicular variant of papillary carcinoma and low-grade lymphomas) show subtle findings and may not be detected with cytology. A positive diagnosis is rendered in 4% to 8% of cases, and the positive predictive value is greater than 96%.[39,40]

The total of the benign and malignant diagnoses accounts for approximately 60% to 70% of thyroid FNA diagnoses. The remaining diagnoses fall into the indeterminate ("gray zone") or unsatisfactory/nondiagnostic categories. The main reasons for this are (1) nonspecific pattern of the lesional cell population (eg, follicular neoplasm), (2) nuclear features concerning but not diagnostic of a neoplastic process, (3) insufficient cellularity, and (4) specimen-processing artifact (eg, blood clotting artifact). Until recently, no standardized categorical systems were available for reporting thyroid cytology diagnoses. The schemes varied most in the reporting and stratification of the indeterminate diagnoses.[40] Some reporting schemes used one or two indeterminate categories, whereas others used three or four.

In an effort to provide a uniform reporting scheme for widespread use, a multidisciplinary conference was held on the campus of the National Cancer Institute in Bethesda, Maryland in October 2007. This conference was attended by 154 cytopathologists, surgical pathologists, endocrinologists, endocrine surgeons, radiologists, and basic scientists. The six major issues addressed were indication, training and

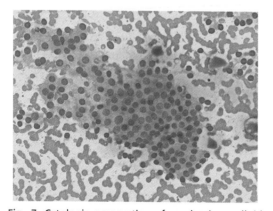

Fig. 7. Cytologic preparations from benign colloid nodules show flat sheets of bland follicular epithelial cells with round uniform nuclei in a background of colloid (which appears pale blue on this image) (Diff-Quik, original magnification ×400).

credentialing, technique, terminology/criteria, ancillary studies, and postthyroid FNA management. Although each issue was important, terminology/criteria received the most attention.[41] Based on a thorough literature review by the Bethesda committee and the ensuing discussions at the Bethesda conference, a six-tiered categorization was established (see Table 2). The proceedings from the meeting were published in *Diagnostic Cytopathology* and the *Cytojournal*.[31,32,41] More recently in December 2009, an atlas was published detailing the definitions, criteria, and explanatory notes of the Bethesda system for reporting thyroid cytopathology diagnoses.[42] This document has become valuable to practicing cytopathologists and trainees in consistently applying the criteria and arriving at diagnoses that may be communicated across multiple institutions.

Of the six categories, the Bethesda system provided the most significant contribution to standardization of the unsatisfactory/nondiagnostic category and three indeterminate categories.

Adequacy of thyroid FNA specimens is a challenging topic. Part of the difficulty in defining adequacy for thyroid lesions is that the various lesions are expected to have different qualitative and quantitative cytologic features. For example, a benign colloid nodule may show only occasional follicular epithelial cell groups in the background of watery colloid. However, a follicular adenoma would yield numerous microfollicular cell clusters without much colloid. Therefore, one may ask, "For what diagnoses are the criteria adequate?" The Bethesda system provides quantitative adequacy criteria of "more than 6 groups of well preserved, well stained follicular cells with 10 or more cells each," which is based on previous studies by Goellner and colleagues.[43] These cell groups should not be entrapped in blood clot or otherwise compromised. Goellner's studies showed a false-negative rate of less than 1% but an unsatisfactory rate of 20%. Therefore, this quantitative adequacy statement is primarily applicable to negative/benign nodules.

In the setting of a typical colloid nodule, watery colloid is abundant in the background and follicular epithelial cells often are sparsely represented. Cytologically, the follicular epithelial cells look like flat sheets with even spacing of nuclei (without crowding) and a honeycomb appearance. The nuclei are round with smooth, even nuclear membranes. The chromatin is evenly distributed and very small inconspicuous nucleoli may be observed. The demonstration of at least 6 well-preserved flat sheets of follicular epithelial cells provides the basis for a negative diagnosis (with an expected false-negative rate of 3%). The false-negative rate is difficult to calculate precisely because patients with negative cytology diagnoses often do not undergo surgery. A recent study by Renshaw[44] using logistical regression analysis estimated the risk of malignancy at approximately 3%.

Although these criteria are appropriate for the diagnosis of negative/benign cases, would the demonstration of just six microfollicular groups be adequate for diagnosis? Microfollicular groups often are associated with follicular neoplasms, which are expected to yield very cellular samples. The Bethesda system states that such a sparsely cellular case may be placed in the category of follicular lesion of undetermined significance (atypia of undetermined significance), which by definition is "satisfactory." However, clinical and radiologic correlation is essential to the evaluation of each case. When considering the clinico-radiologic-cytopathologic features together, these cases may be deemed unsatisfactory/nondiagnostic. The application of adequacy criteria varies among institutions and also among cytopathologists. At institutions where these criteria are applied stringently, the unsatisfactory/nondiagnostic rate approaches 20%.[45]

In support of this practice, studies have shown that the risk of malignancy for unsatisfactory/nondiagnostic cases is greater than the expected risk for a negative/benign diagnosis and is estimated to be 5% to 10%.[46,47] This relatively high risk of malignancy implies that malignant neoplasms (possibly related to increased vascularity) may have a greater likelihood of producing an unsatisfactory specimen. A repeat FNA with immediate evaluation is often recommended after an unsatisfactory diagnosis; 60% of these yield results other than an unsatisfactory/nondiagnostic diagnosis.

Despite best efforts, indeterminate diagnoses (constituting 20% to 30% of diagnoses) are unavoidable using current methods. The indeterminate diagnoses according to the Bethesda Thyroid Classification include suspicious for malignant cells, follicular neoplasm, and follicular lesion (atypical cells) of undetermined significance (FLUS/AUS).[41,42] Among these indeterminate diagnoses, the category of suspicious for malignant cells carries the highest risk for malignancy. This diagnosis is applied to cases with sparse sampling of highly atypical lesional cells or when the specimen may be cellular but the cytologic findings are relatively subtle and do not fulfill malignant criteria.

Most cases of suspicious for malignant cells are suspicious for thyroid papillary carcinoma. However, occasionally, cases suspicious for medullary carcinoma, lymphoma, metastasis, or other neoplasms are found. The suspicious for malignant cells diagnosis is given in 2% to 7% of cases, and the risk of malignancy ranges from 50% to 75%. In general, these figures are inversely related and a higher percentage of suspicious for malignant cells diagnoses usually is associated with a lower positive predictive value and vice versa. Highly atypical reactive changes in hyperplastic nodules or benign neoplasms may mimic malignant cytologic features. However, the positive predictive value of a positive/malignant diagnosis is greater than 98%; therefore, cytopathologists are proficient in distinguishing positive/malignant cases from suspicious for malignant cells cases. At the lower end of the spectrum, the threshold for resulting in the suspicious for malignant cells category is not clearly defined. Cases that show atypia of milder degree border on the FLUS/AUS category.

Follicular neoplasm (suspicious for follicular neoplasm) cases show cellular specimens with numerous microfollicular cell groups composed of tight three-dimensional clusters of follicular cells with very little or no colloid in the lumens. Approximately 15 follicular epithelial cells are identified around the circumference of a microfollicular structure (**Fig. 9**). This category reflects the differential diagnosis of follicular adenoma, follicular carcinoma, follicular variant papillary carcinoma, and a hyperplastic adenomatoid nodule. The distinction between these entities cannot be made because the FNA procedure samples the intranodular cellular population with overlapping cytologic features.

The distinction between follicular adenoma and follicular carcinoma is based on the presence or absence of capsular invasion or vascular invasion. Follicular variant of papillary carcinoma may show

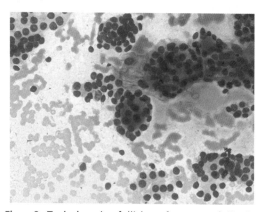

Fig. 9. Typical microfollicles from a follicular neoplasm are composed of approximately 15 follicular cells surrounding a small droplet of colloid (Diff-Quik, original magnification ×400).

the typical cytologic features of papillary carcinoma (ie, nuclear grooves and pseudoinclusions). However, these features may be present only focally, and areas of the neoplasm may show microfollicles composed of relatively bland, uniform nuclei without the characteristic nuclear features of papillary carcinoma. In addition, nodules of cellular hyperplastic adenomatoid nodules (in goiter) also may contain microfollicular structures that are similar to the entities mentioned earlier. Approximately 6% to 10% of FNA cases are entered in the follicular neoplasm category, and the risk of malignancy ranges from 10% to 34%.

By terminology, FLUS/AUS is a new category that was established in the Bethesda Thyroid Classification system.[41,42] Before the establishment of Bethesda criteria, institutions and cytopathologists may have placed these types of cases under different nomenclature, such as "atypical cells present" or "suboptimal specimens." Regardless of the various terms that were previously used for this category, experts understand that these specimens represent a set of cases that do not fulfill criteria for any of the other five categories, and that the significance of the findings is most uncertain.

In general, the FLUS/AUS category shows a mixed conglomerate of cases and does not represent any one entity. Some investigators have advocated subclassifying the FLUS/AUS category. The Bethesda System Atlas has listed nine common situations for which the FLUS/AUS interpretation is appropriate. Overall, the subcategories result from classification issues bordering on other categories except the positive/malignant category. One of the subcategories of FLUS/AUS shows nuclear atypia, borders on the suspicious for malignant cells category, and seems to show the highest positive predictive value for malignant outcome.[48]

The frequency of FLUS/AUS reporting has a rather wide range, from 2% to 20%, and the risk of malignancy reported is also wide, ranging from 6% to 48%.[48–56] The reasons for this heterogeneity may be multifactorial, and the possibilities include differences in patient population characteristics (also regional characteristics), operator and processing techniques (including experience), application of Bethesda classification diagnostic criteria, surgical pathology analysis and diagnostic threshold (eg, frequency of follicular variant papillary carcinoma outcome), contribution of ancillary studies if used, method for data analysis, and threshold for surgical therapy. Setting criteria for the threshold between FLUS/AUS and some of its neighboring diagnoses is a challenge for further refinement.

APPLICATION OF ANCILLARY STUDIES

Conventional thyroid FNA cytology tests yield high sensitivity and specificity for the definitive (negative/benign and positive/malignant) diagnoses. For these cases, the clinical management algorithms are straightforward. However, because the management of 20% to 30% of indeterminate cases is less clear, diagnostic resections often are performed. Currently, approximately 50% of thyroidectomies result in a benign diagnosis, and approximately half of these are for benign neoplasms. Methods that further refine the indeterminate diagnoses will potentially reduce the number of resected benign, nonneoplastic thyroid glands. Ancillary studies most commonly used are immunohistochemistry, fluorescence in situ hybridization (FISH), and polymerase chain reaction (PCR) for nucleic acid. The goal of the application of ancillary studies is to increase the diagnostic sensitivity for malignant thyroid nodules without compromising the specificity. Furthermore, ancillary studies have the potential to determine the malignant potential and specific classification of the neoplasm, guide management, and predict the response to a variety of therapeutic agents.

There are two general applications of ancillary studies to thyroid cytopathology. First, ancillary studies are used when the presence of neoplastic cells is definite but the specific cell lineage is not. Examples include the workup for medullary carcinoma, anaplastic carcinoma, metastatic neoplasms, some lymphomas, and other poorly differentiated neoplasms. Most commonly, immunohistochemical stains are used on cell block sections to identify specific epitopes in the neoplastic cells that help determine the cell lineage. For example, the calcitonin immunopositivity in a neoplastic cell population with a dispersed cell pattern is diagnostic of medullary carcinoma. Occasionally, metastatic neoplasms are encountered in the thyroid gland. In particular, renal cell carcinoma has a propensity to metastasize to the thyroid gland. Immunohistochemical stains for the renal cell carcinoma antigen, CD10, and carbonic anhydrase IX are useful in determining the renal origin of the cell population.

Second, ancillary studies are useful in determining the malignant potential of the lesional cells. This efficacy applies to the indeterminate diagnoses (FLUS/AUS, follicular neoplasm, and suspicious for malignant cells) and the positive/malignant diagnosis. The determination of malignancy is challenging, especially for low-grade neoplasms. In these cases, molecular studies (eg, FISH or PCR) provide a higher degree of

specificity and are preferred over immunohistochemistry. The common primary follicular patterned thyroid lesions for which this type of testing is applicable include cellular adenomatoid nodule in goiter, cellular nodules in lymphocytic thyroiditis, follicular adenoma, follicular carcinoma, follicular variant papillary carcinoma, classic papillary carcinoma, tall cell variant papillary carcinoma, oncocytic adenoma, and oncocytic carcinoma.

For the set of follicular patterned lesions described, the following panel of molecular markers is used at the authors' institution: *BRAF, RAS, RET/PTC,* and *PAX8/PPARgamma* (**Table 5**). Collectively, more than 70% of primary thyroid malignancies show a genetic alteration in one of these markers.[57] *BRAF* is the most common generic alteration in papillary thyroid carcinoma and also may be seen in poorly differentiated carcinoma and anaplastic carcinoma. Generally, it is not seen in follicular carcinoma. The genetic alteration usually results from a T to A transversion at nucleotide 1799, which results in a valine to glutamate substitution at residue 600 and is generally classified as V600E mutation. Papillary carcinomas that harbor *BRAF* mutations usually occur in older patients and often are present in classical papillary carcinoma or the tall cell variant. These papillary carcinomas often show extrathyroidal extension and lymph node metastasis; therefore, patients often present at a higher tumor stage.

Table 5 Molecular markers and their correlates in thyroid pathology	
Molecular Marker	**Pathologic Correlate**
BRAF	Classic papillary carcinoma
	Tall cell variant, papillary carcinoma
	Oncocytic variant, papillary carcinoma
RAS	Follicular variant, papillary carcinoma
	Follicular carcinoma
	Follicular adenoma
RET/PTC	Classic papillary carcinoma
	Solid variant, papillary carcinoma
	Diffuse sclerosing variant, papillary carcinoma
PAX8/PPARgamma	Follicular carcinoma
	Follicular adenoma

The rates of tumor recurrence and related mortality is also higher. There is a propensity for dedifferentiation of the papillary carcinoma in these cases.

However, not all *BRAF*-positive papillary carcinomas are aggressive and not all aggressive papillary carcinomas are *BRAF*-positive. The testing methodology for *BRAF* requires either a fresh sample collected in a nucleic acid preservative solution or microdissected tumor samples from formalin-fixed paraffin-embedded tissue slides. LightCycler realtime PCR is performed and the melting temperature of the PCR products is compared with that of wild-type controls. Otherwise, *BRAF* genetic alterations may be detected with direct sequencing.

Although *BRAF* mutations may be present in other neoplasms (eg, colorectal adenocarcinoma, melanoma, papillary lung adenocarcinoma), *BRAF* mutation among thyroid neoplasms is highly specific (close to 100%) for papillary carcinoma. However, the sensitivity is not nearly as high. Because *BRAF* mutation is often associated with aggressive clinical features, patients who are found to harbor this mutation in their thyroid nodule often undergo central compartment lymph node dissection.

RAS mutation is often found in follicular carcinoma and follicular variant of papillary carcinoma. Occasionally, it may be seen in follicular adenoma. *RAS* mutation has been identified rarely in questionable cases of "atypical hyperplastic nodules." The positive predictive value for malignancy in the presence of *RAS* mutation is approximately 80%. *RAS*-positive neoplasms often show tumor encapsulation without invasion into the surrounding parenchyma. In contrast to *BRAF*-mutated neoplasms, lymph node metastases are uncommon, although distant metastasis and dedifferentiation may be seen. Specific *RAS* mutations found in thyroid neoplasms usually involve *NRAS61*, *HRAS61*, or *KRAS12/13* mutations. The testing methodology for *RAS* is similar to that for *BRAF* and involves the use of a fresh specimen or microdissected tumor samples from formalin-fixed paraffin-embedded tissue slides.

RET/PTC is most often found in classical papillary carcinoma. Other types of papillary carcinoma that show this translocation include the diffuse sclerosing variant and the solid variant. Rare adenomas may harbor *RET/PTC* translocations; however, these cases are considered questionable. Generally, this translocation is not found in follicular carcinoma, poorly differentiated carcinoma, or anaplastic carcinoma. *RET/PTC* translocations are often found in patients who are younger with history of radiation exposure. Lymph node metastases may be identified although the tumor stage is generally low. There is a low risk of progression toward poorly differentiated carcinoma or anaplastic carcinoma.

The most common translocation is *RET/PTC1*, which occurs in approximately two-thirds of the cases and is associated with sporadic occurrence. The other common translocation, *RET/PTC3*, occurs in approximately one-third of the cases and is associated with pediatric radiation exposure and the solid histologic subtype of papillary carcinoma. The testing methodology for the *RET/PTC* translocations involves the use of fresh specimen or frozen tissue. Formalin-fixed paraffin-embedded tissue generally is not used because the testing requires reverse transcription PCR (RT-PCR) from extracted RNA.

PAX8/PPARgamma translocation is often found in follicular neoplasms such as follicular carcinoma, oncocytic carcinoma, and, rarely, in follicular adenoma and papillary carcinoma. This translocation is not present in poorly differentiated carcinoma or anaplastic carcinoma. Affected patients are generally younger with small neoplasms. Histologically, the solid-patterned papillary carcinoma with vascular or angiolymphatic invasion is associated with this genetic alteration. Similar to the *RET/PTC* translocation, the preferred methodology is RT-PCR from extracted RNA; otherwise, FISH may be used. *PAX8/PPARgamma* translocation may be involved in the progression of follicular neoplasms. Follicular adenomas harboring this translocation may have a greater potential to progress to follicular carcinoma, unlike other follicular adenomas, which harbor different genetic alterations and are more indolent.

Currently, testing for these molecular markers is being performed at the clinical level in a few pathology laboratories. Because each laboratory decides on the tests offered and which cases will be tested, standardization of these procedures has not occurred. The costs and resources necessary to perform these tests on all thyroid FNA samples may be prohibitive; therefore, some laboratories have elected to perform these tests primarily on indeterminate and malignant diagnoses. Thus far, results using a panel of these markers have shown that the overall specificity for a malignant diagnosis tends to be very high, especially for *BRAF, RET/PTC*, and *PAX8/PPARgamma*. Although these markers are useful, they must be used in the proper clinico-pathologic context. For example, *BRAF* mutations may be observed in other nonthyroid malignancies, such as malignant melanoma, papillary adenocarcinoma of the lung, colorectal adenocarcinoma, and rare lymphomas/leukemias. Therefore, molecular marker results should be reviewed in conjunction with conventional cytomorphologic features. For the primary follicular patterned lesions of the thyroid, these markers have been helpful in stratifying indeterminate cases, such as those in the FLUS/AUS category. A recent study showed that FLUS/AUS cases with positivity of any these markers showed 100% specificity.[56] However, 7.6% of FLUS/AUS cases without marker positivity resulted in malignancy. Therefore, conventional cytology is still needed, and the best use of these techniques requires the combination of cytomorphologic evaluation for triage and focused application of ancillary studies to address specific issues. The molecular markers discussed, especially those targeting follicular patterned lesions (*BRAF, RAS, RET/PTC*, and *PAX8/PPARgamma*), improve the detection of low-grade thyroid malignancies.

SUMMARY

Advances have been made in the understanding of the pathobiology of thyroid nodules over the recent decades. Most thyroid cancers are low-grade and many share overlapping features with other benign lesions. These features manifest in clinical, radiologic, and pathologic studies. In cytologic evaluation of the thyroid, diagnostic uncertainty is stratified by estimation of risk of malignancy based on specific criteria. The recent development of the Bethesda system for reporting thyroid cytopathology results provides a framework for diagnostic standardization and improved communication. Finally, the application of ancillary studies, particularly molecular studies, provides powerful techniques to improve diagnostic, prognostic, and therapeutic efficacy.

REFERENCES

1. Stoffer RP, Welch JW, Hellwig CA, et al. Nodular goiter. Incidence, morphology before and after iodine prophylaxis, and clinical diagnosis. AMA Arch Intern Med 1960;106:10–4.

2. Vander JB, Gaston EA, Dawber TR. The significance of nontoxic thyroid nodules. Final report of a 15-year study of the incidence of thyroid malignancy. Ann Intern Med 1968;69:537–40.

3. Davies L, Welch HG. Increasing incidence of thyroid cancer in the United States, 1973–2002. JAMA 2006;295:2164–7.

4. Jemal A, Siegel R, Ward E, et al. Cancer statistics, 2008. CA Cancer J Clin 2008;58:71–96.

5. Muddegowda PH, Lingegowda J, Natesan R, et al. Divide and rule: cytodiagnosis of thyroid lesions using pattern analysis: a study of 233 cases. Diagn Cytopathol, in press.

6. Knudsen N, Bulow I, Laurberg P, et al. High occurrence of thyroid multinodularity and low occurrence of subclinical hypothyroidism among tobacco smokers in a large population study. J Endocrinol 2002;175:571–6.

7. Krohn K, Fuhrer D, Bayer Y, et al. Molecular pathogenesis of euthyroid and toxic multinodular goiter. Endocr Rev 2005;26:504–24.

8. Bignell GR, Canzian F, Shayeghi M, et al. Familial nontoxic multinodular thyroid goiter locus maps to chromosome 14q but does not account for familial nonmedullary thyroid cancer. Am J Hum Genet 1997;61:1123–30.

9. Levy A. Monoclonality of endocrine tumours: what does it mean? Trends Endocrinol Metab 2001;12: 301–7.

10. Szkudlinski MW, Fremont V, Ronin C, et al. Thyroid-stimulating hormone and thyroid-stimulating hormone receptor structure-function relationships. Physiol Rev 2002;82:473–502.

11. Dayan CM, Daniels GH. Chronic autoimmune thyroiditis. N Engl J Med 1996;335:99–107.

12. Harach HR, Soubeyran I, Brown A, et al. Thyroid pathologic findings in patients with Cowden disease. Ann Diagn Pathol 1999;3:331–40.

13. Stratakis CA, Courcoutsakis NA, Abati A, et al. Thyroid gland abnormalities in patients with the syndrome of spotty skin pigmentation, myxomas, endocrine overactivity, and schwannomas (Carney complex). J Clin Endocrinol Metab 1997;82:2037–43.

14. McCord EL, Geonka S. Development of thyroid follicular adenoma on simvastatin therapy. Tenn Med 2000;93:210–2.

15. Beige G, Roque L, Soares J, et al. Cytogenetic investigations of 340 thyroid hyperplasias and adenomas revealing correlations between cytogenetic findings and histology. Cancer Genet Cytogenet 1998;10:42–8.

16. Teyssier JR, Liautaud-Roger F, Ferre D, et al. Chromosomal changes in thyroid tumors. Relation with DNA content, karyotypic features, and clinical data. Cancer Genet Cytogenet 1990;50:249–63.

17. Roque L, Gomes P, Correia C, et al. Thyroid nodular hyperplasia: chromosomal studies in 14 cases. Cancer Genet Cytogenet 1993;69:31–4.

18. Ward LS, Brenta G, Medvedovic M, et al. Studies of allelic loss in thyroid tumors reveal major differences in chromosomal instability between papillary and follicular carcinomas. J Clin Endocrinol Metab 1998;83:525–30.

19. Esapa CT, Johnson SJ, Kendall-Taylor P, et al. Prevalence of Ras mutations in thyroid neoplasia. Clin Endocrinol (Oxf) 1999;50:529–35.

20. Nikiforova MN, Biddinger PW, Caudill CM, et al. PAX8-PPARgamma rearrangement in thyroid tumors: RT-PCR

and immunohistochemical analyses. Am J Surg Pathol 2002;26:1016–23.

21. Meiboom M, Beige G, Bol S, et al. Does conventional cytogenetics detect the real frequency of 19q13 aberrations in benign thyroid lesions? A survey of 38 cases. Cancer Genet Cytogenet 2003;146:70–2.

22. Hemminki K, Eng C, Chen B. Familial risks for non-medullary thyroid cancer. J Clin Endocrinol Metab 2005;90:5747–53.

23. Wreesman VB, Sieczka EM, Socci ND, et al. Genome-wide profiling of papillary thyroid cancer identifies MUC1 as an independent prognostic marker. Cancer Res 2004;64:3780–9.

24. Rodrigues R, Roque L, Espadinha C, et al. Comparative genomic hybridization, BRAF, RAS, RET, and oligo-array analysis in aneuploid papillary thyroid carcinomas. Oncol Rep 2007;18:917–26.

25. Kjellman P, Lagercrantz S, Hoog A, et al. Gain of 1q and loss of 9q21.3-q32 are associated with a less favorable prognosis in papillary thyroid carcinoma. Genes Chromosomes Cancer 2001;32:43–9.

26. Gillespie JW, Nasir A, Kaiser HE. Loss of heterozygosity in papillary and follicular thyroid carcinoma: a mini review. In Vivo 2000;14:139–40.

27. Hunt JL, Fowler M, Lomago D, et al. Tumor suppressor gene allelic loss profiles of the variants of papillary thyroid carcinoma. Diagn Mol Pathol 2004;13:41–6.

28. Robinson MJ, Cobb MH. Mitogen-activated protein kinase pathways. Curr Opin Cell Biol 1997;9:180–6.

29. Nikiforov YE, Steward DL, Robinson-Smith TM, et al. Molecular testing for mutations in improving the fine-needle aspiration diagnosis of thyroid nodules. J Clin Endocrinol Metab 2009;94:2092–8.

30. Baloch ZW, LiVolsi VA. Our approach to follicular-patterned lesions of the thyroid. J Clin Pathol 2007; 60:244–50.

31. Pittman MB, Abele J, Ali SZ, et al. Techniques for thyroid FNA: a synopsis of the National Cancer Institute Thyroid Fine-Needle Aspiration State of the Science Conference. Diagn Cytopathol 2008;36: 407–24.

32. Ljung BM, Langer J, Mazzaferri EL, et al. Training, credentialing and re-credentialing for the performance of a thyroid FNA: a synopsis of the National Cancer Institute Thyroid Fine-Needle Aspiration State of the Science Conference. Diagn Cytopathol 2008;36:400–6.

33. Rizvi SA, Husain M, Khan S, et al. A comparative study of fine needle aspiration cytology versus non-aspiration technique in thyroid lesions. Surgeon 2005;3:273–6.

34. Oertel YC. Thyroid fine-needle aspiration. Am J Clin Pathol 2009;132:308.

35. Renshaw AA, Pinnar N. Comparison of thyroid fine-needle aspiration and core needle biopsy. Am J Clin Pathol 2007;128:370–4.

36. Zhang S, Ivanovic M, Nemcek AA, et al. Thin core needle biopsy crush preparations in conjuction with fine-needle aspiration for the evaluation of thyroid nodules: a complementary approach. Cancer 2008;114:512–8.

37. Layfield LJ, Bentz JS, Gopez EV. Immediate on-site interpretation of fine-needle aspiration smears: a cost and compensation analysis. Cancer 2001;93:319–22.

38. Ljung BM. Thyroid fine-needle aspiration: smears versus liquid-base preparations. Cancer 2008;114: 114–8.

39. Yang J, Schnadig V, Logrono R, et al. Fine-needle aspiration of thyroid nodules: a study of 4703 patients with histologic and clinical correlations. Cancer 2007;111:306–15.

40. Wang HH. Reporting thyroid fine-needle aspiration: literature review and a proposal. Diagn Cytopathol 2006;34:67–76.

41. Baloch ZW, LiVolsi VA, Asa SL, et al. Diagnostic terminology and morphologic criteria for cytologic diagnosis of thyroid lesions: a synopsis of the National Cancer Institute Thyroid Fine-Needle Aspiration State of the Science Conference. Diagn Cytopathol 2008;36:425–37.

42. Baloch ZW, Alexander EK, Gharib H, et al. Overview of diagnostic terminology and reporting. In: Ali SZ, Cibas ES, editors. The Bethesda System for reporting thyroid cytopathology. Definitions, criteria and explanatory notes. New York: Springer; 2010. p. 1–4.

43. Goellner JR, Gharib H, Grant CS, et al. Fine needle aspiration cytology of the thyroid, 1980 to 1986. Acta Cytol 1987;31:587–90.

44. Renshaw A. An estimate of risk of malignancy for a benign diagnosis in thyroid fine-needle aspirates. Cancer Cytopathol 2010;118:190–5.

45. Alexander EK, Heering JP, Benson CB, et al. Assessment of nondiagnostic ultrasound-guided fine needle aspirations of thyroid nodules. J Clin Endocrinol Metab 2002;87:4924–7.

46. McHenry CR, Walfish PG, Rosen IB. Non-diagnostic fine needle aspiration biopsy: a dilemma in management of nodular thyroid disease. Am Surg 1993;59: 415–9.

47. Chow LS, Gharib H, Goellner JR, et al. Nondiagnostic thyroid fine-needle aspiration cytology: management dilemmas. Thyroid 2001;11:1147–51.

48. Renshaw AA. Should "atypical follicular cells" in thyroid fine-needle aspirates be subclassified? Cancer Cytopathol 2010;118:186–9.

49. Layfield LJ, Morton MJ, Cramer HM, et al. Implications of the proposed thyroid fine-needle aspiration category of "follicular lesion of undetermined significance": a five-year multi-institutional analysis. Diagn Cytopathol 2009;37:710–4.

50. Nayar R, Ivanovic M. The indeterminate thyroid fine-needle aspiration: experience from an academic center using terminology similar to that proposed in the 2007 National Cancer Institute Thyroid Fine

Needle Aspiration State of the Science Conference. Cancer Cytopathol 2009;117:195–202.

51. Marchevsky AM, Walts AE, Bose S, et al. Evidence-based evaluation of the risks of malignancy predicted by thyroid fine-needle aspiration biopsies. Diagn Cytopathol 2010;38:252–9.

52. Shi Y, Ding X, Klein M, et al. Thyroid fine-needle aspiration with atypia of undetermined significance: a necessary or optional category? Cancer Cytopathol 2009;117:298–304.

53. Theoharis CG, Schofield KM, Hammers L, et al. The Bethesda thyroid fine-needle aspiration classification system: year 1 at an academic institution. Thyroid 2009;19:1215–23.

54. Jo VY, Stelow EB, Dustin SM, et al. Malignancy risk for fine-needle aspiration of thyroid lesions according to the Bethesda System for Reporting Thyroid Cytopathology. Am J Clin Pathol 2010; 134:450–6.

55. Faquin WC, Baloch ZW. Fine-needle aspiration of follicular patterned lesions of the thyroid: diagnosis, management, and follow-up according to National Cancer Institute (NCI) recommendations. Diagn Cytopathol 2010;38:731–9.

56. Ohori NP, Nikiforova MN, Schoedel KE, et al. Contribution of molecular testing to thyroid fine-needle aspiration cytology of "follicular lesion of undetermined significance/atypia of undetermined significance". Cancer Cytopathol 2010;118:17–23.

57. Nikiforov YE. Thyroid carcinoma: molecular pathways and therapeutic targets. Mod Pathol 2008;21(Suppl 2): S37–43.

Diagnosis and Treatment of Differentiated Thyroid Carcinoma

Amy E. Cox, MD[a], Shane O. LeBeau, MD[b],*

KEYWORDS

- Thyroid cancer • FNA • Radioiodine • Thyroglobulin
- Surveillance testing

EPIDEMIOLOGY

Thyroid cancer is the most common endocrine malignancy in the United States, with a prevalence of more than 400,000.[1] There are 4 main histologic types of thyroid cancer: papillary, follicular, medullary, and anaplastic. Papillary is the most prevalent and accounts for 80% to 90% of reported thyroid cancer diagnoses.[1,2] The second most common type of thyroid cancer, follicular carcinoma, accounts for 5% to 10% of all thyroid carcinoma. Finally, medullary and anaplastic carcinoma account for 2% and 1%, respectively, of new thyroid carcinoma diagnoses.[2] For this discussion, the authors focus on well-differentiated thyroid cancer of follicular cell origin (ie, papillary and follicular thyroid carcinoma).

According to the National Cancer Institute Surveillance, Epidemiology, and End Results (SEER) program, there has been a steady increase in the incidence of thyroid cancer over the past 30 years. The annual incidence rate reported for 1980 was 4.3 cases per 100,000 people.[1] By 2007 the annual incidence rate had increased to 10.2 cases per 100,000 people.[1] This increase translates to approximately 37,000 new thyroid cancer cases in the United States during 2009.[3]

The reason behind this increase in thyroid cancer incidence is not entirely clear. In an analysis of the SEER database, there was a significant increase in the detection of small papillary thyroid cancers over time.[2] Specifically, between 1988 and 2002 a total of 49% of reported thyroid cancers were less than 1 cm in size; whereas, 87% were less than 2 cm in size. A separate birth cohort analysis of the same SEER data found that recent birth cohorts have a higher incidence of papillary thyroid cancer than older ones. This increase was present in both men and women and encompassed all sizes of thyroid cancer, from subcentimeter to greater than 5 cm.[4] A French study from 1980 to 2000 revealed a 3-fold increase in thyroid cancer prevalence among subjects undergoing surgery.[5] There was a significant increase in the percentage of subjects evaluated with thyroid ultrasound and fine-needle aspiration (FNA), but no change in the total number of subjects having surgery. Only thyroid nodule FNA was significantly associated with thyroid cancer. Collectively, these studies suggest that the increased incidence of thyroid cancer may be explained, at least in part, by the detection of small, subclinical thyroid cancers as a result of improved imaging capabilities, FNA, pathological techniques, and surgical practices.[4,5] However, environmental exposures, such as increased exposure to diagnostic X rays or radiation, may also play a role.[4] Despite the increased incidence of thyroid cancer, the overall mortality

The authors have nothing to disclose.
[a] Division of Endocrinology and Metabolism, University of Pittsburgh Medical Center, 200 Lothrop Street, E 1140 BST, Pittsburgh, PA 15261, USA
[b] Division of Endocrinology and Metabolism, University of Pittsburgh Medical Center, 3601 Fifth Avenue, Falk Medical Building, Suite 581, Pittsburgh, PA 15213, USA
* Corresponding author.
E-mail address: lebeauso4@upmc.edu

Radiol Clin N Am 49 (2011) 453–462
doi:10.1016/j.rcl.2011.02.006
0033-8389/11/$ – see front matter © 2011 Elsevier Inc. All rights reserved.

has remained quite low, with a 5-year survival for all stages of approximately 95%.[1]

DIAGNOSIS

Fine-needle aspiration via ultrasound guidance or palpation is the gold standard for evaluating thyroid nodules for malignancy. However, ultrasound guidance, as opposed to palpation, allows for the sampling of nodules that cannot be felt and permits specific targeting within nodules. For instance, in the case of a complex nodule, one can visualize and direct the needle into the solid portion of the nodule. Selective ultrasound targeting improves the adequacy of the sample and the diagnostic accuracy. A study of nearly 10,000 thyroid nodules reported a nondiagnostic rate of only 3.5% with ultrasound guidance, but nearly 9.0% with palpation-directed FNA.[6] Furthermore, ultrasound guidance had a significantly lower false-negative rate when compared to palpation-directed FNA.

FNA cytology has historically been the primary method of preoperatively evaluating thyroid nodules for malignancy. Although studies vary based on clinical practice type, roughly 60% to 70% of nodules are found to be benign on FNA and therefore require only serial follow-up.[7] Conversely, 3% to 7% of nodules are shown to be malignant; fine-needle aspirates of the remaining nodules are either nondiagnostic or indeterminate.[7] Repeat ultrasound-guided FNA of nondiagnostic specimens results in a definitive diagnosis in most cases.[8] The greatest shortcoming of FNA evaluation is the approximately 20% of all cases that are deemed indeterminate.[8,9] In this instance (ie, an indeterminate nodule), the differentiation between a benign and malignant process is not possible on cytology and surgical resection is recommended because of the increased risk of cancer. This practice results in unnecessary surgeries or surgical resections that may be inadequate, leading to frequent reoperation.

Testing of FNA specimens for the molecular mutations known to occur in thyroid cancer has recently become a useful adjunct tool. The molecular mutations most frequently identified in thyroid cancer are BRAF, RAS, RET/PTC, and PAX8/PPAR gamma.[10] In a recent study, testing FNA samples for the mutational panel BRAF, RAS, RET/PTC, and PAX8/PPAR gamma significantly increased the diagnostic accuracy and ability to predict malignancy in nodules with indeterminate cytology.[11] Of the 52 indeterminate nodules, all 15 that were positive for mutations on FNA were malignant on final histology. Therefore, a positive mutation in an FNA sample with indeterminate

cytology had a positive predictive value for malignancy of 100%. Additionally, the presence of a mutation was strongly correlated with cancer independent of the cytological diagnosis. Of the 32 mutation-positive nodules examined, only 13 had a definitive cytological diagnosis. However, 31 of the 32 mutation-positive nodules (97%) were malignant on final histology. Among the molecular mutations, BRAF is the most commonly identified, occurring in 45% of papillary thyroid cancers, and possesses the most robust data.[11–13] A summary of all available data reports a positive predictive value for thyroid cancer of 99.8% when a BRAF mutation is detected in any thyroid nodule FNA specimen.[10] These data highlight the importance of preoperative molecular testing of FNA specimens in the diagnosis and surgical management of patients with thyroid nodules.

TREATMENT
Preoperative Evaluation

Appropriate treatment for thyroid cancer begins before patients enter the operating room. Once a malignant diagnosis has been established, patients should undergo a preoperative evaluation for cervical lymph node metastases. Several imaging modalities (eg, ultrasonography, computed tomography, magnetic resonance imaging, and positron emission tomography) have been used to detect cervical lymph node metastases of thyroid cancer.[14–20] Although the results of studies vary, ultrasound is at least as accurate as the other more expensive modalities and is currently the preoperative staging tool of choice among most thyroidologists.[14,21]

The advantage of ultrasonography in comparison to other radiologic techniques is its ability to differentiate benign and suspicious-appearing nodes morphologically. Benign reactive lymph nodes are typically oblong and possess a central hyperechogenic hilum.[22] When neoplastic infiltration occurs, lymph nodes often become round in shape and the central hilum disappears.[23] Additionally, benign lymph nodes are usually hypoechoic with an organized pattern of blood flow within the central hilum. Conversely, metastatic nodes may be hypoechoic, heterogeneous, or hyperechoic with disorganized, peripherally located vascularity.[23] Cystic changes and the presence of intranodal calcifications are highly specific for thyroid cancer.[22,23]

The incidence of lymph node metastases identified by preoperative neck ultrasound ranges from 20% to 31%.[24,25] The central neck compartment (level VI) is the most common anatomic location of lymph node metastases in thyroid cancer.[26] Lymph nodes in the lateral neck, levels II to IV, are also common locations of metastases and occur on the side ipsilateral to the primary tumor more often than contralaterally.[26,27] Lymph nodes in the supraclavicular and submental regions (levels V and I, respectively) may also be involved, although much less commonly than the central and lateral compartments.[27]

The American Thyroid Association Task Force on Thyroid Nodules and Differentiated Thyroid Cancer recommends ultrasound-guided FNA of suspicious-appearing lymph nodes that are greater than 5 to 8 mm in the smallest diameter if positive results would alter management.[21] Like thyroid nodules, cytologic evaluation of potential lymph node metastases may be limited, particularly when they appear cystic on ultrasound.[28-32] Fine-needle aspiration specimens may be suboptimal or even false negative because of a paucity of cellular material. Thyroglobulin (Tg) measurement from FNA washout specimens of suspicious lymph nodes is more sensitive and has a greater negative predictive value than cytology alone.[28,31-34] Further, the presence of serum Tg antibodies does not appear to affect the measurement of Tg in lymph node washout specimens.[34,35] Therefore, suspicious-appearing lymph nodes that meet the aforementioned size threshold should be evaluated with both cytological specimens and Tg washout measurement.[21]

vIdentifying lymph node metastases preoperatively is important because it may alter the initial surgical approach and as such prevent future operations.[36] The impact of lymph node involvement on both recurrence and survival has been examined. In a retrospective study of nearly 10,000 subjects, the overall survival was significantly affected by lymph node metastases with a 79% long-term survival in node-positive subjects compared to 82% in node-negative subjects.[29] This adverse effect of lymph node involvement was independent of age.[29] A second study of approximately 33,000 subjects revealed a significant increased risk of death associated with lymph node involvement among subjects aged 45 years and older with papillary thyroid cancer, but no increased risk among subjects aged less than 45 years.[37] In subjects with follicular thyroid cancer from the same study, the presence of lymph node metastases was associated with an increased risk of death in all subjects independent of age.

Surgery

Multiple retrospective studies have shown a decreased risk of recurrence and improved overall survival among subjects treated with total or near total thyroidectomy.[38-41] For instance, a study of approximately 52,000 subjects from the National Cancer Database showed that subjects who underwent total or near-total thyroidectomy had a lower risk of both recurrent disease and death compared to those who underwent only lobectomy.[38] Conversely, a prospective study of 3000 subjects followed by the National Thyroid Cancer Treatment Cooperative Study Group reported an overall survival benefit with total/near-total thyroidectomy in all high-risk subjects, but only some low-risk subjects, and found no disease-specific survival benefit related to surgery in either high-risk or low-risk subjects.[42] Despite this recent prospective study, most thyroidologists recommend total or near-total thyroidectomy for cancers greater than 1 cm in size and reserve thyroid lobectomy for small cancers (<1 cm) that are unifocal, intrathyroidal, and low-risk histopathologically.[21]

The extent of surgery as it pertains to lymph node dissection is more controversial. Central compartment (level VI) dissection with total thyroidectomy is recommended for patients with preoperative detection of central or lateral neck lymph node involvement.[21] However, the role for prophylactic central node dissection in patients without preoperatively identified lymph node disease is not clear and outcomes may be influenced by surgical expertise.[43,44] The utility of prophylactic dissection may be further defined in the future with the use of molecular markers (ie, BRAF, RAS, RET/PTC, and PAX8/PPAR gamma mutations). In a recent study of subjects with papillary thyroid cancer, central compartment lymph node metastases were more common in BRAF-positive cancers (47%) compared to those that were BRAF negative (19%).[45] Additionally, reoperation for persistent or recurrent metastatic disease was also more common in subjects who were BRAF positive.[45] As research evolves and the risk of metastases associated with specific molecular markers is better defined, the decision regarding prophylactic central compartment dissection may be dictated by molecular test results.

Similar to the central compartment, patients with biopsy-proven lateral compartment lymph node involvement should undergo a lateral compartment surgery at the time of initial treatment.[21] Patients with preoperatively identified lateral disease frequently possess multilevel disease.[27] Therefore, a compartmental en-bloc resection may be more beneficial than a simple resection of individually identified metastatic lymph nodes.[21]

Staging and Risk Stratification

As with other malignancies, clinical staging of thyroid cancer is imperative. Currently, the American Joint Commission on Cancer (AJCC) classification system, which utilizes TNM parameters and age, is recommended for thyroid cancer.[46,47] This system enables health care providers to affectively communicate about patients, establishes a standard format that may be utilized in cancer registries and clinical research, and ultimately predicts patient mortality.[21] The AJCC reports a 5-year observed survival for papillary thyroid carcinoma of 97%, 93%, 82%, and 41% for stages I, II, III, and IV, respectively. With respect to patients with follicular thyroid carcinoma the 5-year observed survivals rates are similar at 97%, 89%, 58%, and 41%.[48] Accordingly, the AJCC stage assigned to a particular patient is useful in tailoring both immediate adjuvant treatment as well as short-term and long-term surveillance testing.

Although the mortality rate of thyroid cancer is quite low, a significant proportion of patients (approximately 14%–35%) experience disease recurrence.[1,49,50] Therefore, additional concerns for patients and health care providers revolve around persistent or recurrent disease and include minimizing morbidity associated with over-aggressive treatment, early detection and appropriate therapy of recurrence, and minimizing excess health care expenditures related to surveillance testing. In order to achieve these goals, patients with thyroid cancer are further risk stratified into 1 of 3 categories (low risk, intermediate risk, or high risk) based on the extent of tumor and final histology.[21] Patients who are low risk have undergone complete macroscopic tumor resection and have no evidence of local or distant metastases, no invasion of vascular or locoregional structures, and the absence of aggressive histologic variants (eg, tall cell, insular, or columnar). Patients who are intermediate risk demonstrate cervical lymph node metastases via surgical pathology or post-treatment whole-body radioiodine scan, vascular or microscopic invasion into perithyroidal soft tissue, or an aggressive histology.[21] Finally, patients who are high risk have incomplete tumor resection, the presence of distant metastases, macroscopic tumor invasion, or thyroglobulin concentrations higher than one would expect based on the outcome of post-treatment whole-body radioiodine scan.

Radioiodine

Postoperative radioiodine (^{131}I) therapy following thyroidectomy is performed for 3 theoretical reasons. First, it may detect previously unrecognized metastases and therefore functions as the final staging tool in patients with thyroid cancer. Second, ^{131}I is used to ablate any residual normal thyroid tissue remaining after total or near-total thyroidectomy, which increases the sensitivity of follow-up testing. Third, ^{131}I serves as adjuvant treatment of thyroid cancer, which may exist following surgery.

The use of ^{131}I in the management of thyroid cancer is currently evolving. Convincing prospective data regarding its effectiveness is limited. A retrospective analysis of outcomes in subjects with papillary thyroid cancer treated at the Mayo Clinic (1940–1999), found that despite increasing use of ^{131}I in recent decades, there was no improvement in disease-specific mortality or tumor recurrence in either high-risk or low-risk subjects treated with radioiodine.[50] However, in the only prospective study to date examining postoperative ^{131}I therapy, radioiodine improved overall survival, disease-specific survival, and disease-free survival in high-risk subjects.[42] Among low-risk subjects, ^{131}I appeared to improve overall survival in some subjects, but did not impact disease-specific or disease-free survival in any low-risk individuals.[42] It is also important to recognize that radioiodine is not innocuous; risks include salivary gland and duct damage, nasolacrimal duct obstruction, bone marrow suppression, and possibly secondary malignancies.[51–58]

In light of these data, most thyroidologists are becoming more judicious with the use of postoperative radioiodine.[21] Accordingly, postoperative ^{131}I therapy is recommended for all patients with primary tumors greater than 4 cm and for patients with extrathyroidal extension or distant metastases. It is also recommended for selected patients with cancers 1 to 4 cm in size, when confounding factors exist, such as worrisome histologic subtype, BRAF positivity, lymph node metastases, or other features that place patients into intermediate-risk or high-risk stratification. Postoperative radioiodine is not recommended for patients with tumors less than 1 cm in size or multifocal cancers that measure less than 1 cm in size unless a concomitant high-risk feature exists.[21]

When performed, radioiodine therapy requires thyrotropin (TSH) stimulation of thyroid cells in order to be effective. This stimulatory process increases the passage of ^{131}I into thyroid cells through the sodium-iodine symporter and promotes organification thereby trapping iodine in thyroid tissue. As ^{131}I decays it emits beta particle radiation that is capable of destroying both normal and malignant thyroid tissue. TSH stimulation can be achieved by either thyroid hormone withdrawal, which entails the discontinuation of thyroid hormone for 2 to 4 weeks depending on the thyroid hormone preparation used, or via the administration of recombinant human TSH (rhTSH) while patients continue to take thyroid hormone therapy.

Prospective studies comparing the efficacy of thyroid hormone withdrawal and rhTSH-stimulated thyroid ablation have been conducted in low-risk patients and reveal no significant difference in ablative success between the 2 methods.[59,60] In a study evaluating the effectiveness of different radioiodine doses, there was no difference between subjects receiving 100 mCi or 50 mCi of [131]I.[61] Collectively, these studies indicate that low-risk patients can be successfully ablated with low doses of ^{131}I, (ie, 50 mCi), via either thyroid hormone withdrawal or rhTSH. However, because quality-of-life measures are significantly higher in patients receiving rhTSH, this is the preferred stimulatory method in low-risk patients.[60,62] Data supporting the use of rhTSH-stimulated ablation in intermediate and high-risk patients is limited to a single retrospective study.[63] In this study, the effectiveness of radioiodine therapy in nearly 400 subjects treated at a single institution with either thyroid hormone withdrawal or rhTSH was reviewed. Subjects from all AJCC/UICC stages were included. A total of 18.5% of the subjects were either stage III or IV. After nearly 2.5 years of follow-up there was no difference in recurrence rates based on age, stage, or histology of primary tumor between the thyroid hormone withdrawal and rhTSH group when diagnostic whole body scan (WBS), stimulated thyroglobulin level of less than 10 ng/mL, and suppressed thyroglobulin level of less than 2 ng/mL were used to define no evidence of disease. However, when more stringent criteria where used (ie, a stimulated thyroglobulin level of <2 ng/mL and a suppressed thyroglobulin level of <1 ng/mL) the group prepared with rhTSH fared better with 74% showing no evidence of disease compared to 55% in the thyroid hormone withdrawal group.[63] This finding suggests that rhTSH may be superior to thyroid hormone withdrawal in treating higher-risk patients; however, prospective data would be much more convincing.

TSH Suppression

Exogenous thyroid hormone suppression of pituitary TSH production (ie, TSH suppression) is the final step of routine thyroid cancer treatment. The hypothesis behind this therapy is that thyroid cancer cells that have not been successfully treated via surgical excision and radioiodine, may respond to TSH stimulation, and as such grow or metastasize. This hypothesis has yet to be definitively proven and assumes that thyroid cancer cells possess TSH receptors that are functional and responsible for thyroid cancer growth.[64–67]

Several groups have evaluated the benefit of TSH suppression in patients with thyroid cancer. A retrospective study of 141 subjects with thyroid cancer followed for an average of 8 years revealed that subjects with TSH concentrations of less than 0.1 had a significantly longer relapse-free survival than those whose TSH concentrations were not suppressed.[68] However, a more recent prospective publication indicates that aggressive suppression for all patients with thyroid cancer may not be beneficial.[42] In this study, researchers found a benefit in overall survival when TSH levels were suppressed to the undetectable range only in high-risk subjects. Some low-risk subjects had an increase in overall survival when their TSH levels were suppressed to just below normal, but detectable; whereas, the lowest-risk subjects did not appear to benefit from any thyroid hormone suppression. These data indicate that the degree of TSH suppression should be tailored to the individual patient because of the fact that a proven benefit does not exist in all patients and excessive TSH suppression may have adverse consequences. Studies have shown that TSH concentrations persistently lower than 0.1 mg/dL are associated with bone loss in postmenopausal women as well as atrial fibrillation.[69–71]

FOLLOW-UP/SURVEILLANCE TESTING

Once treated, patients with thyroid cancer must be monitored for recurrence with clinical follow-up and surveillance testing. The rate of long-term recurrence ranges from 14% to 35% with the majority occurring during the first decade following initial treatment.[49,50] Patients with persistent/recurrent disease after initial treatment have a 40% reduction in life expectancy when compared to an age-matched normal population.[72] In contrast, patients free of disease have a normal life expectancy.[72] Intuitively, one would expect that detecting recurrent disease earlier rather than later would be associated with better treatment outcomes and long-term prognosis, although this has yet to be proven.

There are 3 general modalities used to monitor for recurrent disease: clinical examination, biochemical testing, and radiological imaging. Currently, there is no data to validate appropriate time intervals for clinical follow-up. However, it seems reasonable to perform clinical examinations every 6 to 12 months to assess for evidence of disease. This follow-up should be tailored to individual patients based on risk stratification, with higher-risk patients being seen at shorter follow-up intervals than low-risk patients.

Thyroglobulin, a glycoprotein produced by both normal and malignant thyroid tissue, is the primary biochemical test utilized in the surveillance of patients with thyroid cancer. Under normal physiologic TSH stimulation, small quantities of Tg are released into the circulation along with thyroid hormones. Most reference laboratories use immunometric assays as opposed to radioimmunoassays to measure Tg concentration. Despite international standardization (CRM-457), significant interassay variability exists.[73] Therefore, Tg assessment in individual patients should be measured serially on the same assay so that differences in reported values can be interpreted correctly.

Thyroglobulin measurement has a high sensitivity and specificity for detecting patients with thyroid cancer recurrence.[74–76] A meta-analysis of 46 studies found that Tg measurement following thyroid hormone withdrawal in subjects previously treated with thyroid remnant ablation had a sensitivity of 96% and a specificity of 95% for tumor recurrence.[75] Importantly, the sensitivity was significantly lower (77%) in subjects tested without stimulation and the specificity significantly lower (76%) in subjects who had not undergone remnant ablation.[75]

The degree of Tg elevation appears to be an important predictor of the extent of recurrent disease.[77] Research has found that tumor mass, assessed by total surface area and volume, was directly related to serum Tg/TSH ratio.[77] It has been reported that a rhTSH-stimulated Tg level of greater than or equal to 2 ng/mL predicted recurrence in 100% of subjects with distantly metastatic disease.[74] In a separate study, 107 subjects with thyroid cancer were followed and stratified according to their initial rhTSH-stimulated Tg concentrations: less than or equal to 0.5 ng/mL, 0.6 to 2.0 ng/mL, and greater than 2.0 ng/mL.[76] In this study, a stimulated Tg concentration greater than 2 ng/mL was highly sensitive for identifying subjects with disease. A total of 80% of subjects (16 of 20) who were clinically free of disease but had a stimulated Tg concentration greater than 2 ng/ml were found to have discrete disease radiologically over the next 3 to 5 years. However, a discrete metastatic foci was identified in only 5% of subjects (1 of 18) with a stimulated Tg of 0.6 to 2.0 ng/mL. In fact, in half of these subjects (9 of 18), repeat stimulated

Tg levels became undetectable over time. Finally, a stimulated Tg concentration of less than or equal to 0.5 ng/mL had a negative predictive value for recurrent disease of 98.5% (62 of 63). Other researchers have found similar results in subjects with undetectable stimulated Tg concentrations.[78] A total of 98% of subjects (67 of 68) with an undetectable stimulated Tg level (defined as <1.0 ng/mL) on initial surveillance testing continued to be clinically free of disease over the course of 3 years based on repeat Tg stimulation and neck sonography.[78] The recent development of highly sensitive Tg assays, with a clinical detection limit of 0.1 ng/mL, raises the question of whether stimulated Tg measurement will be necessary for the follow-up of all patients with thyroid cancer in the future. A recent study found that only 2 of 80 subjects (2.5%) with suppressed Tg levels less than 0.1 ng/mL had stimulated Tg levels greater than 2.0 ng/mL and only 1 subject was found to have recurrent disease with anatomic imaging.[79]

The utility of Tg measurement in the follow-up of patients with thyroid cancer is adversely affected by the presence of Tg antibodies. The presence of Tg antibodies can both overestimate or underestimate the actual Tg concentration present depending on the specific assay being used.[80] In these cases, serial measurement of Tg antibodies may be useful for disease monitoring.[80] Subjects who were disease free following initial treatment showed a decline in antibody concentrations to low or undetectable levels; whereas, those with persistent or recurrent disease continued to have detectable antibodies in follow-up.[80]

Radiologic evaluation is the third and final surveillance modality used in following patients with thyroid cancer. The majority of recurrent disease is local, with 68% occurring in the neck versus 32% distantly.[49] Therefore, evaluating the neck (ie, central [level VI], lateral [levels II–IV], supraclavicular [level V], and submental [level I] compartments) is imperative. As previously outlined, ultrasonography has an advantage over other imaging modalities of differentiating benign and suspicious-appearing lymph nodes morphologically. In a study of 456 subjects with low-risk thyroid cancer, all 38 subjects with histologically proven recurrence disease were identified by neck ultrasound and subsequent fine-needle aspiration.[81] Of these 38 subjects, 18% (7 of 38) had undetectable (≤1.0 ng/mL) stimulated Tg concentrations.[81]

The combination of stimulated Tg and neck ultrasound has proven to be more powerful than either alone, particularly in patients with low-risk disease.[76,81,82] In a retrospective study of 340 subjects with thyroid cancer, stimulated Tg measurement combined with neck ultrasound had a positive predictive value of 100% for detecting persistent/recurrent disease and negative predictive value of 99.5% in low-risk subjects.[82] A second study confirmed these findings reporting a negative predictive value of 98.8% in low-risk subjects with an undetectable stimulated Tg concentration and neck ultrasound 1 year following initial treatment.[81]

Diagnostic whole body scan, once the standard for following patients for persistent/recurrent disease, is gradually falling out of favor. In a study of low-risk subjects, only 41% of the subjects with recurrent disease on ultrasound were successfully identified by WBS, and no subjects with positive WBS were missed by neck ultrasound.[81] In a second study, the sensitivity of rhTSH-stimulated WBS was 20% with a false-negative rate of 79%.[82] When combined with stimulated Tg concentrations, WBS had an overall sensitivity of 92.7%, compared to 96.3% for stimulated Tg combined with ultrasound. Therefore, diagnostic WBS is not helpful in identifying recurrent disease among low-risk patients. In contrast, diagnostic WBS does have value in the surveillance of high-risk patients, where it can detect distant metastases that are not adequately screened for with neck ultrasound.[82]

The American Thyroid Association Guidelines Taskforce on Thyroid Nodules and Differentiated Thyroid Cancer recently published recommendations regarding follow up and surveillance testing of patients with differentiated thyroid cancer.[21] These guidelines recommend measuring Tg every 6 to 12 months on the same immunometric assay with simultaneous Tg antibody concentrations. Ultrasound of the thyroid bed and cervical lymph node compartments should be performed 6 to 12 months following initial therapy and then periodically based on patients' risk stratification. Patients who have undetectable Tg concentrations on thyroid hormone suppression and negative neck ultrasound during the first year following treatment should undergo stimulated Tg assessment approximately 1 year following initial radioiodine ablation. In low-risk patients with negative neck ultrasound and undetectable stimulated Tg concentrations at 1 year follow-up, there is rarely benefit from performing additional stimulated Tg testing.[78] Therefore, such low-risk patients may be followed with yearly clinical examinations, suppressed Tg measurement, and periodic neck ultrasounds.[21] Diagnostic WBS is not necessary in these low-risk patients unless uptake outside the thyroid bed was visualized on the initial post-therapy WBS. However, diagnostic WBS is recommended 6 to 12 months following initial radioiodine remnant ablation in patients with intermediate-risk or high-risk disease.

SUMMARY

Thyroid cancer is the most common endocrine malignancy. Historically, the diagnosis has been made via fine-needle aspiration cytology; however, molecular marker analysis, particularly of indeterminant specimens, is beginning to play a more prominent role. Once the diagnosis of thyroid cancer is established, patients should undergo preoperative ultrasound evaluation followed by appropriate surgical resection, radioiodine ablation, and TSH suppression. After the initial treatment, patients must be monitored regularly for recurrent disease utilizing clinical examination, thyroglobulin measurement, and radiological imaging.

REFERENCES

1. Altekruse SF, Kosary CL, Krapcho M, et al, editors. SEER Cancer Statistics Review. Bethesda (MD): National Cancer Institue. Available at: http://seer.cancer.gov/csr/1975_2007/, based on November 2009 SEER data submission, posted to the SEER web site, 2010, 1975–2007. Accessed July, 2010.
2. Davies L, Welch HG. Increasing incidence of thyroid cancer in the United States, 1973–2002. JAMA 2006;295:2164.
3. Jemal A, Siegel R, Ward E, et al. Cancer statistics, 2009. CA Cancer J Clin 2009;59:225.
4. Zhu C, Zheng T, Kilfoy BA, et al. A birth cohort analysis of the incidence of papillary thyroid cancer in the United States, 1973–2004. Thyroid 2009;19:1061.
5. Leenhardt L, Bernier MO, Boin-Pineau MH, et al. Advances in diagnostic practices affect thyroid cancer incidence in France. Eur J Endocrinol 2004;150:133.
6. Danese D, Sciacchitano S, Farsetti A, et al. Diagnostic accuracy of conventional versus sonography-guided fine-needle aspiration biopsy of thyroid nodules. Thyroid 1998;8:15.
7. Cibas ES, Ali SZ. The Bethesda system for reporting thyroid cytopathology. Thyroid 2009;19:1159.
8. Yassa L, Cibas ES, Benson CB, et al. Long-term assessment of a multidisciplinary approach to thyroid nodule diagnostic evaluation. Cancer 2007; 111:508.
9. Gharib H, Goellner JR, Johnson DA. Fine-needle aspiration cytology of the thyroid. A 12-year experience with 11,000 biopsies. Clin Lab Med 1993;13:699.
10. Nikiforova MN, Nikiforov YE. Molecular diagnostics and predictors in thyroid cancer. Thyroid 2009;19:1351.

11. Nikiforov YE, Steward DL, Robinson-Smith TM, et al. Molecular testing for mutations in improving the fine-needle aspiration diagnosis of thyroid nodules. J Clin Endocrinol Metab 2009;94:2092.

12. Xing M. BRAF mutation in thyroid cancer. Endocr Relat Cancer 2005;12:245.

13. Xing M, Clark D, Guan H, et al. BRAF mutation testing of thyroid fine-needle aspiration biopsy specimens for preoperative risk stratification in papillary thyroid cancer. J Clin Oncol 2009;27:2977.

14. Jeong HS, Baek CH, Son YI, et al. Integrated 18F-FDG PET/CT for the initial evaluation of cervical node level of patients with papillary thyroid carcinoma: comparison with ultrasound and contrast-enhanced CT. Clin Endocrinol (Oxf) 2006;65:402.

15. Gross ND, Weissman JL, Talbot JM, et al. MRI detection of cervical metastasis from differentiated thyroid carcinoma. Laryngoscope 2001;111:1905.

16. Kim E, Park JS, Son KR, et al. Preoperative diagnosis of cervical metastatic lymph nodes in papillary thyroid carcinoma: comparison of ultrasound, computed tomography, and combined ultrasound with computed tomography. Thyroid 2008;18:411.

17. Choi JS, Kim J, Kwak JY, et al. Preoperative staging of papillary thyroid carcinoma: comparison of ultrasound imaging and CT. AJR Am J Roentgenol 2009;193:871.

18. Kouvaraki MA, Shapiro SE, Fornage BD, et al. Role of preoperative ultrasonography in the surgical management of patients with thyroid cancer. Surgery 2003;134:946.

19. King AD, Ahuja AT, To EW, et al. Staging papillary carcinoma of the thyroid: magnetic resonance imaging vs ultrasound of the neck. Clin Radiol 2000;55:222.

20. Stulak JM, Grant CS, Farley DR, et al. Value of preoperative ultrasonography in the surgical management of initial and reoperative papillary thyroid cancer. Arch Surg 2006;141:489.

21. Cooper DS, Doherty GM, Haugen BR, et al. Revised American Thyroid Association management guidelines for patients with thyroid nodules and differentiated thyroid cancer. Thyroid 2009;19:1167.

22. Solbiati L, Osti V, Cova L, et al. Ultrasound of thyroid, parathyroid glands and neck lymph nodes. Eur Radiol 2001;11:2411.

23. Leboulleux S, Girard E, Rose M, et al. Ultrasound criteria of malignancy for cervical lymph nodes in patients followed up for differentiated thyroid cancer. J Clin Endocrinol Metab 2007;92:3590.

24. Solorzano CC, Carneiro DM, Ramirez M, et al. Surgeon-performed ultrasound in the management of thyroid malignancy. Am Surg 2004;70:576.

25. Shimamoto K, Satake H, Sawaki A, et al. Preoperative staging of thyroid papillary carcinoma with ultrasonography. Eur J Radiol 1998;29:4.

26. Machens A, Hinze R, Thomusch O, et al. Pattern of nodal metastasis for primary and reoperative thyroid cancer. World J Surg 2002;26:22.

27. Kupferman ME, Patterson M, Mandel SJ, et al. Patterns of lateral neck metastasis in papillary thyroid carcinoma. Arch Otolaryngol Head Neck Surg 2004;130:857.

28. Cignarelli M, Ambrosi A, Marino A, et al. Diagnostic utility of thyroglobulin detection in fine-needle aspiration of cervical cystic metastatic lymph nodes from papillary thyroid cancer with negative cytology. Thyroid 2003;13:1163.

29. Podnos YD, Smith D, Wagman LD, et al. The implication of lymph node metastasis on survival in patients with well-differentiated thyroid cancer. Am Surg 2005;71:731.

30. Leboulleux S, Rubino C, Baudin E, et al. Prognostic factors for persistent or recurrent disease of papillary thyroid carcinoma with neck lymph node metastases and/or tumor extension beyond the thyroid capsule at initial diagnosis. J Clin Endocrinol Metab 2005;90:5723.

31. Cunha N, Rodrigues F, Curado F, et al. Thyroglobulin detection in fine-needle aspirates of cervical lymph nodes: a technique for the diagnosis of metastatic differentiated thyroid cancer. Eur J Endocrinol 2007;157:101.

32. Uruno T, Miyauchi A, Shimizu K, et al. Usefulness of thyroglobulin measurement in fine-needle aspiration biopsy specimens for diagnosing cervical lymph node metastasis in patients with papillary thyroid cancer. World J Surg 2005;29:483.

33. Pacini F, Fugazzola L, Lippi F, et al. Detection of thyroglobulin in fine needle aspirates of nonthyroidal neck masses: a clue to the diagnosis of metastatic differentiated thyroid cancer. J Clin Endocrinol Metab 1992;74:1401.

34. Boi F, Baghino G, Atzeni F, et al. The diagnostic value for differentiated thyroid carcinoma metastases of thyroglobulin (Tg) measurement in washout fluid from fine-needle aspiration biopsy of neck lymph nodes is maintained in the presence of circulating anti-Tg antibodies. J Clin Endocrinol Metab 2006;91:1364.

35. Borel AL, Boizel R, Faure P, et al. Significance of low levels of thyroglobulin in fine needle aspirates from cervical lymph nodes of patients with a history of differentiated thyroid cancer. Eur J Endocrinol 2008;158:691.

36. Ito Y, Tomoda C, Uruno T, et al. Ultrasonographically and anatomopathologically detectable node metastases in the lateral compartment as indicators of worse relapse-free survival in patients with papillary thyroid carcinoma. World J Surg 2005;29:917.

37. Zaydfudim V, Feurer ID, Griffin MR, et al. The impact of lymph node involvement on survival in patients with papillary and follicular thyroid carcinoma. Surgery 2008;144:1070.

38. Bilimoria KY, Bentrem DJ, Ko CY, et al. Extent of surgery affects survival for papillary thyroid cancer. Ann Surg 2007;246:375.

39. DeGroot LJ, Kaplan EL, McCormick M, et al. Natural history, treatment, and course of papillary thyroid carcinoma. J Clin Endocrinol Metab 1990;71:414.

40. Mazzaferri EL, Young RL. Papillary thyroid carcinoma: a 10-year follow-up report of the impact of therapy in 576 patients. Am J Med 1981;70:511.

41. Samaan NA, Schultz PN, Hickey RC, et al. The results of various modalities of treatment of well differentiated thyroid carcinomas: a retrospective review of 1599 patients. J Clin Endocrinol Metab 1992;75:714.

42. Jonklaas J, Sarlis NJ, Litofsky D, et al. Outcomes of patients with differentiated thyroid carcinoma following initial therapy. Thyroid 2006;16:1229.

43. Sosa JA, Bowman HM, Tielsch JM, et al. The importance of surgeon experience for clinical and economic outcomes from thyroidectomy. Ann Surg 1998;228:320.

44. Yim JH, Carty SE. Thyroid surgery and surgeons: the common interest. Thyroid 2010;20:357.

45. Yip L, Nikiforova MN, Carty SE, et al. Optimizing surgical treatment of papillary thyroid carcinoma associated with BRAF mutation. Surgery 2009;146: 1215.

46. Brierley JD, Panzarella T, Tsang RW, et al. A comparison of different staging systems predictability of patient outcome. Thyroid carcinoma as an example. Cancer 1997;79:2414.

47. Loh KC, Greenspan FS, Gee L, et al. Pathological tumor-node-metastasis (pTNM) staging for papillary and follicular thyroid carcinomas: a retrospective analysis of 700 patients. J Clin Endocrinol Metab 1997;82:3553.

48. Edge SB, Byrd DR, Compton CC, et al. AJCC Cancer Staging Manual. 7th edition. Springer; 2010. p. 87.

49. Mazzaferri EL, Kloos RT. Clinical review 128: current approaches to primary therapy for papillary and follicular thyroid cancer. J Clin Endocrinol Metab 2001;86:1447.

50. Hay ID, Thompson GB, Grant CS, et al. Papillary thyroid carcinoma managed at the Mayo Clinic during six decades (1940–1999): temporal trends in initial therapy and long-term outcome in 2444 consecutively treated patients. World J Surg 2002; 26:879.

51. Walter MA, Turtschi CP, Schindler C, et al. The dental safety profile of high-dose radioiodine therapy for thyroid cancer: long-term results of a longitudinal cohort study. J Nucl Med 2007;48:1620.

52. Kloos RT, Duvuuri V, Jhiang SM, et al. Nasolacrimal drainage system obstruction from radioactive iodine therapy for thyroid carcinoma. J Clin Endocrinol Metab 2002;87:5817.

53. Benua RS, Cicale NR, Sonenberg M, et al. The relation of radioiodine dosimetry to results and complications in the treatment of metastatic thyroid cancer. Am J Roentgenol Radium Ther Nucl Med 1962;87:171.

54. Brown AP, Chen J, Hitchcock YJ, et al. The risk of second primary malignancies up to three decades after the treatment of differentiated thyroid cancer. J Clin Endocrinol Metab 2008;93:504.

55. Sandeep TC, Strachan MW, Reynolds RM, et al. Second primary cancers in thyroid cancer patients: a multinational record linkage study. J Clin Endocrinol Metab 2006;91:1819.

56. Rubino C, de Vathaire F, Dottorini ME, et al. Second primary malignancies in thyroid cancer patients. Br J Cancer 2003;89:1638.

57. Sawka AM, Thabane L, Parlea L, et al. Second primary malignancy risk after radioactive iodine treatment for thyroid cancer: a systematic review and meta-analysis. Thyroid 2009;19:451.

58. Subramanian S, Goldstein DP, Parlea L, et al. Second primary malignancy risk in thyroid cancer survivors: a systematic review and meta-analysis. Thyroid 2007;17:1277.

59. Chianelli M, Todino V, Graziano FM, et al. Low-activity (2.0 GBq; 54 mCi) radioiodine post-surgical remnant ablation in thyroid cancer: comparison between hormone withdrawal and use of rhTSH in low-risk patients. Eur J Endocrinol 2009;160:431.

60. Pacini F, Ladenson PW, Schlumberger M, et al. Radioiodine ablation of thyroid remnants after preparation with recombinant human thyrotropin in differentiated thyroid carcinoma: results of an international, randomized, controlled study. J Clin Endocrinol Metab 2006;91:926.

61. Pilli T, Brianzoni E, Capoccetti F, et al. A comparison of 1850 (50 mCi) and 3700 MBq (100 mCi) 131-iodine administered doses for recombinant thyrotropin-stimulated postoperative thyroid remnant ablation in differentiated thyroid cancer. J Clin Endocrinol Metab 2007;92:3542.

62. Lee J, Yun MJ, Nam KH, et al. Quality of life and effectiveness comparisons of thyroxine withdrawal, triiodothyronine withdrawal, and recombinant thyroid-stimulating hormone administration for low-dose radioiodine remnant ablation of differentiated thyroid carcinoma. Thyroid 2010;20:173.

63. Tuttle RM, Brokhin M, Omry G, et al. Recombinant human TSH-assisted radioactive iodine remnant ablation achieves short-term clinical recurrence rates similar to those of traditional thyroid hormone withdrawal. J Nucl Med 2008;49:764.

64. Cai WY, Lukes YG, Burch HB, et al. Analysis of human TSH receptor gene and RNA transcripts in patients with thyroid disorders. Autoimmunity 1992;13:43.

65. Goretzki PE, Koob R, Koller T, et al. The effect of thyrotropin and cAMP on DNA synthesis and cell

growth of human thyrocytes in monolayer culture. Surgery 1986;100:1053.

66. Tanaka K, Inoue H, Miki H, et al. Relationship between prognostic score and thyrotropin receptor (TSH-R) in papillary thyroid carcinoma: immunohistochemical detection of TSH-R. Br J Cancer 1997; 76:594.

67. Sheils OM, Sweeney EC. TSH receptor status of thyroid neoplasms–TaqMan RT-PCR analysis of archival material. J Pathol 1999;188:87.

68. Pujol P, Daures JP, Nsakala N, et al. Degree of thyrotropin suppression as a prognostic determinant in differentiated thyroid cancer. J Clin Endocrinol Metab 1996;81:4318.

69. Mikosch P, Obermayer-Pietsch B, Jost R, et al. Bone metabolism in patients with differentiated thyroid carcinoma receiving suppressive levothyroxine treatment. Thyroid 2003;13:347.

70. Uzzan B, Campos J, Cucherat M, et al. Effects on bone mass of long term treatment with thyroid hormones: a meta-analysis. J Clin Endocrinol Metab 1996;81:4278.

71. Sawin CT, Geller A, Wolf PA, et al. Low serum thyrotropin concentrations as a risk factor for atrial fibrillation in older persons. N Engl J Med 1994;331:1249.

72. Links TP, van Tol KM, Jager PL, et al. Life expectancy in differentiated thyroid cancer: a novel approach to survival analysis. Endocr Relat Cancer 2005;12:273.

73. Spencer CA, Bergoglio LM, Kazarosyan M, et al. Clinical impact of thyroglobulin (Tg) and Tg autoantibody method differences on the management of patients with differentiated thyroid carcinomas. J Clin Endocrinol Metab 2005;90:5566.

74. Haugen BR, Pacini F, Reiners C, et al. A comparison of recombinant human thyrotropin and thyroid hormone withdrawal for the detection of thyroid remnant or cancer. J Clin Endocrinol Metab 1999; 84:3877.

75. Eustatia-Rutten CF, Smit JW, Romijn JA, et al. Diagnostic value of serum thyroglobulin measurements in the follow-up of differentiated thyroid carcinoma, a structured meta-analysis. Clin Endocrinol (Oxf) 2004;61:61.

76. Kloos RT, Mazzaferri EL. A single recombinant human thyrotropin-stimulated serum thyroglobulin measurement predicts differentiated thyroid carcinoma metastases three to five years later. J Clin Endocrinol Metab 2005;90:5047.

77. Bachelot A, Cailleux AF, Klain M, et al. Relationship between tumor burden and serum thyroglobulin level in patients with papillary and follicular thyroid carcinoma. Thyroid 2002;12:707.

78. Castagna MG, Brilli L, Pilli T, et al. Limited value of repeat recombinant human thyrotropin (rhTSH)-stimulated thyroglobulin testing in differentiated thyroid carcinoma patients with previous negative rhTSH-stimulated thyroglobulin and undetectable basal serum thyroglobulin levels. J Clin Endocrinol Metab 2008;93:76.

79. Smallridge RC, Meek SE, Morgan MA, et al. Monitoring thyroglobulin in a sensitive immunoassay has comparable sensitivity to recombinant human tsh-stimulated thyroglobulin in follow-up of thyroid cancer patients. J Clin Endocrinol Metab 2007;92:82.

80. Spencer CA, Takeuchi M, Kazarosyan M, et al. Serum thyroglobulin autoantibodies: prevalence, influence on serum thyroglobulin measurement, and prognostic significance in patients with differentiated thyroid carcinoma. J Clin Endocrinol Metab 1998;83:1121.

81. Torlontano M, Attard M, Crocetti U, et al. Follow-up of low risk patients with papillary thyroid cancer: role of neck ultrasonography in detecting lymph node metastases. J Clin Endocrinol Metab 2004; 89:3402.

82. Pacini F, Molinaro E, Castagna MG, et al. Recombinant human thyrotropin-stimulated serum thyroglobulin combined with neck ultrasonography has the highest sensitivity in monitoring differentiated thyroid carcinoma. J Clin Endocrinol Metab 2003; 88:3668.

Thyroid Carcinoma: The Surgeon's Perspective

Linwah Yip, MD*, Michael T. Stang, MD, Sally E. Carty, MD

KEYWORDS

- Thyroid carcinoma • Thyroidectomy • Lymphadenectomy
- Fine-needle aspiration biopsy

The incidence of thyroid cancer is increasing, with an estimated 44,670 new cases diagnosed in 2010. Approximately 1 in 111 men and women will develop thyroid cancer in their lifetime. The incidence in women is threefold higher than in men, and the median age is 49 years. However, the prognosis is excellent, with an overall 5-year survival of 97.3% and stable mortality rates over time.[1]

The increase in incidence was recently studied by analysis of Surveillance, Epidemiology, and End Results (SEER) data, and may be due to improved detection of small (<2 cm) papillary thyroid cancers.[2] Coincident with the increase is widespread use of ultrasonography and fine-needle aspiration biopsy (FNAB). Long-term follow-up is needed to determine whether early detection will eventually have a beneficial impact.

Although up to 70% of people will have a thyroid mass visualized on ultrasonography, the overall risk of thyroid cancer in a nodule is only approximately 5%. As discussed in other articles in this issue, evidence-based clinical management algorithms guide the evaluation. FNAB is highly accurate and specific, but 10% to 15% of the results will fall into the indeterminate category, which now includes 3 subsets: follicular lesion of undetermined significance (FLUS), follicular or oncocytic neoplasm, and suspicious for malignancy results.[3] Thyroidectomy is currently often required for definitive diagnosis of indeterminate cytology results. The risks of thyroid surgery include morbidity and associated health care costs.

Imaging characteristics in addition to other diagnostic modalities can help define malignancy risk and guide the extent of surgery.

INDICATIONS FOR SURGERY

A surgical evaluation is usually prompted by clinical history, FNAB results, and/or patient request. Radiation exposure and family history in first-degree relatives are two well-documented risk factors for differentiated thyroid cancer. Exposure to nuclear fallout or therapeutic ionizing radiation to the head and neck are two of the most common types of radiation exposure that increase the risk of thyroid cancer. The latency period is usually 25 to 30 years, but the effects can be significant for up to 40 years.[4,5] Radiation exposure can also increase the risk of primary hyperparathyroidism, and affected patients should be screened for both disorders. Several inherited syndromes can be associated with thyroid cancer, including Cowden syndrome (macrocephaly, mucocutaneous lesions, and breast cancer), Carney complex type 1 (cardiac myxoma, skin and mucosal pigmentations), and familial adenomatous polyposis (colon cancer).[6] In addition, if there is a family history of thyroid cancer, hypercalcemia, mucosal lesions, and/or hypertension secondary to pheochromocytoma, multiple endocrine neoplasia type 2 is a consideration. A fasting serum calcitonin should be obtained preoperatively to evaluate for C-cell hyperplasia and medullary thyroid carcinoma.

Section of Endocrine Surgery, Department of Surgery, University of Pittsburgh School of Medicine, Pittsburgh, PA, USA
* Corresponding author. University of Pittsburgh School of Medicine, Suite 101 Kaufmann Building, 3471 Fifth Avenue, Pittsburgh, PA 15213.
E-mail address: yipl@upmc.edu

Radiol Clin N Am 49 (2011) 463–471
doi:10.1016/j.rcl.2011.02.007
0033-8389/11/$ – see front matter © 2011 Elsevier Inc. All rights reserved.

A clinical history of an enlarging thyroid mass increases the concern for malignancy. On physical examination, an immobile and firm thyroid nodule is also worrisome. Routine evaluation should also assess for dysphagia, positional dyspnea, orthopnea, anterior neck discomfort, hoarseness, tracheal deviation, lymphadenopathy, and the presence of contralateral thyroid nodules. Supine dyspnea that is relieved by positional change and/or an inability to palpate the inferior aspect of the thyroid gland should raise the concern for a substernal component. A computed tomography (CT) scan of the neck without intravenous contrast is usually obtained to assess the caudal extent of the thyroid gland (**Fig. 1**). Goiter extending below the aortic arch may require a partial sternal split for complete resection. A history of sleep apnea or significant thyromegaly at the thoracic outlet on examination should also prompt a noncontrasted CT scan to evaluate for tracheal compression that could affect both extent of surgery and method of anesthesia induction (**Fig. 2**). A neck CT scan with contrast is helpful only if the relationship of the thyroid mass to adjacent vascular structures needs to be better delineated.

As discussed in other articles in this issue, a neck ultrasound is routinely obtained to evaluate thyroid nodule size and characteristics. Cervical lymphadenopathy should also be concurrently evaluated. FNAB is the initial diagnostic test and determines subsequent clinical management. Diagnostic thyroidectomy is indicated for FNAB results in either the indeterminate or positive for malignancy categories (**Fig. 3**). Persistently inadequate FNAB

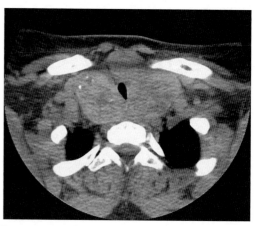

Fig. 2. Transverse section of a CT scan of the neck without intravenous contrast obtained for a 49-year-old woman who presented with a large cervical goiter that was noted on routine physical examination. Although she was asymptomatic, her enlarged thyroid gland was causing 65% tracheal compression, and she required a fiberoptic intubation while awake prior to general anesthesia for her thyroidectomy.

results also prompt diagnostic thyroid surgery. In addition, clinically or sonographically suspicious nodules should be further evaluated, even if FNAB results are initially benign. Patients with significant risk factors for thyroid cancer who have a dominant (>1 cm) thyroid nodule, symptomatic thyromegaly, tracheal compression, and/or substernal goiter that is unable to be evaluated completely with FNAB or ultrasonography should also be considered for thyroidectomy.[7]

Size has been shown in several studies to be associated with both malignancy and false-negative benign FNAB results. Meko and Norton[8] first reported an overall malignancy rate of 21% for thyroid nodules of 3 cm or larger and a 30% false-negative rate for benign FNAB results. Using a study design recently described to be more accurate at determining the true false-negative FNAB results,[9] a larger investigation described 223 consecutive patients for whom the presence of a thyroid mass 4 cm or larger was considered an independent indication for thyroidectomy, and found that 26% had clinically significant thyroid cancer. Among the patients with thyroid nodules of 4 cm or larger who had benign preoperative FNAB results, 13% had a clinically significant thyroid cancer within the biopsied nodule.[10] Because of the high false-negative rate associated with benign FNAB in large nodules, the authors currently perform thyroidectomy for nodules 4 cm or larger, regardless of FNAB results.

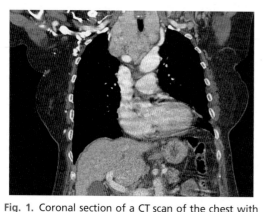

Fig. 1. Coronal section of a CT scan of the chest with intravenous contrast obtained for a 72-year-old woman who presented with acute shortness of breath. Her large thyroid goiter is predominantly substernal and not appreciated on physical examination. Although a thoracic surgeon was available for a possible sternotomy, her thyroid was successfully mobilized and resected through a 5-cm cervical incision.

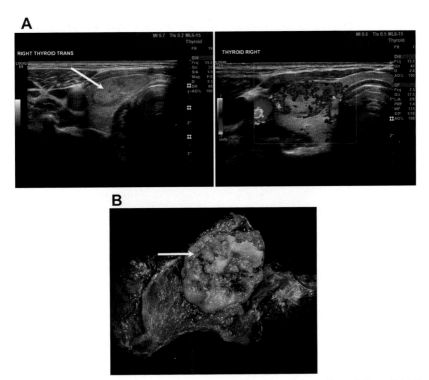

Fig. 3. (*A*) A transverse neck ultrasound image of a 38-year-old woman with a solitary 2.5-cm right thyroid nodule (*arrow*) that has a hypoechoic rim and hypervascularity. A follicular neoplasm was diagnosed after FNAB. (*B*) Following thyroid lobectomy, a 2-cm follicular variant papillary thyroid carcinoma (*arrow*) was diagnosed, and she went on to receive completion thyroidectomy within 2 weeks.

EXTENT OF INITIAL THYROIDECTOMY

The extent of initial thyroidectomy depends on whether the diagnosis of thyroid cancer can be determined on FNAB. Patients with FNAB results positive for thyroid carcinoma should be counseled about the associated low but real false-positive rate.[3] In the absence of an FNAB result positive for malignancy, the decision for thyroid lobectomy versus total/near-total thyroidectomy depends on clinical characteristics and risk of malignancy as outlined herein. The minimum operation at initial operation should be a complete lobectomy and isthmusectomy, with the margin of resection being the junction of the isthmus to the contralateral lobe. A partial lobectomy or "nodulectomy" puts the ipsilateral recurrent laryngeal nerve at increased risk if a reoperation is required, and partial lobectomy has thus been abandoned. Although the main benefit of an initial thyroid lobectomy is to potentially prevent chronic postoperative hypothyroidism, replacement L-thyroxine therapy is still required in 25% to 40% of patients.[11] Initial lobectomy also prevents the risk of postoperative hypoparathyroidism. However,

if thyroid cancer is diagnosed on final histopathology, a completion thyroidectomy may be necessary. Completion thyroidectomy unfortunately exposes the patient to a second general anesthetic as well as to the higher complication risks associated with reoperation (**Table 1**).

Total or near-total thyroidectomy leaves less than 50 mg of tissue at the ligament of Berry, and is considered the initial surgical procedure of choice for known thyroid cancers greater than 1 cm in size. In all patients with thyroid cancer, the purpose of thyroidectomy is to remove the primary tumor, minimize treatment-related morbidity, determine accurate staging, facilitate treatment with radioactive iodine when indicated, facilitate long-term surveillance, and minimize the risk of recurrence and metastatic disease.[7] Associated abnormal lymphadenopathy is also resected, if present. A subtotal thyroidectomy that leaves more than 1 g of tissue is not a desirable procedure for thyroid cancer.

Initial total thyroidectomy should also be considered if there is a high risk of thyroid cancer, such as with suspicious findings or significant atypia seen on biopsy, a close family history of thyroid cancer,

Table 1
Operative risks associated with thyroid surgery

	Total Thyroidectomy	Thyroid Lobectomy	Completion Thyroidectomy
Recurrent laryngeal nerve injury			
Unilateral	1%–3%	1%–3%	1%–3%
Bilateral	<1%	0%	0%
Superior laryngeal nerve injury	5%–10%	5%–10%	5%–10%
Permanent hypoparathyroidism	0.5%–3%	0%	0.5%–3%
Cervical hematoma	0.5%–1%	0.5%–1%	0.5%–1%
Hypothyroidism	100%	20%–40%	100%

a history of therapeutic radiation exposure such as whole body radiation for lymphoma, and nodules larger than 4 cm with indeterminate (either oncocytic cell or follicular neoplasm) FNAB results. Other relative indications for an initial total thyroidectomy include a preexisting history of hypothyroidism, a contralateral dominant (>1 cm) nodule, an elevated calcitonin, or a family history of a genetic predisposition syndrome. After adequate counseling, patients may also elect to undergo an up-front total thyroidectomy and avoid the potential for a second operation.[7]

If thyroid cancer is diagnosed after thyroid lobectomy, completion thyroidectomy is subsequently performed to facilitate use of radioactive iodine ablation for therapy and staging, and is also recommended for tumor types with a high risk of multifocality.[7] Unifocal papillary thyroid microcarcinoma (<1 cm) is associated with excellent long-term survival and, in the absence of aggressive histopathologic factors such as extrathyroidal extension or lymph node metastasis, a lobectomy alone is currently considered adequate treatment. In a retrospective study of more than 50,000 papillary thyroid carcinoma patients from the National Cancer Database, total thyroidectomy as compared with lobectomy was associated with improved 10-year local recurrence rates (7.7% vs 9.8%) and 10-year survival (98.4% vs 97.1%) except among patients with papillary thyroid carcinoma smaller than 1 cm.[12] At present, the recommendation of the American Thyroid Association is to perform completion thyroidectomy for all patients who would have undergone total thyroidectomy if the diagnosis of thyroid cancer was known prior to initial surgery.[7]

Follicular carcinoma that is diagnosed in older (>40 years old) patients, has vascular invasion, or is widely invasive is associated with a poorer prognosis, and patients should undergo completion thyroidectomy.[13,14] Oncocytic (Hürthle cell)

carcinoma can be multifocal, and several small studies have suggested that prognosis is improved following total thyroidectomy.[15] Completion thyroidectomy is usually performed either immediately (<2 weeks) after lobectomy, or 6 to 8 weeks following the initial procedure, to allow resolution of early postoperative inflammatory changes. Completion surgery should always be preceded by laryngoscopy to evaluate vocal cord function.

LYMPHADENECTOMY

Cervical lymph node metastasis in thyroid cancer is present in 20% to 90% of patients at the time of presentation, depending on the detection method. However, clinically apparent metastases are seen in 10% of patients, at most.[16,17] The prognostic significance of lymph node metastases is controversial, but it is clear that the presence of gross nodal disease is associated with local recurrence.[18] Cervical lymph node disease is best evaluated by preoperative ultrasonography and, when present, is confirmed by FNAB for cytology and/or thyroglobulin measurement of the aspirate. If indicated, a functional, compartment-oriented neck dissection is thought to reduce the risk of local recurrence, and is the surgical approach favored over "berry-picking."

Central Compartment

Studies have shown that the central compartment (level VI) is usually the first site of metastatic disease. The central compartment is defined by the boundaries of the hyoid bone (superiorly), carotid arteries (laterally), superficial layer of the deep cervical fascia (anteriorly), and deep layer of the deep cervical fascia (posteriorly). On the right, the innominate artery defines the inferior boundary while the equivalent plane defines this boundary on the left. A unilateral central compartment lymph node dissection includes the prelaryngeal (Delphian), pretracheal, in addition to either the right or left paratracheal lymph nodes, while a bilateral dissection includes both paratracheal nodal basins.[19]

In the presence of clinically evident metastases, a therapeutic central compartment lymph node dissection is recommended. Because the thyroid gland itself can obscure an accurate assessment, imaging can frequently miss abnormal lymph nodes. Routine intraoperative assessment of central compartment lymph nodes by palpation and visual inspection is usually performed.

Whether a prophylactic central compartment lymph node dissection should be performed is controversial. Routine ipsilateral central compartment dissection has been shown to reduce postoperative thyroglobulin levels, but long-term prospective studies have yet to show that routine dissection leads to improvements in either recurrence or disease-specific mortality.[20] Prophylactic central neck dissection may lead to more accurate staging and risk stratification, allowing in the future for a selective approach to radioactive iodine ablation.[21] However, the risk of hypoparathyroidism appears to be more frequent after thyroidectomy with central compartment neck dissection than after thyroidectomy alone, and this risk, as well as the risk of recurrent laryngeal nerve injury, should be considered when deciding whether to perform prophylactic central neck dissection.[22]

Lateral Compartment

The lateral compartment can have metastatic disease, even in the absence of central compartment disease.[23] The lateral compartment is defined by the boundaries of the internal jugular vein (medially), trapezoid muscle (laterally), subclavian vein (inferiorly), and hypoglossal nerve (superiorly). The lymph nodes within the lateral compartment are further separated by anatomic boundaries defining levels I to V. The most common levels involved with metastatic thyroid cancer are II to IV. In the absence of gross involvement, a modified neck dissection that preserves the internal jugular vein and sternocleidomastoid, spinal accessory, and phrenic nerves is usually performed for thyroid cancer.

Little controversy exists in the management of the lateral compartment. Therapeutic lateral neck dissection is indicated for patients with clinically or radiographically evident lymph node metastases. Prophylactic lateral neck dissection has never been shown to improve long-term outcomes and is not recommended for patients with differentiated thyroid cancers.[7]

SURGICAL TECHNIQUES

Thyroidectomy is usually performed under general anesthesia, although some centers perform thyroidectomy in selected patients after cervical block and intravenous sedation only.[24] After induction of anesthesia, the neck is gently extended to expose the anterior surface. Patients with a history of cervical stenosis or symptoms such as peripheral radiculopathy after prolonged neck extension should undergo preoperative magnetic resonance imaging of the neck to evaluate the cervical spine for possible cord compression. During patient positioning, somatosensory evoked potential monitoring can be used to evaluate for position-related cord compression after neck extension.

Recurrent laryngeal nerve monitoring can be used during thyroidectomy; however, large studies have not shown that routine use reduces nerve injury rates.[25] Nerve monitoring may be most helpful in reoperative cases or in massive goiter resections where the anatomy may be obscured. Some clinicians advocate a baseline laryngeal examination for all patients prior to surgery. Absolute indications for preoperative assessment of vocal cord function include preoperative voice changes, massive goiter, and a history of prior surgery of any type associated with recurrent laryngeal nerve injury, such as (in approximate decreasing order of occurrence) anterior cervical spine fusion, carotid surgery, thoracic or cardiac surgery, and prior thyroid or parathyroid resection.

A standard thyroidectomy incision is short, measuring 4 to 5 cm, although this can vary widely by patient body mass index and thyroid volume.[26] Parathyroid glands are gently preserved in situ on their vascular pedicle, but if they are found to be adherent to the thyroid and resected, or if they appear nonviable, they should be autotransplanted into the ipsilateral sternocleidomastoid muscle. Intraoperative frozen section is used selectively if results could change the operative management, such as during lobectomy if there is suspicion for thyroid cancer or if there is concern for anaplastic thyroid cancer or thyroid lymphoma. Meticulous hemostasis is obligatory. A cervical drain is no longer routinely placed except after lateral neck dissection, because of the risk of lymphatic and/or chylous leak with that procedure.

Minimally invasive thyroidectomy is a type of surgical approach that can reduce the surgical incision to 1.5 to 2 cm in selected patients. Candidates for this technique include patients with solitary nodules smaller than 3 cm or a small multinodular goiter (total estimated thyroid volume on ultrasonography of ≤ 25 mL). Absolute contraindications include patients undergoing re-operation or with large multinodular goiter, locally invasive thyroid cancer, or prior neck radiation. The presence of Graves' disease and Hashimoto's thyroiditis are relative contraindications, due to the higher risk of intraoperative bleeding and associated inflammatory changes. Miccoli, who pioneered the most commonly used technique, recently estimated that only 10% to 15% of patients undergoing thyroidectomy in his practice are candidates for this approach.[27]

To avoid a cervical incision completely, another option is use of robotic assistance to endoscopically resect the thyroid through either a transaxillary and/or periareolar approach. The largest series is from Ryu and colleagues,[28] who have performed transaxillary robot-assisted thyroidectomy in more than 1000 patients using either a single axillary incision or an anterior chest wall counterincision. These investigators report hematoma, hypoparathyroidism, and recurrent laryngeal nerve injury rates that are equivalent to standard thyroidectomy, but because the technique requires elevation of subcutaneous tissue flaps to approach the thyroid, additional reported complications include brachial plexus injury, chyle leak, seroma formation, and lengthy operation. Candidates for the robotic approach include thin patients with an anteriorly situated thyroid nodule 2 cm or smaller, and this approach is inappropriate for patients with a body mass index greater than 35 kg/m^2, deep or large thyroid lesions, prior neck surgery, Graves' disease, extrathyroidal tumor invasion, or bulky lateral lymph node metastases.

After standard thyroid lobectomy, patients can be safely discharged on the same day as surgery as long as no cervical hematoma is evident on examination. Length of stay after total thyroidectomy is generally about 1 day. Postoperative L-thyroxine supplementation is initiated either immediately after surgery or after pathology results are available. The dose depends on the method and need for postoperative radioactive iodine ablation.

COMPLICATIONS

Complication rates after thyroidectomy are typically low. Sosa and colleagues[29] demonstrated inverse relationships between surgeon volume and complication rate, length of hospital stay, and hospital charges. Overall complication rates after thyroidectomy are 5% to 7%. The most concerning and acute complications compromise the patient's airway and include either bilateral recurrent laryngeal nerve injury or postoperative hematoma.

A unilateral recurrent laryngeal nerve injury occurs in 1% to 3% of patients in most surgical series. If there is intraoperative concern for a nerve injury, a lobectomy alone should be performed until a functional assessment of the nerve can be performed. If transected, primary neurorrhaphy of the recurrent laryngeal nerve may preserve laryngeal muscle tone and prevent atrophy of the vocal fold. The majority of recurrent laryngeal nerve palsies are transient. Postoperative symptoms after unilateral paresis depend on the degree of medialization of the immobile vocal fold, which can change over time. Occasionally, patients can be asymptomatic but other symptoms include hoarseness, weak cough, dyspnea especially while speaking, and dysphagia to thin liquids. Laryngeal electromyography can provide some prognostic information. Temporizing procedures include noninvasive strategies such as a chin tuck maneuver to the ipsilateral side to prevent aspiration and/or more invasive procedures to medialize the vocal fold, such as injection with calcium hydroxyapatite. If the palsy does not recover in 6 months, a permanent intervention can be considered, such as an autologous fat laryngoplasty or surgical thyroplasty. Although rare, bilateral recurrent laryngeal nerve paralysis is a serious life-threatening problem in which hoarseness and aspiration are inversely proportional to obstruction of the tracheal air column. If a patient has significant stridor immediately after total thyroidectomy and the airway is found to be compromised, a tracheostomy is necessary.

Neck hematoma occurs in 0.5% to 1% of patients following thyroidectomy. To avoid this potentially life-threatening complication, anticoagulants and antiplatelet medications including low-dose aspirin are routinely stopped before surgery. Patients who resume these medications after surgery do not have a significantly higher rate of hematoma. The diagnosis of cervical hematoma requiring operative evacuation can be determined by physical examination and should be apparent well before airway compromise is clinically evident. Hematoma is never observed nonoperatively. Following urgent or emergent reoperation for hematoma, upper airway edema can be significant, and careful assessment of airway patency should be performed before extubation. Imaging such as ultrasonography can sometimes be helpful in the delayed postoperative setting to differentiate between seroma formation and routine incisional changes.

Permanent hypoparathyroidism rates after total thyroidectomy are 0.5% to 3%, but transient hypocalcemia can be seen in up to 15% of postoperative patients. To diminish the usually temporary effects of parathyroid gland dissection, calcium supplementation is routinely prescribed for all patients after total thyroidectomy, and this intervention also cushions the management of the rare patient who goes on to develop hypoparathyroidism. Peripheral or perioral paresthesias are the most sensitive indicator of hypocalcemia. Chvostek's sign is less sensitive, as it is frequently seen preoperatively and in patients with normal calcium levels after thyroidectomy. The diagnosis of hypoparathyroidism requires the combined presence of severe hypocalcemia, hyperphosphatemia, and undetectable parathyroid hormone levels. Patients with hypoparathyroidism and poor oral calcium absorption from prior gastric bypass surgery, celiac sprue, or chronic vitamin D deficiency from other causes may require readmission for intravenous calcium supplementation until optimal oral calcium and vitamin D supplementation doses can be determined.

Voice changes in the absence of recurrent laryngeal nerve paresis have been documented after thyroid surgery in up to 30% of patients.[30] The most common cause is injury to the external branch of the superior laryngeal nerve (the "opera-singer's nerve"). Ligation of the superior pole vessels close to the thyroid capsule can help prevent this injury. Fibrosis of the cricothyroid muscle can also contribute to voice alterations, but is difficult to diagnose. Rarely, acute dysphagia may result from pharyngeal perforation caused by esophageal instrumentation by temperature probes or oral-gastric tubes. Crepitance is suggestive; in addition to urgent cross-sectional imaging, a swallow study and bronchoscopy should be performed. Dysphagia described as a globus sensation can be observed and may persist for up to a year after surgery. For chronic dysphagia, a multidisciplinary management approach is effective and includes careful patient counseling, voice therapy, and exclusion of other possible causes. The authors have found that firm daily anterior cervical massage performed for 3 to 6 months postoperatively not only minimizes globus sensation but also markedly improves the cosmetic appearance of the scar. Wound infection is rare.

RECURRENT DISEASE

Cancer recurrence occurs in 5% to 20% of thyroid cancer patients, and is typically diagnosed by detectable thyroglobulin levels following thyroidectomy and radioactive iodine ablation. Surgery is indicated if the recurrence is (1) large enough

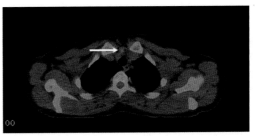

Fig. 4. Transverse section of a fused CT-PET scan obtained for a 29-year-old woman with a history of metastatic papillary thyroid cancer initially treated with total thyroidectomy, bilateral central compartment and bilateral lateral compartment lymphadenectomies, followed by radioactive iodine ablation. A rising thyroglobulin level prompted whole-body ^{131}I scan and neck ultrasonography, both of which were negative. Subsequent PET scan demonstrated a single focus of FDG avidity in the upper mediastinum. After an uneventful reoperative cervical exploration and resection of the nodule, recurrent papillary thyroid cancer (*arrow*) was confirmed.

to be radiographically apparent and (2) confirmed by cytologic findings after FNAB or elevated thyroglobulin levels in the aspirate. The most common location of surgically resectable disease is in the central compartment. Because of fibrosis and anatomy alterations in a previously operated field, the risks of reoperation including nerve injury and permanent hypoparathyroidism are significantly higher. Needle localization can be one method of preventing operative failure.[31] The use of ultrasound localization in the preoperative holding area to directly mark the area of recurrence is another less invasive technique to help guide the reoperation, and can effectively reduce postoperative thyroglobulin levels.[32] Lateral neck recurrences should be managed with a compartment-oriented dissection, if not previously performed.

^{18}F-Fluorodeoxyglucose positron emission tomography (FDG-PET) can be useful in patients with thyroglobulin elevation who do not have evidence of disease on either ultrasonography or whole-body iodine scan (**Fig. 4**). FDG-PET has an overall sensitivity of 50% to 70% and the sensitivity increases as the thyroglobulin level increases. No significant differences appear to occur when the study is obtained with or without thyroid-stimulating hormone stimulation.[33]

SUMMARY

Surgery is often needed to diagnose thyroid cancer, but is also the initial therapeutic modality. Several current imaging techniques are important for the appropriate management of patients undergoing thyroid surgery and are particularly informative for thyroid nodule characterization to assist in risk stratification and to determine the extent of surgery.

REFERENCES

1. Altekruse SF, Kosary CL, Krapcho M, et al, editors. SEER cancer statistics review, 1975–2007. Based on November 2009 SEER data submission, posted to the SEER web site, 2010. National Cancer Institute. Bethesda (MD). Available at: http://seer.cancer.gov/csr/1975_2007/. Accessed November, 2010.

2. Davies L, Welch HG. Increasing incidence of thyroid cancer in the United States, 1973-2002. JAMA 2006; 295:2164–7.

3. Baloch ZW, LiVolsi VA, Asa SL, et al. Diagnostic terminology and morphologic criteria for cytologic diagnosis of thyroid lesions: a synopsis of the national cancer institute thyroid fine-needle aspiration state of the science conference. Diagn Cytopathol 2008;36:425–37.

4. Schneider AB, Ron E, Lubin J, et al. Dose-response relationships for radiation-induced thyroid cancer and thyroid nodules: evidence for the prolonged effects of radiation on the thyroid. J Clin Endocrinol Metab 1993;77:362–9.

5. Kikuchi S, Perrier ND, Ituarte P, et al. Latency period of thyroid neoplasia after radiation exposure. Ann Surg 2004;239:536–43.

6. Hemminki K, Eng C, Chen B. Familial risks for non-medullary thyroid cancer. J Clin Endocrinol Metab 2005;90:5747–53.

7. American Thyroid Association (ATA) Guidelines Taskforce on Thyroid Nodules and Differentiated Thyroid Cancer, Cooper DS, Doherty GM, Haugen BR, et al. Revised American Thyroid Association management guidelines for patients with thyroid nodules and differentiated thyroid cancer. Thyroid 2009;19:1167–214.

8. Meko JB, Norton JA. Large cystic/solid thyroid nodules: a potential false-negative fine-needle aspiration. Surgery 1995;118:996–1003 [discussion: 1003–4].

9. Tee YY, Lowe AJ, Brand CA, et al. Fine-needle aspiration may miss a third of all malignancy in palpable thyroid nodules: a comprehensive literature review. Ann Surg 2007;246:714–20.

10. McCoy KL, Jabbour N, Ogilvie JB, et al. The incidence of cancer and rate of false-negative cytology in thyroid nodules greater than or equal to 4 cm in size. Surgery 2007;142:837–44 [discussion: 844.e1–3].

11. McHenry CR, Slusarczyk SJ. Hypothyroidism following hemithyroidectomy: incidence, risk factors, and management. Surgery 2000;128:994–8.

12. Bilimoria KY, Bentrem DJ, Linn JG, et al. Utilization of total thyroidectomy for papillary thyroid cancer in the United States. Surgery 2007;142:906–13.

13. Chow SM, Law SC, Mendenhall WM, et al. Follicular thyroid carcinoma: prognostic factors and the role of radioiodine. Cancer 2002;95:488–98.

14. Carling T, Udelsman R. Follicular neoplasms of the thyroid: what to recommend. Thyroid 2005;15: 583–7.

15. McDonald MP, Sanders LE, Silverman ML, et al. Hürthle cell carcinoma of the thyroid gland: prognostic factors and results of surgical treatment. Surgery 1996;120:1000–4.

16. Grebe SK, Hay ID. Thyroid cancer nodal metastases: biologic significance and therapeutic considerations. Surg Oncol Clin N Am 1996;5:43–63.

17. Loh KC, Greenspan FS, Gee L, et al. Pathological tumor-node-metastasis (pTNM) staging for papillary and follicular thyroid carcinomas: a retrospective analysis of 700 patients. J Clin Endocrinol Metab 1997;82:3553–62.

18. Zavdfudim V, Feurer ID, Griffin MR, et al. The impact of lymph node involvement on survival in patients with papillary and follicular thyroid carcinoma. Surgery 2008;144:1070–7.

19. American Thyroid Association Surgery Working Group, American Association of Endocrine Surgeons, American Academy of Otolaryngology-Head and Neck Surgery, American Head and Neck Society. Carty SE, Cooper DS, Doherty GM, et al. Consensus statement on the terminology and classification of central neck dissection for thyroid cancer. Thyroid 2009;19:1153–8.

20. Sywak M, Cornford L, Roach P, et al. Routine ipsilateral level VI lymphadenectomy reduces postoperative thyroglobulin levels in papillary thyroid cancer. Surgery 2006;140:1000–5.

21. Bonnet S, Hartl D, LebOulleux S, et al. Prophylactic lymph node dissection for papillary thyroid cancer less than 2 cm: implications for radioiodine treatment. J Clin Endocrinol Metab 2009;94:1162–7.

22. Mazzaferri EL, Doherty GM, Steward DL. The pros and cons of prophylactic central compartment lymph node dissection for papillary thyroid carcinoma. Thyroid 2009;19:683–9.

23. Gimm O, Rath FW, Dralle H. Pattern of lymph node metastases in papillary thyroid carcinoma. Br J Surg 1998;85:252–4.

24. LoGerfo P, Ditkoff BA, Shabot J, et al. Thyroid surgery using monitored anesthesia care: an alternative to general anesthesia. Thyroid 1994;4:437–9.

25. Angelos P. Recurrent laryngeal nerve monitoring: state of the art, ethical, and legal issues. Surg Clin North Am 2009;89:1157–69.

26. Brunaud L, Zarnegar R, Wada N, et al. Incision length for standard thyroidectomy and parathyroidectomy: when is it minimally invasive? Arch Surg 2003;138:1140–3.

27. Miccoli P, Materazzi G, Berti P. Minimally invasive thyroidectomy in the treatment of well differentiated

thyroid cancers: indications and limits. Curr Opin Otolaryngol Head Neck Surg 2010;18:114–8.

28. Ryu HR, Kang SW, Lee SH, et al. Feasibility and safety of a new robotic thyroidectomy through a gasless, transaxillary single-incision approach. J Am Coll Surg 2010;211:e13–9.

29. Sosa JA, Bowman HM, Tielsch JM, et al. The importance of surgeon experience for clinical and economic outcomes from thyroidectomy. Ann Surg 1998;228:320–30.

30. Stojadinovic A, Shaha AR, Orlikoff RF, et al. Prospective functional voice assessment in patients undergoing thyroid surgery. Ann Surg 2002;236:823–32.

31. Triponez F, Poder L, Zarnegar R, et al. Hook needle-guided excision of recurrent differentiated thyroid cancer in previously operated neck compartments: a safe technique for small, nonpalpable recurrent disease. J Clin Endocrinol Metab 2006;91:4943–7.

32. McCoy KL, Yim JH, Tublin ME, et al. Same-day ultrasound guidance in reoperation for locally recurrent papillary thyroid cancer. Surgery 2007;142: 965–72.

33. Shammas A, Degirmenci B, Mountz JM, et al. 18F-FDG PET/CT in patients with suspected recurrent or metastatic well-differentiated thyroid cancer. J Nucl Med 2007;48:221–6.

Imaging Surveillance of Differentiated Thyroid Cancer

Nathan A. Johnson, MD[a],*, Shane O. LeBeau, MD[b], Mitchell E. Tublin, MD[a]

KEYWORDS

- Differentiated thyroid cancer • Imaging • Surveillance
- Sonography • PET/CT • Radioiodine • Thyroglobulin

Differentiated thyroid cancer (DTC) is typically an indolent disease with a very low disease-specific mortality. Although most cases are cured with a combination of surgical resection and radioiodine therapy, tumor recurrence, predominantly within the local-regional cervical lymph nodes, occurs in 15% to 30% of patients, usually within the first 10 years following initial diagnosis.[1,2] This high rate of recurrence, along with the potential to develop recurrent disease many years following initial therapy, has led to the adoption of intensive post-treatment surveillance strategies. Current surveillance strategies rely primarily on serial serum thyroglobulin (Tg) measurements in combination with cervical sonography to identify local-regional nodal recurrence and image-guided fine needle aspiration (FNA) of suspicious lesions.[3–5] Whole-body iodine 131 scintigraphy (WBS), once the mainstay of post-therapy imaging surveillance, has largely been replaced by cervical sonography as the modality of choice for long-term imaging surveillance, although it still may be used for the detection of occult or distant metastases, particularly in the setting of a newly elevated serum Tg level. Positron emission tomography with fluorine 18-fluorodeoxyglucose (FDG-PET) and PET/CT are currently used primarily to assess for metastases in the setting of non-iodine-avid tumors.

This intensive imaging surveillance has resulted in the ability to detect small-volume, often clinically occult, residual or recurrent disease. For most patients with DTC, such findings are unlikely to have an impact on disease-specific survival but our ability to predict which patients are at greatest risk and should receive the most aggressive therapies is surpassed by our ability to detect recurrence. Thus, the optimal treatment and surveillance regimens will surely continue to evolve as our ability to predict tumor behavior and aggressiveness improves. A familiarity with the rationale underlying current surveillance strategies, and an understanding of the utility and implications of imaging findings are critical for the appropriate care of patients with DTC.

OVERVIEW OF DTC EPIDEMIOLOGY, STAGING, AND INITIAL THERAPY

The incidence of thyroid cancer is approximately 10 per 100,000 and has been steadily increasing for decades, up from 3.6 per 100,000 in 1973.[6] In 2010, there were an estimated 44,670 new cases of thyroid cancer and 1690 deaths.[7] Over the past 3 decades, the incidence of thyroid cancer has increased approximately 2.4-fold with nearly all of this increase attributable to an increased incidence of papillary thyroid cancer.[8] During this same period the size of the tumor at initial diagnosis has steadily decreased while mortality as a result of DTC has remained essentially

Financial Disclosure/Conflicts of Interest: None.

[a] Division of Abdominal Imaging, Department of Radiology, University of Pittsburgh School of Medicine, 200 Lothrop Street, Suite 3950 PST, Pittsburgh, PA 15213, USA

[b] Division of Endocrinology and Metabolism, University of Pittsburgh Medical Center, 3601 Fifth Avenue, Falk Medical Building, Suite 581, Pittsburgh, PA 15213, USA

* Corresponding author.

E-mail address: johnsonna2@upmc.edu

Radiol Clin N Am 49 (2011) 473–487
doi:10.1016/j.rcl.2011.02.008
0033-8389/11/$ – see front matter © 2011 Elsevier Inc. All rights reserved.

unchanged. These findings suggest that increased detection related to the concurrent increase in imaging and sampling of thyroid nodules may be a major factor accounting for this increase, although the concurrent increase in the incidence of larger cancers, even those larger than 5 cm and unlikely to be clinically occult, suggests other unrecognized factors may contribute to the rising incidence.[9]

The vast majority of cases consist of the differentiated subtypes with papillary carcinomas accounting for 88% of cases and follicular carcinomas accounting for 8%. Medullary thyroid cancer and poorly differentiated histologies (eg, anaplastic) account for only 3%.[8] Although several histologic variants and subtypes exist, papillary and follicular carcinomas are commonly grouped together as DTC because both tumors share a typically indolent course and very similar treatment and surveillance strategies.

DTC can occur at any age but has a median age at diagnosis of 49 years. Approximately 39% of new cases are diagnosed before the age of 45, an important criterion in the current TNM classification system.[6] The prevalence in women is 3 times that in men for unclear reasons. Most cases are sporadic but risk factors include a family history and a history of prior neck irradiation.

Several tumor-staging systems have been developed for DTC in an attempt to include factors with prognostic value to guide the appropriate intensity of treatment and surveillance. Staging of thyroid cancer is covered in further detail elsewhere in this issue but several staging criteria are particularly important for the imager to keep in mind when reporting imaging findings for patients undergoing surveillance. The most relevant factors include patient age, tumor size and extent, regional nodal involvement, and distant metastases. A younger age at diagnosis is associated with a much more favorable prognosis because these tumors tend to be the more indolent histologic subtypes and are typically highly radioiodine responsive. The American Joint Committee on Cancer TNM staging system categorizes all patients younger than 45 years as stage I irrespective of tumor size or the presence of local-regional metastases. Patients younger than 45 years are considered to have stage II disease if distant metastases are identified. A distinction between the central and lateral cervical lymph node compartments is also important for staging. The TNM staging categorizes the location of cervical lymph node metastases into central compartment (level VI) lymph nodes (lymph node stage N1a) and lateral compartment (levels II–V) nodes (stage N1b), reflecting the improved outcomes for patients with adenopathy limited to the central compartment.

For cases of biopsy-proven thyroid cancer, surgical therapy usually consists of a near-total thyroidectomy in which all gross thyroidal tissue is removed with the possible exception of a small amount of tissue required to preserve the recurrent laryngeal nerves and the parathyroid glands. A hemilobectomy may be performed in those cases in which biopsy results are indeterminate with the patient returning for completion thyroidectomy in the case of malignancy being diagnosed within the hemilobectomy specimen. Some controversy exists as to the necessity for completion thyroidectomy in patients with unifocal micropapillary carcinoma (<1 cm) confined to the resected lobe in the absence of any high-risk features, but if treatment plans include radioiodine ablation, completion thyroidectomy will first be performed. Total thyroidectomy is typically followed by radioiodine ablation with ^{131}I for the treatment of any residual disease, a specific and effective therapy given that the vast majority of DTC concentrates iodine. There is controversy as to the appropriate use of radioiodine ablation for patients with tumors confined to the thyroid gland but it is generally recommended for patients with nodal metastases or patients whose tumor histology or clinical factors suggest a higher risk for recurrent cancer.

SURVEILLANCE OF DTC
Overview

Long-term surveillance strategies continue to evolve but the mainstay of current surveillance regimens for most patients with DTC includes serial serum Tg measurements coupled with cervical ultrasound with an aim toward identifying residual or recurrent disease, most commonly within the thyroidectomy bed and cervical lymph node chains. Although many variations exist with regard to the optimal surveillance, the imaging surveillance regimen discussed here comes from the guidelines of the American Thyroid Association (ATA), based on an evidence-based review by a multidisciplinary group of leaders in the field of thyroid cancer. Surveillance is guided by the following therapeutic principles for the treatment of recurrent or residual disease: (1) surgical resection for cure of detected local-regional metastases in the absence of distant metastases; and (2) repeated radioiodine therapy for persistent disease, local recurrence, or distant metastatic disease that is not resectable until a treatment effect is no longer detected or bone marrow reserve is compromised. Thus, the primary goal of imaging surveillance is to identify and localize local-regional recurrence for possible surgical excision.

The intensity of surveillance may also be tailored by a risk assessment of recurrence based on clinical and pathologic factors. A proposed 3-level stratification by the ATA includes the following criteria: (1) low risk: no local or distant metastases, all macroscopic tumor resected, no local tumor invasion, no aggressive histology (eg, tall cell, insular, columnar subtypes), and no vascular invasion; (2) intermediate risk: microscopic tumor invasion, cervical lymph node metastases, tumor with aggressive histology or vascular invasion, or uptake outside of thyroidectomy bed on post-therapy [131]IWBS; (3) high risk: macroscopic tumor invasion, incomplete tumor resection, distant metastases, or thyroglobulinemia out of proportion to what is seen on posttreatment [131]IWBS.

Serum Thyroglobulin Surveillance

Tg is ideally suited to the surveillance of DTC given that it is a protein unique to thyroid tissue but also secreted by well-differentiated malignancies. The serum levels of Tg are most useful as a marker of recurrence after the patient has undergone total thyroidectomy and radioiodine ablation so that the patient no longer has functioning normal thyroid tissue. Baseline serum Tg measurements obtained following initial therapy provide evidence regarding the presence of any persistent disease. A baseline Tg above 2.0 ng/mL predicts persistent disease or the subsequent development of metastases, whereas a level of less than 0.5 ng/mL indicates the absence of persistent disease for 98% of patients.[10,11] Follow-up Tg measurements have been shown to be an accurate predictor of the development of recurrence or metastatic disease. The negative predictive value of a normal Tg level (< 0.5 ng/mL) exceeds 90% in low-risk patients.[10]

There are additional factors that are important to consider when interpreting Tg results including the presence of Tg antibodies and whether the Tg measurement was performed as a stimulated or unstimulated study. Circulating Tg antibodies can falsely lower or elevate serum Tg measurements rendering them unreliable for the assessment of recurrence. These antibodies can be found in approximately 10% of the general population and 25% of patients with thyroid cancer.[12] Additionally, antibody levels can fluctuate substantially over time, particularly in the 3 years following thyroidectomy, so it is recommended that anti-Tg antibodies are measured each time a Tg measurement is obtained.[13,14]

It is also important to know whether the Tg level was obtained while thyroid stimulating hormone (TSH) was stimulated. This refers to whether the TSH level is elevated at the time the Tg is measured. One feature of DTC is that it may be stimulated to grow by circulating TSH. Therefore, patients are on thyroid hormone replacement following thyroidectomy, which keeps the TSH stimulus low. In fact, depending on tumor aggressiveness, thyroid hormone replacement may be titrated to keep TSH levels below the usual euthyroid range to minimize any stimulus of tumor growth by TSH.[15,16] Thus, the sensitivity of a Tg measurement increases when the examination is performed under TSH stimulation. A meta-analysis of studies of follow-up Tg measurements in patients with DTC found a sensitivity of 96% for stimulated Tg versus 78% for unstimulated measurements.[17] The specificity also improves with stimulated measurements with a 98% negative predictive value for a negative stimulated measurement (<2 ng/mL) versus an 86% negative predictive value for a negative unstimulated measurement (<0.5 ng/mL).[18] In the unstimulated setting, Tg produced by small-volume metastases may be masked given the lack of TSH stimulus, resulting in a false-negative study.[17] Stimulation can be obtained by thyroid hormone withdrawal, allowing the patient to become clinically hypothyroid over several weeks. This process is generally poorly tolerated by patients. Alternatively, recombinant TSH can be injected intramuscularly several days before the serum Tg is measured, in effect stimulating any potential tumor without making the patient hypothyroid. There is only a small reduction in the sensitivity for the detection of residual disease using thyrotropin alfa stimulation (93%) versus thyroid hormone withdrawal (96%).[17]

[131]Iodine Whole Body Scintigraphy

Once the mainstay of DTC surveillance imaging, diagnostic [131]Iodine whole body scintigraphy (WBS) has been replaced by other techniques, predominantly cervical ultrasound, as the primary imaging modality. In a large series in which patients with DTC were followed with both WBS and cervical ultrasound, WBS had a sensitivity of 20% for the detection of local recurrence versus 70% for cervical ultrasound.[3] Furthermore, the ability of cervical ultrasound to accurately localize local-regional recurrence to guide potential surgical resection is superior.

A theoretical disadvantage of diagnostic WBS is an effect known as stunning, which refers to a diminished capacity for the metastatic disease to take up radioiodine should a subsequent therapy be necessary. However, a negative impact on radioiodine therapy has not been demonstrated at the low doses of ^{131}I typically used for these studies.[19,20] Routine use of diagnostic WBS for surveillance is not recommended for low-risk patients who did not show evidence of disease outside of the thyroidectomy bed on their initial post-therapy WBS. However, diagnostic WBS is still used in patients with intermediate or high risk of recurrence, as well as to assess any patient for evidence of recurrence in the setting of an elevated Tg level with negative cervical ultrasound. WBS performed after empiric treatment with radioiodine is more sensitive than diagnostic scanning. This is typically performed 1 week following administration of the therapeutic dose of radioiodine and is referred to as therapeutic WBS (**Fig. 1**).

Ultrasound Surveillance

Ultrasound has emerged as the dominant imaging modality in the imaging surveillance regimen for patients with DTC given the many advantages suited to the detection of DTC recurrence. Most metastases occur within the thyroidectomy bed and anterior cervical lymph nodes; both are areas well evaluated with cervical sonography. Technical advances allow for the routine identification and tissue sampling of metastases as small as 5 mm (**Fig. 2**). Widespread availability, lack of radiation,

and relatively low cost are additional advantages of ultrasound that make this modality well suited for long-term surveillance. Revised ATA thyroid cancer guidelines recommend a baseline follow-up cervical ultrasound 6 to 12 months following surgery and radioablation (if performed), followed by periodic surveillance ultrasound depending on the risk status of the patient and Tg status.[21] The most recent guidelines include a recommendation for ultrasound- guided FNA of any suspicious lesions greater than 5 to 8 mm if this would alter clinical management, with follow-up sonography reserved for smaller lesions or those not safely accessible percutaneously because of their anatomic location.

Cervical ultrasound should be performed with a high-frequency linear transducer (12–15 MHz), although lower frequencies may be necessary for increased depth of acoustic penetration depending on the patient's body habitus. The neck should be slightly hyperextended; hyperextension can be facilitated by placing a towel beneath the patient's neck. Compound imaging and gentle compression may improve the resolution of small lesions and may increase the conspicuity of subtle findings such as microcalcifications. The neck should be scanned systematically and in multiple imaging planes; at our institution we begin in the thyroidectomy bed. Axial and sagittal images of both thyroidectomy beds are obtained with cine images

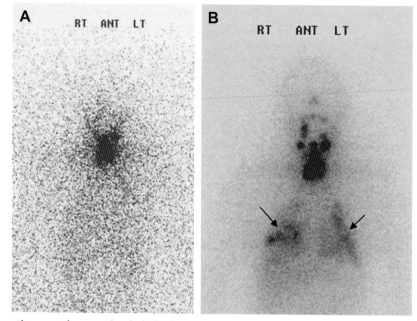

Fig. 1. Diagnostic versus therapeutic whole body scintigraphy. (*A*) Diagnostic WBS image of the neck and chest shows the relatively poor scintigraphic counts associated with WBS at the diagnostic dose. No convincing extracervical activity is shown. (*B*) Therapeutic WBS in the same patient performed 1 week following administration of a therapeutic dose of radioiodine shows bilateral lung metastases (*arrows*) not detected on the diagnostic WBS.

extension. Attention is then turned to the lateral compartment lymph nodes. We report the location of abnormal findings according to the now widely used neck imaging classification scheme published by Som and colleagues,[22] but reporting the position relative to adjacent anatomic structures may also be helpful to referring endocrinologists and thyroid surgeons (**Fig. 3**).

The normal post-thyroidectomy bed site appears as an inverted triangle of heterogeneous echogenic tissue reflecting the proliferation of fibrofatty tissues within the operative bed.[23] This triangle is bounded anteriorly by the overlying strap muscles, medially by the trachea, and laterally by the carotid and internal jugular vessels. In the immediate postoperative period, evaluation of the thyroidectomy bed can be difficult because of the distortion of tissue planes by postoperative edema, seromas, and possibly hematomas. Absorbable hemostatic material in the operative bed may be confused with other pathology but has a distinctive uniform echogenic appearance (**Fig. 4**).[24] Before treatment with radioiodine,

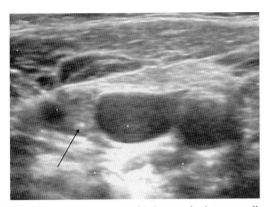

Fig. 2. Transverse sonographic image depicts a needle tip (*arrow*) within small volume cervical nodal metastasis. Ultrasound-guided sampling of nodules as small as 5 mm is feasible with current imaging platforms.

obtained of suspicious lesions. Small lobectomy bed recurrences may be better visualized with movement of the patient's head away from the transducer, whereas pretracheal lesions near the sternal notch are often better visualized with neck

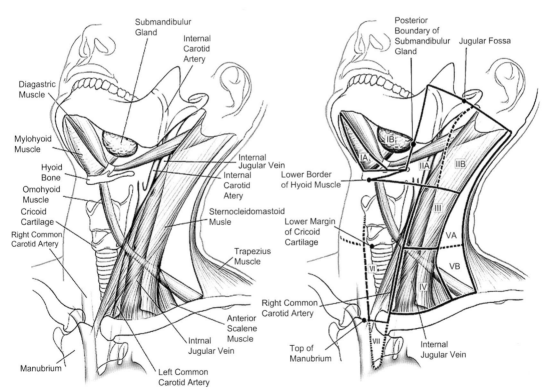

Fig. 3. Commonly used imaging-based scheme for classification of cervical nodal stations. In the setting of DTC, nodal stations are commonly grouped together as central compartment (level VI) and lateral compartment (levels II–V). Central compartment nodal dissection is typically done at the time of thyroidectomy if there is known malignancy, whereas dissection of the lateral compartment lymph nodes requires more extensive surgery. (*From* Som PM, Curtin HD, Mancuso AA. An imaging-based classification for the cervical nodes designed as an adjunct to recent clinically based nodal classifications. Arch Otolaryngol Head Neck Surg 1999;125(4):388–96. Copyright © 1999 American Medical Association; with permission.)

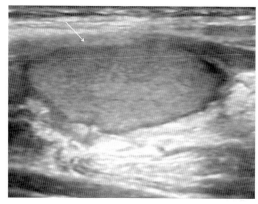

Fig. 4. Surgical hemostatic material mimicking thyroidectomy bed recurrence. Longitudinal sonographic image of the thyroidectomy bed obtained several weeks following thyroidectomy showing a uniform hypoechoic nodule representing residual surgical hemostatic material (arrow).

thyroid remnant tissue may be present within the thyroidectomy bed and appear as vascular lobules of tissue equal in echogenicity to the thyroid gland. Following radioablation, macroscopic thyroid remnants typically appear as hypoechoic heterogeneous nodules without internal vascularity.[25]

Thyroidectomy bed recurrence typically appears as well-defined hypoechoic oval nodules within the resection bed (Fig. 5). A small proportion of recurrent nodules may contain microcalcifications; this is a specific feature of recurrence when identified. Otherwise, the sonographic appearance is commonly nonspecific and serial sonograms can be helpful to evaluate small nodules for interval growth. The size of thyroidectomy bed recurrence

is typically small with one series reporting an average size of biopsied nodules of 7 mm; this is near the lower limit of size for which a reliable FNA can be performed.[26] Given the nonspecific sonographic features, a variety of entities may be mistaken for recurrence. One retrospective series of thyroidectomy bed nodule biopsies found multiple entities in the samples negative for recurrent tumor including remnant thyroid, fibrosis, suture granuloma, strap muscle, reactive lymph nodes, and fat necrosis.[26] Suture granulomas are a chronic granulomatous foreign body reaction that can be seen within the surgical bed with a sonographic appearance that potentially can be confused with disease recurrence, as they can be present years following surgery (Fig. 6). One specific sonographic sign that can suggest this diagnosis is the presence of central linear echogenic lines within a hypoechoic nodule; double parallel lines greater than 1 mm in width are particularly characteristic.[27,28]

Gray-scale sonographic features of metastatic lymph nodes include microcalcifications, cystic change, round shape, hyperechogenicity, absence of a fatty hilum, and an increased short-axis diameter (Fig. 7).[23,26,29–35] Nodal microcalcifications and cystic change are highly specific signs of malignant adenopathy with reported specificities at or near 100% in several series.[29–35] These findings are not found in most nodal metastases; thus, the low reported sensitivities for cystic change (10%–34%) and microcalcifications (32%–50%).[31,34,35] A round shape, in contradistinction to the oval shape of benign lymph nodes, can also be a helpful discriminating feature with 57% to 80% of malignant lymph nodes versus

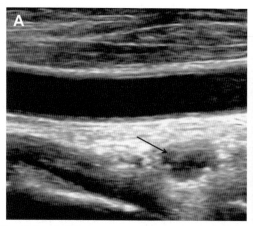

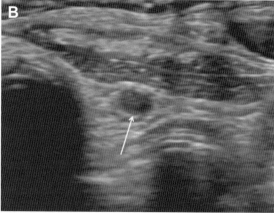

Fig. 5. Local DTC recurrence. (A) Longitudinal sonographic image of the right lobectomy bed showing a 7-mm nodule (arrow) with cystic change, a highly specific feature for nodal recurrence in the setting of DTC. (B) Transverse image of the left thyroidectomy bed with a 5-mm rounded hypoechoic nodule (arrow) that represented recurrent tumor. Small-volume recurrence such as shown here commonly does not have specific sonographic features indicating malignancy and assessment of the clinical importance of such findings depends on serial imaging and correlation with serum Tg levels.

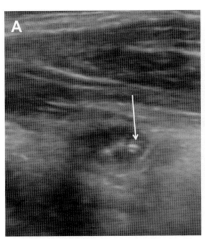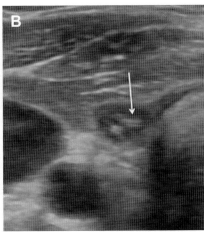

Fig. 6. Suture granuloma mimicking central compartment recurrence. Longitudinal (*A*) and axial (*B*) sonographic images of the right thyroidectomy bed show a hypoechoic nodule containing several central echogenic foci. The parallel echogenic lines (*arrows*) reflects the presence of suture material central to the granulomatous reaction and can be a specific sign for suture granuloma in the appropriate clinical setting.

12% to 30% of reactive lymph nodes having a short axis to long axis measurement ratio of more than 0.5.[31,32] Hyperechogenicity of the lymph node has also been reported to be a specific sign of metastases with specificities ranging from 85% to 100%.[31,34,35] Reported sensitivities for the absence of a fatty hilum range considerably, between 32% and 100%; the specificity of this sonographic feature ranges from 48% to 71%.[31,34,35] One of the largest series to date found short axis size to be the best discriminator between benign and malignant nodes but this has not been replicated in other series.[32]

The color-Doppler vascularity of cervical lymph nodes may be an additional discriminatory feature between benign and malignant nodes. Normal lymph node vascularity tends to enter the hilum of the lymph node and ramify peripherally, whereas flow within malignant lymph nodes may be distributed in the capsule (**Fig. 8**).[35–37] Doppler ultrasound of cervical lymph nodes has been most extensively studied in the setting of squamous cell carcinoma and other more common neck malignancies. One recent study comparing DTC nodal metastasis to reactive lymph nodes found peripheral nodal vascularity to be a statistically significant sign of malignancy.[35]

No single sonographic feature can be relied on in isolation, and assessment for malignancy should be based on all ultrasound discriminatory criteria. For example, lymph nodes are routinely found in which a demonstrable fatty hilum is not identified but all other sonographic features are normal. As an isolated finding in the neck, this is less suspicious for a nodal metastasis. On the other hand, the index of suspicion is raised if multiple lymph nodes lacking a fatty hilum are clustered or if additional features of malignancy are identified in adjacent nodes.

Although ultrasound findings alone can be highly suggestive of malignancy, the overlap in the appearance of benign and malignant lymph nodes makes ultrasound-guided FNA necessary for pathologic confirmation in many cases. FNA is typically performed with ultrasound guidance using a 27-gauge to 22-gauge needle. Collection techniques include capillary action and suction and multiple passes are generally performed to improve sample adequacy. Measurement of Tg levels within fine-needle aspirates can improve the diagnostic accuracy of this technique. This may be particularly useful when sampling small or partially cystic lymph nodes in which cellular yield may be minimal. An elevated Tg level is diagnostic of nodal metastasis even when cytopathologic results are inconclusive.[38–40] The importance of Tg aspirates when sampling cervical lymph nodes is highlighted by one recent study in which all suspicious cervical lymph nodes were sampled before resection: nodal metastases were found in 34% of suspicious nodes despite a negative cytology.[34]

Surgical resection remains the standard therapy for local-regional recurrences in the absence of distant metastases but ultrasound also has the potential to guide percutaneous therapy for recurrence in patients who may be considered high surgical risks because of prior neck surgeries or medical comorbidities. The safety and efficacy of ultrasound-guided ethanol ablation therapy has been demonstrated in small series with

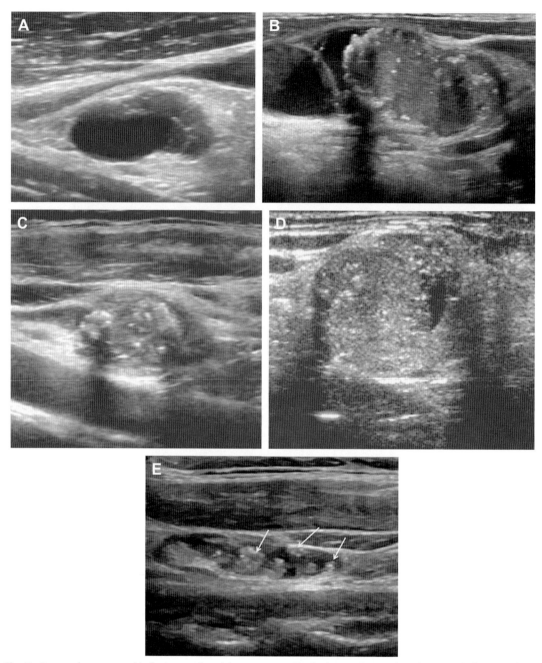

Fig. 7. Gray-scale sonographic features of nodal metastases. Cystic change (*A, B, D*) and microcalcifications (*A–E*) are highly specific signs of nodal metastasis. Other features include round shape (*C, D*), loss of fatty hilum (*A–D*), and hyperechogenicity (*B, C, D*). (*E*) Small echogenic foci (*arrows*) represent small metastatic foci within an otherwise normal-appearing cervical lymph node.

short-term follow-up.[41,42] A limited experience with ultrasound-guided radiofrequency ablation suggests this may be another potential therapeutic option. Potential complications limiting the use of these techniques include damage to the recurrent laryngeal nerve, which may occur even with

precise technique and continuous monitoring of the ablation with ultrasound.[42]

PET and PET/CT

The tumor biology of DTC defines the role of PET and PET/CT in imaging surveillance. The inverse

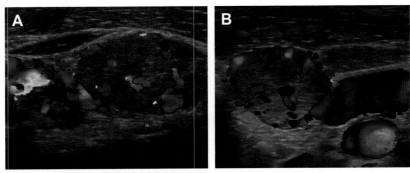

Fig. 8. Color Doppler of nodal metastases. At color Doppler interrogation, nodal metastases (*A, B*) may be hypervascular and show peripheral vascularity compared with normal lymph node vascularity, which tends to arise centrally from a hilar vessel and ramify peripherally.

relationship between the ability of DTC to take up iodine and its FDG-avidity is explained by a decrease in sodium-iodide symporter expression and an increase in glucose transporter-1 expression (the transporter by which FDG is taken up by cells), which occurs with tumor dedifferentiation.[43] This so-called "flip-flop" phenomenon likely accounts for the increased prevalence of FDG-avid DTC in the setting of negative WBS. It may also explain the poorer prognosis attributed to FDG-avidity because these cancers tend to be less responsive to radioiodine therapy (**Fig. 9**).[44] Thus, the primary role of PET is for the detection of local recurrence and distant metastatic disease in the setting of Tg-positive, but cervical ultrasound–negative and WBS-negative disease.

The sensitivity of PET for the detection of DTC recurrence in part depends on the indications used for patient selection. The largest series report sensitivities between 50% and 75%.[45–49] A positive correlation between PET positivity and serum Tg levels shown in several studies suggests an increased sensitivity for detection of metastases in the setting of an elevated Tg. In a multicenter European trial for PET in thyroid cancer, the sensitivity for detection of metastasis was 85% for the subset of patients with negative WBS versus 65% for patients with WBS positivity.[45] Similarly, in a study of 51 patients with elevated Tg and normal WBS, reported sensitivities for PET were 50%, 62%, and 83% for unstimulated Tg levels of less than 1.0 mg/dL, 1.0 to 10.0 mg/dL, and greater than 10 mg/dL, respectively.[49] As Tg levels have been shown to correlate with the number of metastases,[50] this relationship may simply reflect the greater detection of larger-volume tumor. Other confounding variables that might affect reported sensitivities include varying imaging indications (eg, WBS positivity or negativity), and the extent of other imaging (cervical ultrasound, chest

CT) performed before the decision was made to perform a PET scan.

More recently, combined PET/CT has been used for similar indications. The sensitivity of PET/CT is similar to PET alone for the detection of local-regional and distant metastases.[51–56] PET/CT improves specificity, however. The ability to correlate scintigraphic findings with anatomic imaging makes it possible to identify potential false positives caused by FDG uptake in muscle, brown fat, and surgical bed inflammatory changes. CT also increases the ability to accurately localize local-regional metastasis should surgical resection be necessary. In a series of 124 patients who underwent PET/CT to evaluate for post-ablation residual or recurrent disease, the sensitivity for the detection of metastases was 81% and the specificity was 89%. In part because of the added utility of CT, the results of the PET/CT reportedly changed the treatment of the patient in 28% of cases and provided important information for subsequent surgical intervention in 21% of cases.[51] Other series using PET/CT reported alterations of patient management in 32% to 44% of cases and changes in surgical management in 32% to 33%.[53–55]

There is the potential for expansion of the indications for PET/CT beyond the localization of disease in Tg-positive and WBS-negative patients with DTC. Potential indications include initial staging of patients with high-risk tumor histologies, such as tall-cell or insular subtypes, as well as Hurthle cell variants. Additionally, given the relatively poor prognosis of FDG-avid thyroid malignancies compared with iodine-avid tumors, there is potential for further refinement of PET/CT as a prognostic tool.[21,57]

CT and MR Imaging

CT and MR imaging are rarely used for DTC surveillance given the advantages and efficacy of

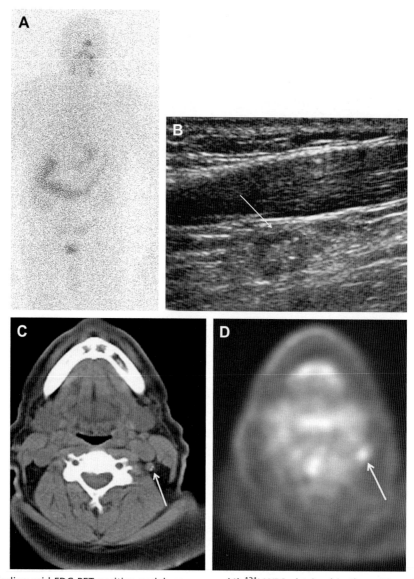

Fig. 9. Non-iodine-avid FDG-PET positive nodal recurrence. (*A*) ^{131}I WBS obtained in the setting of elevated Tg reveals no abnormal uptake within the neck. (*B*) Sonographic image of a small left level IV nodal recurrence (*arrow*) containing microcalcifications. (*C*) CT of the neck shows corresponding nodal microcalcifications (*arrow*) and concurrent PET (*D*) confirms FDG-avidity within this lymph node (*arrow*). FDG-PET and PET/CT are commonly used in the setting of a negative WBS and elevated Tg, as there is an inverse relationship between iodine avidity and FDG-avidity.

ultrasound as a technique for the detection of local-regional recurrence. CT of the neck can also be limited because iodinated contrast may be contraindicated in many patients with DTC; iodine can interfere with future radioiodine therapy and may also potentially cause false-negative WBS studies. Many of the features of nodal metastases (cystic change, fine calcifications, round shape) are applicable to CT, although there is little recent literature on the role of CT in the surveillance of DTC beyond that included as a part of PET/CT studies. The primary role for CT in posttreatment surveillance is the evaluation of patients with positive Tg and negative cervical ultrasound, although PET-CT may be preferred if available for this indication. CT of the chest is also commonly used in the evaluation for metastases, as lung metastases are the most common site of disease outside of the neck. Both micronodular and macronodular lung metastases are readily

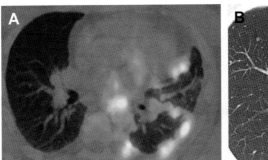
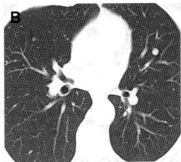

Fig. 10. Patterns of lung metastases. (*A*) Fused FDG-PET image of the chest in a patient with extensive left-sided pleural-based metastases. (*B*) Axial unenhanced CT image of the chest in a patient with disseminated pulmonary metastases shows both the micronodular and macronodular patterns of lung metastases. A miliary pattern of lung metastases has been described in DTC with individual lung nodules below the resolution of FDG-PET.

detectible with chest CT (**Fig. 10**). A miliary pattern of lung metastases is also described, which may not be detectible on diagnostic WBS or PET images because of their limited resolution.[58]

MR imaging is also not generally a part of surveillance imaging strategies for DTC. With more aggressive tumors, MR imaging may be used to evaluate the extent of local tumor invasion of structures such as the trachea or recurrent laryngeal nerve and may aid surgical planning in selected cases.[59,60] Small series have shown sensitivities for the detection of cervical metastases similar to that of ultrasound but the practical advantages of ultrasound, including the added benefit of ultrasound guidance for FNA, has prevented the widespread use of MR imaging (**Fig. 11**).[61–63] MR imaging of the neck and mediastinum can be helpful in the setting of an elevated Tg and negative ultrasound to look for tumor that may be obscured or inaccessible at ultrasound. Retroesophageal/retrotracheal tumor as well as mediastinal disease may be particularly well shown by MR imaging.

CLINICAL SIGNIFICANCE OF SMALL-VOLUME LOCAL-REGIONAL METASTATIC DISEASE IN DTC

As the number of patients undergoing imaging surveillance increases and the ability of our imaging technologies to depict smaller and smaller foci of tumor improves, imagers should be mindful of the clinical implications of such findings. Several lines of evidence illustrate the indolent nature of DTC and call into question the clinical impact of tiny foci of local-regional recurrent tumor. Autopsy studies demonstrate that a large proportion of the population harbors subclinical foci of thyroid cancer with prevalence ranging from 5% to 24%.[64–66] In a study of more than 700 patients with known incidental micropapillary carcinomas (<1 cm) who opted for clinical observation over surgical treatment, only 1% of patients developed lateral compartment metastases over a 5-year period, whereas 70% the of patients' lesions remained stable or even decreased in size.[67] Several large surgical series from Japan, in which nearly all patients with DTC underwent extensive

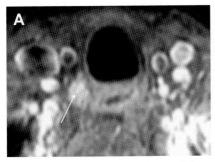
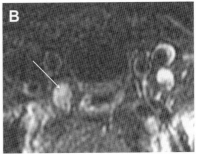

Fig. 11. MR imaging depiction of right level VI nodal recurrence. (*A*) Axial T2-weighted MR image of the inferior neck demonstrates a T2-hyperintense (*arrow*) nodule within the right thyroidectomy bed. (*B*) Brisk enhancement of this nodule is shown on the axial T1-postgadolinium image (*arrow*).

modified neck dissection irrespective of preoperative clinical evidence of lateral compartment metastases, found tiny (<3 mm) foci of nodal metastasis in up to 90% of patients.[68,69] The fact that the prognosis is so favorable despite the very high prevalence of nodal metastasis suggests that most of these findings are clinically occult. Recent improvements in ultrasound platforms have made possible the identification of tiny abnormal foci within cervical lymph nodes (see **Fig. 7E**) and tiny thyroidectomy bed nodules, a common occurrence in patients undergoing imaging surveillance. The revised ATA guidelines now recommend ultrasound-guided biopsy of suspicious lymph nodes as small as 5 mm if it will change clinical management. Whether the application of such aggressive surveillance strategies will have a measurable positive impact on patient outcomes awaits further study and probably will require a better understanding of the tumor biology of DTC. Until such time, close collaboration with referring endocrinologists, thyroid surgeons, and, ultimately, the patient, is necessary to define reasonable surveillance and treatment strategies.

SUMMARY

Imaging surveillance of DTC relies predominantly on cervical ultrasound to evaluate for local-regional recurrence in combination with serial serum Tg. Sonographic features of nodal metastases include a round shape, absence of a fatty hilum, hyperechogenicity, cystic change, and microcalcifications. When necessary to confirm the presence of metastases, ultrasound-guided FNA is safe and effective, particularly when combined with a Tg assay of the aspirate. Evaluation of distant metastases can be performed with WBS and chest CT, as the lungs and skeleton are the most common sites of distant metastases. PET and PET/CT are currently used primarily in the evaluation for metastases in patients with tumors that do not concentrate iodine, but there is the potential for additional uses including prognosis and surveillance of specific tumor subtypes. The appropriate intensity of post-therapy surveillance will likely continue to evolve as our understanding of tumor biology improves the ability to predict outcomes.

REFERENCES

1. Mazzaferri EL, Jhiang SM. Long-term impact of initial surgical and medical therapy on papillary and follicular thyroid cancer. Am J Med 1994; 97(5):418–28.

2. Hay ID, Thompson GB, Grant CS, et al. Papillary thyroid carcinoma managed at the Mayo Clinic during six decades (1940–1999): temporal trends in initial therapy and long-term outcome in 2444 consecutively treated patients. World J Surg 2002; 26(8):879–85.

3. Pacini F, Molinaro E, Castagna MG, et al. Recombinant human thyrotropin-stimulated serum thyroglobulin combined with neck ultrasonography has the highest sensitivity in monitoring differentiated thyroid carcinoma. J Clin Endocrinol Metab 2003;88(8): 3668–73.

4. Schlumberger M, Berg G, Cohen O, et al. Follow-up of low-risk patients with differentiated thyroid carcinoma: a European perspective. Eur J Endocrinol 2004;150(2):105–12.

5. Torlontano M, Crocetti U, Augello G, et al. Comparative evaluation of recombinant human thyrotropin-stimulated thyroglobulin levels, 131I whole-body scintigraphy, and neck ultrasonography in the follow-up of patients with papillary thyroid microcarcinoma who have not undergone radioiodine therapy. J Clin Endocrinol Metab 2006;91(1):60–3.

6. Surveillance epidemiology and end results. Available at: http://www.seer.cancer/gov. Accessed September 1, 2010.

7. Jemal A, Siegel R, Xu J, et al. Cancer statistics, 2010. CA Cancer J Clin 2010;60:277–300.

8. Davies L, Welch HG. Increasing incidence of thyroid cancer in the United States, 1973–2002. JAMA 2006;295(18):2164–7.

9. Zhu C, Zheng T, Kilfoy BA, et al. A birth cohort analysis of the incidence of papillary thyroid cancer in the United States, 1973–2004. Thyroid 2009; 19(10):1061–6.

10. Mazzaferri EL, Robbins RJ, Spencer CA, et al. A consensus report of the role of serum thyroglobulin as a monitoring method for low-risk patients with papillary thyroid carcinoma. J Clin Endocrinol Metab 2003;88(4):1433–41.

11. Kim TY, Kim WB, Kim ES, et al. Serum thyroglobulin levels at the time of 131I remnant ablation just after thyroidectomy are useful for early prediction of clinical recurrence in low-risk patients with differentiated thyroid carcinoma. J Clin Endocrinol Metab 2005; 90(3):1440–5.

12. Hollowell JG, Staehling NW, Flanders WD, et al. Serum TSH, T(4), and thyroid antibodies in the United States population (1988 to 1994): National Health and Nutrition Examination Survey (NHANES III). J Clin Endocrinol Metab 2002; 87(2):489–99.

13. Gorges R, Maniecki M, Jentzen W, et al. Development and clinical impact of thyroglobulin antibodies in patients with differentiated thyroid carcinoma during the first 3 years after thyroidectomy. Eur J Endocrinol 2005;153(1):49–55.

14. Rubello D, Casara D, Girelli ME, et al. Clinical meaning of circulating antithyroglobulin antibodies in differentiated thyroid cancer: a prospective study. J Nucl Med 1992;33(8):1478–80.

15. Pujol P, Daures JP, Nsakala N, et al. Degree of thyrotropin suppression as a prognostic determinant in differentiated thyroid cancer. J Clin Endocrinol Metab 1996;81(12):4318–23.

16. Cooper DS, Specker B, Ho M, et al. Thyrotropin suppression and disease progression in patients with differentiated thyroid cancer: results from the National Thyroid Cancer Treatment Cooperative Registry. Thyroid 1998;8(9):737–44.

17. Eustatia-Rutten CF, Smit JW, Romijn JA, et al. Diagnostic value of serum thyroglobulin measurements in the follow-up of differentiated thyroid carcinoma, a structured meta-analysis. Clin Endocrinol (Oxf) 2004;61(1):61–74.

18. Kloos RT, Mazzaferri EL. A single recombinant human thyrotropin-stimulated serum thyroglobulin measurement predicts differentiated thyroid carcinoma metastases three to five years later. J Clin Endocrinol Metab 2005;90(9):5047–57.

19. Dam HQ, Kim SM, Lin HC, et al. 131I therapeutic efficacy is not influenced by stunning after diagnostic whole-body scanning. Radiology 2004; 232(2):527–33.

20. Silberstein EB. Comparison of outcomes after (123)I versus (131)I pre-ablation imaging before radioiodine ablation in differentiated thyroid carcinoma. J Nucl Med 2007;48(7):1043–6.

21. Cooper DS, Doherty GM, Haugen BR, et al. Revised American Thyroid Association management guidelines for patients with thyroid nodules and differentiated thyroid cancer. Thyroid 2009;19(11):1167–214.

22. Som PM, Curtin HD, Mancuso AA. An imaging-based classification for the cervical nodes designed as an adjunct to recent clinically based nodal classifications. Arch Otolaryngol Head Neck Surg 1999; 125(4):388–96.

23. Simeone JF, Daniels GH, Hall DA, et al. Sonography in the follow-up of 100 patients with thyroid carcinoma. AJR Am J Roentgenol 1987;148(1):45–9.

24. Tublin ME, Alexander JM, Ogilvie JB. Appearance of absorbable gelatin compressed sponge on early post-thyroidectomy neck sonography: a mimic of locally recurrent or residual thyroid carcinoma. J Ultrasound Med 2010;29(1):117–20.

25. Ko MS, Lee JH, Shong YK, et al. Normal and abnormal sonographic findings at the thyroidectomy sites in postoperative patients with thyroid malignancy. AJR Am J Roentgenol 2010;194(6): 1596–609.

26. Shin JH, Han BK, Ko EY, et al. Sonographic findings in the surgical bed after thyroidectomy: comparison of recurrent tumors and nonrecurrent lesions. J Ultrasound Med 2007;26(10):1359–66.

27. Kim JH, Lee JH, Shong YK, et al. Ultrasound features of suture granulomas in the thyroid bed after thyroidectomy for papillary thyroid carcinoma with an emphasis on their differentiation from locally recurrent thyroid carcinomas. Ultrasound Med Biol 2009;35(9):1452–7.

28. Rettenbacher T, Macheiner P, Hollerweger A, et al. Suture granulomas: sonography enables a correct preoperative diagnosis. Ultrasound Med Biol 2001; 27(3):343–50.

29. Wunderbaldinger P, Harisinghani MG, Hahn PF, et al. Cystic lymph node metastases in papillary thyroid carcinoma. AJR Am J Roentgenol 2002; 178(3):693–7.

30. Kessler A, Rappaport Y, Blank A, et al. Cystic appearance of cervical lymph nodes is characteristic of metastatic papillary thyroid carcinoma. J Clin Ultrasound 2003;31(1):21–5.

31. Rosario PW, de Faria S, Bicalho L, et al. Ultrasonographic differentiation between metastatic and benign lymph nodes in patients with papillary thyroid carcinoma. J Ultrasound Med 2005;24(10): 1385–9.

32. Kuna SK, Bracic I, Tesic V, et al. Ultrasonographic differentiation of benign from malignant neck lymphadenopathy in thyroid cancer. J Ultrasound Med 2006;25(12):1531–7 [quiz: 1538–40].

33. Lee JH, Lee HK, Lee DH, et al. Ultrasonographic findings of a newly detected nodule on the thyroid bed in postoperative patients for thyroid carcinoma: correlation with the results of ultrasonography-guided fine-needle aspiration biopsy. Clin Imaging 2007;31(2):109–13.

34. Sohn YM, Kwak JY, Kim EK, et al. Diagnostic approach for evaluation of lymph node metastasis from thyroid cancer using ultrasound and fine-needle aspiration biopsy. AJR Am J Roentgenol 2010;194(1):38–43.

35. Park JS, Son KR, Na DG, et al. Performance of preoperative sonographic staging of papillary thyroid carcinoma based on the sixth edition of the AJCC/UICC TNM classification system. AJR Am J Roentgenol 2009;192(1):66–72.

36. Ahuja AT, Ying M, Yuen HY, et al. Power Doppler sonography of metastatic nodes from papillary carcinoma of the thyroid. Clin Radiol 2001;56(4): 284–8.

37. Lyshchik A, Higashi T, Asato R, et al. Cervical lymph node metastases: diagnosis at sonoelastography—initial experience. Radiology 2007;243(1):258–67.

38. Cignarelli M, Ambrosi A, Marino A, et al. Diagnostic utility of thyroglobulin detection in fine-needle aspiration of cervical cystic metastatic lymph nodes from papillary thyroid cancer with negative cytology. Thyroid 2003;13(12):1163–7.

39. Baskin HJ. Detection of recurrent papillary thyroid carcinoma by thyroglobulin assessment in the

needle washout after fine-needle aspiration of suspicious lymph nodes. Thyroid 2004;14(11):959–63.

40. Uruno T, Miyauchi A, Shimizu K, et al. Usefulness of thyroglobulin measurement in fine-needle aspiration biopsy specimens for diagnosing cervical lymph node metastasis in patients with papillary thyroid cancer. World J Surg 2005;29(4):483–5.

41. Lewis BD, Hay ID, Charboneau JW, et al. Percutaneous ethanol injection for treatment of cervical lymph node metastases in patients with papillary thyroid carcinoma. AJR Am J Roentgenol 2002; 178(3):699–704.

42. Monchik JM, Donatini G, Iannuccilli J, et al. Radiofrequency ablation and percutaneous ethanol injection treatment for recurrent local and distant well-differentiated thyroid carcinoma. Ann Surg 2006; 244(2):296–304.

43. Lazar V, Bidart JM, Caillou B, et al. Expression of the Na+/I– symporter gene in human thyroid tumors: a comparison study with other thyroid-specific genes. J Clin Endocrinol Metab 1999;84(9):3228–34.

44. Wang W, Larson SM, Fazzari M, et al. Prognostic value of [18F]fluorodeoxyglucose positron emission tomographic scanning in patients with thyroid cancer. J Clin Endocrinol Metab 2000;85(3):1107–13.

45. Grunwald F, Kalicke T, Feine U, et al. Fluorine-18 fluorodeoxyglucose positron emission tomography in thyroid cancer: results of a multicentre study. Eur J Nucl Med 1999;26(12):1547–52.

46. Dietlein M, Scheidhauer K, Voth E, et al. Fluorine-18 fluorodeoxyglucose positron emission tomography and iodine-131 whole-body scintigraphy in the follow-up of differentiated thyroid cancer. Eur J Nucl Med 1997;24(11):1342–8.

47. Schluter B, Bohuslavizki KH, Beyer W, et al. Impact of FDG PET on patients with differentiated thyroid cancer who present with elevated thyroglobulin and negative 131I scan. J Nucl Med 2001;42(1):71–6.

48. Alzahrani AS, Mohamed GE, Al Rifai A, et al. Role of [18F]fluorodeoxyglucose positron emission tomography in follow-up of differentiated thyroid cancer. Endocr Pract 2006;12(2):152–8.

49. Giammarile F, Hafdi Z, Bournaud C, et al. Is [18F]-2-fluoro-2-deoxy-d-glucose (FDG) scintigraphy with non-dedicated positron emission tomography useful in the diagnostic management of suspected metastatic thyroid carcinoma in patients with no detectable radioiodine uptake? Eur J Endocrinol 2003; 149(4):293–300.

50. Robbins RJ, Srivastava S, Shaha A, et al. Factors influencing the basal and recombinant human thyrotropin-stimulated serum thyroglobulin in patients with metastatic thyroid carcinoma. J Clin Endocrinol Metab 2004;89(12):6010–6.

51. Razfar A, Branstetter BF, Christopoulos A, et al. Clinical usefulness of positron emission tomography-computed tomography in recurrent thyroid carcinoma. Arch Otolaryngol Head Neck Surg 2010;136(2):120–5.

52. Saab G, Driedger AA, Pavlosky W, et al. Thyroid-stimulating hormone-stimulated fused positron emission tomography/computed tomography in the evaluation of recurrence in 131I-negative papillary thyroid carcinoma. Thyroid 2006;16(3): 267–72.

53. Shammas A, Degirmenci B, Mountz JM, et al. 18F-FDG PET/CT in patients with suspected recurrent or metastatic well-differentiated thyroid cancer. J Nucl Med 2007;48(2):221–6.

54. Nahas Z, Goldenberg D, Fakhry C, et al. The role of positron emission tomography/computed tomography in the management of recurrent papillary thyroid carcinoma. Laryngoscope 2005;115(2): 237–43.

55. Palmedo H, Bucerius J, Joe A, et al. Integrated PET/CT in differentiated thyroid cancer: diagnostic accuracy and impact on patient management. J Nucl Med 2006;47(4):616–24.

56. Jeong HS, Baek CH, Son YI, et al. Integrated 18F-FDG PET/CT for the initial evaluation of cervical node level of patients with papillary thyroid carcinoma: comparison with ultrasound and contrast-enhanced CT. Clin Endocrinol (Oxf) 2006;65(3): 402–7.

57. Pryma DA, Schoder H, Gonen M, et al. Diagnostic accuracy and prognostic value of 18F-FDG PET in Hurthle cell thyroid cancer patients. J Nucl Med 2006;47(8):1260–6.

58. Zoller M, Kohlfuerst S, Igerc I, et al. Combined PET/CT in the follow-up of differentiated thyroid carcinoma: what is the impact of each modality? Eur J Nucl Med Mol Imaging 2007;34(4):487–95.

59. Takashima S, Takayama F, Wang J, et al. Using MR imaging to predict invasion of the recurrent laryngeal nerve by thyroid carcinoma. AJR Am J Roentgenol 2003;180(3):837–42.

60. Wang JC, Takashima S, Takayama F, et al. Tracheal invasion by thyroid carcinoma: prediction using MR imaging. AJR Am J Roentgenol 2001; 177(4):929–36.

61. King AD, Ahuja AT, To EW, et al. Staging papillary carcinoma of the thyroid: magnetic resonance imaging vs ultrasound of the neck. Clin Radiol 2000;55(3):222–6.

62. Takashima S, Sone S, Takayama F, et al. Papillary thyroid carcinoma: MR diagnosis of lymph node metastasis. AJNR Am J Neuroradiol 1998;19(3): 509–13.

63. Gross ND, Weissman JL, Talbot JM, et al. MRI detection of cervical metastasis from differentiated thyroid carcinoma. Laryngoscope 2001;111(11 Pt 1): 1905–9.

64. Harach HR, Franssila KO, Wasenius VM. Occult papillary carcinoma of the thyroid. A "normal"

finding in Finland. A systematic autopsy study. Cancer 1985;56(3):531–8.

65. Komorowski RA, Hanson GA. Occult thyroid pathology in the young adult: an autopsy study of 138 patients without clinical thyroid disease. Hum Pathol 1988;19(6):689–96.

66. Kovacs GL, Gonda G, Vadasz G, et al. Epidemiology of thyroid microcarcinoma found in autopsy series conducted in areas of different iodine intake. Thyroid 2005;15(2):152–7.

67. Ito Y, Uruno T, Nakano K, et al. An observation trial without surgical treatment in patients with papillary microcarcinoma of the thyroid. Thyroid 2003;13(4): 381–7.

68. Ito Y, Tomoda C, Uruno T, et al. Ultrasonographically and anatomopathologically detectable node metastases in the lateral compartment as indicators of worse relapse-free survival in patients with papillary thyroid carcinoma. World J Surg 2005; 29(7):917–20.

69. Ito Y, Tomoda C, Uruno T, et al. Clinical significance of metastasis to the central compartment from papillary microcarcinoma of the thyroid. World J Surg 2006;30(1):91–9.

Parathyroid Imaging

Nathan A. Johnson, MD[a],*, Sally E. Carty, MD[b],
Mitchell E. Tublin, MD[a]

KEYWORDS

- Hyperparathyroidism • Parathyroid adenoma • Sonography
- Ultrasonography • Sestamibi • SPECT/CT

Primary hyperparathyroidism is a common endocrine disorder caused by the overproduction of parathyroid hormone (PTH) by either a single adenomatous gland (85%) or, less commonly, by multiple adenomatous or hyperplastic glands (15%). Surgical resection of the abnormal parathyroid glands is the standard treatment, and the goal of initial parathyroidectomy is durable biochemical cure. The traditional operative approach consists of bilateral cervical exploration, during which all parathyroid glands are identified and the enlarged glands are resected. Cure rates with this approach exceed 95% in experienced hands.[1]

Recently surgeons have shifted to more minimally invasive and selective techniques for parathyroid exploration.[2] Aided by advancements including rapid intraoperative PTH assay, cure rates have remained similarly high.[3–6] The more selective surgical approaches rely on accurate preoperative imaging techniques to localize the abnormal parathyroid glands. Intraoperative PTH monitoring is used as a functional indicator of focused and adequate resection. Thus, for many patients with primary hyperparathyroidism preoperative imaging has become a standard part of management, making it imperative for radiologists interpreting these studies to be familiar with the imaging features of the parathyroid glands as well as the role of imaging in patient care.

ANATOMY AND EMBRYOLOGY

There is wide variability in parathyroid gland anatomic location, shape, and number. This simple reality is the reason why successful parathyroid surgery can be challenging and requires specific skills and experience. Most people have 4 parathyroid glands: 2 superior glands derived from the fourth branchial pouch along with the lateral portions of the thyroid gland, and 2 inferior glands derived from the third branchial pouch along with the thymus (**Fig. 1**). Their separate embryologic origins help account for the variable positions and anatomic relationships encountered.

The superior parathyroid glands are less variable in location. Approximately 80% are located posterior to the mid-portion of the thyroid lobe at the level of the cricothyroid junction and along the tracheoesophageal groove. Most of the remaining glands are positioned posterior to the upper pole of the lobe. Most glands are separate from the overlying thyroid capsule (a discriminating sonographic feature if the adenoma is not mobile along with the thyroid when the patient is asked to swallow), though a small number may be within the thyroid capsule or completely within thyroid parenchyma. Rarely, superior parathyroid glands are found in a deep retropharyngeal or retroesophageal location.[7,8]

Most inferior parathyroid glands are positioned inferior, posterior, or lateral to the lower pole of the ipsilateral thyroid lobe. Those glands not immediately adjacent to the lower pole of the thyroid are commonly found more caudally in the thyrothymic ligament (connective tissue between the thyroid and thymus glands), the thymic tongue (the superior extension of the thymus into the inferior neck), or within the thymus gland of the anterior superior mediastinum. Rarely, inferior glands can fail to descend, and are found in the carotid

Financial disclosure/Conflicts of interest: None.
[a] Division of Abdominal Imaging, Department of Radiology, University of Pittsburgh School of Medicine, 200 Lothrop Street, Suite 3950 PST, Pittsburgh, PA 15213, USA
[b] Section of Endocrine Surgery, Department of Surgery, University of Pittsburgh School of Medicine, 3471 Fifth Avenue, Kaufmann Building, Suite 101, Pittsburgh, PA 15213, USA
* Corresponding author.
E-mail address: johnsonna2@upmc.edu

Radiol Clin N Am 49 (2011) 489–509
doi:10.1016/j.rcl.2011.02.009
0033-8389/11/$ – see front matter © 2011 Elsevier Inc. All rights reserved.

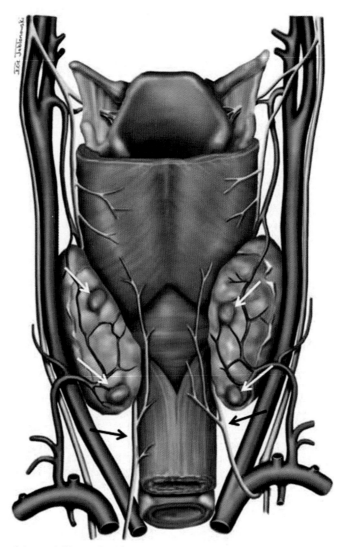

Fig. 1. Posterior view of the neck illustrating the most common location of the parathyroid glands (*white arrows*) deep to the midpole of the thyroid lobes (superior glands) and inferior or deep to the lower poles (inferior glands). Also, note the close relationship of the recurrent laryngeal nerves (*black arrows*), which must be carefully preserved during parathyroid exploration. One of the benefits of a more focused surgical approach is a diminished risk of recurrent laryngeal nerve injury. (*From* Johnson NA, Tublin ME, Ogilvie JB. Parathyroid imaging: technique and role in the preoperative evaluation of primary hyperparathyroidism. AJR Am J Roentgenol 2007;188(6):1706–15; with permission from the American Roentgen Ray Society.)

sheath near the carotid bifurcation or near the upper pole of the thyroid gland. Rarer still are inferior glands that descend below the thymus into the anterior mediastinum. Given their separate embryological origin from the thyroid gland, inferior parathyroid glands are unlikely to be found in a true intrathyroidal location, but this does occur in fewer than 1% of patients.[7,8]

More than 4 glands are present in 2% to 9% of individuals. Supernumerary glands are commonly located inferiorly within the thyrothymic ligament or deep to the thyroid between the 2 other glands.[7] The average normal parathyroid gland is small, measuring $5 \times 3 \times 1$ mm with an average weight of 35 mg (25–50 mg),[9] but in primary hyperparathyroidism, suppressed normal glands can be even smaller (20 mg). Most glands (83%) have an oval, rounded, or bean shape, but they can be elongated (11%) particularly when the relatively noncompressible gland is positioned within the thyroid capsule. Not uncommonly (5%), glands may be bilobed or even multilobulated (1%).[8]

PATHOPHYSIOLOGY OF HYPERPARATHYROIDISM

The parathyroid glands play a key role in calcium homeostasis via the production of PTH. PTH has several actions including promoting renal tubular calcium absorption, decreasing tubular absorption of phosphate, and promoting the stimulation of osteoclasts, which increases the release of cationic calcium from mineralized calcium within the bony matrix. PTH also stimulates vitamin D production by the kidneys, which increases intestinal absorption of dietary calcium.

Primary hyperparathyroidism is diagnosed when the serum PTH is increased or inappropriately high-normal in the setting of an elevated serum calcium level.[10] Imaging studies have no role in diagnosis. Approximately 85% of cases are caused by a single parathyroid adenoma with, 15% caused by multiglandular disease (either 4-gland hyperplasia or multiple adenomata). Rarely (<1%), the disease is caused by parathyroid carcinoma. Most cases are sporadic, but primary hyperparathyroidism may also be seen in the setting of multiple endocrine neoplasia (MEN) syndromes including MEN-1 and MEN-2a. In a recent study, MEN-1 was surprisingly common, occurring in 4.5% of patients referred for surgery of presumed sporadic hyperparathyroidism; the use of a simple 6-question panel was effective in uncovering unrecognized MEN-1, which was even more likely in male patients younger than 30 years.[11] Familial hypocalciuric hypercalcemia (FHH) is an autosomal dominant disorder that causes a change in the renal set-point for calcium excretion and PTH-dependent hypercalcemia; the primary morbidity of FHH is unnecessary parathyroid surgery. FHH can be distinguished from primary hyperparathyroidism by a low urinary calcium to urinary creatinine ratio (measured by 24-hour urine collection), a modestly elevated or normal serum PTH concentration, an early age of onset, and in some cases an associated family history.

Primary hyperparathyroidism is a common disorder affecting between 1 and 4 people per 1000 in population-based screening studies, with a twofold increased prevalence in women.[12] The peak incidence is in women between the ages of 50 and 60 years. Approximately 75% of cases are asymptomatic, with many patients initially diagnosed incidentally by routine blood tests that reveal an elevated serum calcium level.[12] Clinical symptoms are often nonspecific, and neuropsychiatric symptoms are common; they include fatigue, malaise, irritability, mood swings, anxiety, and depression.[13] Hypertension, renal stone disease, bone pain, and osteoporosis are additional conditions that prompt surgical treatment. Given that many of these symptoms and conditions are difficult to measure objectively, it is uncertain how many patients with primary hyperparathyroidism are truly asymptomatic. Guidelines from a 2002 National Institutes of Health (NIH) Consensus Conference recommend parathyroidectomy for asymptomatic patients unlikely or unwilling to comply with long-term medical follow-up as well as for those with serum calcium concentration 1.0 mg/dL above normal, 24-hour urine calcium excretion greater than 400 mg/d, T-score less than −2.5, age less than 50, or creatinine clearance reduced by more than 30%.[14] A consensus workshop in 2008 noted that many asymptomatic patients have neuropsychiatric symptoms relieved by successful parathyroidectomy (evidence that supports surgical treatment), but acknowledged that further objective study is certainly needed.[13] Imaging studies play no role in the decision for initial parathyroid exploration.

Secondary hyperparathyroidism is diagnosed when an elevation of PTH occurs in response to the metabolic derangements of chronic kidney disease, including hyperphosphatemia, diminished vitamin D production, vitamin D deficiency, and decreased PTH clearance. The majority of cases of secondary hyperparathyroidism are treated medically; when parathyroidectomy is indicated, parathyroid imaging is not routinely performed because bilateral exploration is always performed. Tertiary hyperparathyroidism is thought to occur when the continued physiologic stimulation of secondary hyperparathyroidism causes autonomous function of parathyroid tissue. Tertiary hyperparathyroidism is defined by hypercalcemia and is always associated with a history of renal failure. This condition generally resolves within 12 months of renal transplantation, but uncommonly does not resolve, prompting bilateral parathyroid exploration. Although a single adenoma does occur occasionally in this patient population, in most cases multiglandular disease is present and is treated with subtotal parathyroidectomy, or total parathyroidectomy with autotransplantation.[15] For patients who are poor surgical candidates, image-guided ethanol ablation techniques have been used in the treatment of tertiary hyperparathyroidism.[16,17]

INITIAL SURGICAL APPROACH TO PRIMARY HYPERPARATHYROIDISM

Before the widespread use of minimally invasive approaches, bilateral parathyroid exploration was the gold standard and procedure of choice for all patients undergoing initial surgery. Bilateral exploration is performed through a transverse cervical incision, and involves the identification of all (4 or more) parathyroid glands including those in the most common ectopic sites. When a single or double adenoma is identified, the enlarged gland(s) is/are resected, whereas if multiglandular disease is identified (15%) a subtotal 3.5-gland resection is performed, generally with cryopreservation. When initial bilateral exploration is planned for any reason, preoperative parathyroid imaging is usually not performed as it rarely changes the operative approach. However, thyroid ultrasonography is often helpful in identifying and managing concurrent thyroid disease, which has been found in up to 40% of patients being evaluated for hyperparathyroidism.[18–20]

Over the past 10 to 15 years, the development of several minimally invasive surgical approaches to parathyroidectomy has made preoperative localization imaging studies essential. One 2008 survey of surgeons who perform parathyroidectomy found that only 10% routinely employed bilateral neck exploration compared with 74% of respondents to a similar survey in 1998.[2,21] In selected patients, these focused techniques are reported to have several advantages over the traditional use of routine bilateral exploration, including decreased operative time, shorter incision, faster recovery, shorter hospital stay, and the possible benefit of focused dissection in reducing morbidity should future cervical surgery be necessary for any reason.[5,6,22,23] Unfortunately, parathyroid imaging does not reliably identify or exclude multiglandular disease.[24–26] The use of intraoperative PTH monitoring is well established to produce results equivalent to routine bilateral exploration.[27,28] Based on functional, rather than visual, assessment of operative cure, the use of PTH monitoring facilitates a focused dissection in patients whose intraoperative data suggest a single adenoma, and signals the conversion to bilateral exploration in patients whose intraoperative findings suggest multiglandular disease. In general, parathyroid imaging informs the surgeon where to begin the exploration and intraoperative PTH monitoring lets the surgeon know when to end the operation. Negative parathyroid imaging results do not affect the decision for initial surgery, but do predict a higher likelihood of multiglandular disease.[24]

PARATHYROID REOPERATION

When initial parathyroid exploration fails and reoperation is clinically required, the risks are higher because of the dense scar tissue that forms. This change in the risk to benefit ratio accounts for the very different management strategy of parathyroid reoperation. Surgery is not contemplated unless the patient has major symptoms or pronounced biochemical disease and parathyroid imaging is always performed. Surgery is not offered unless an imaging test is positive (some experts require two concordantly positive studies), and when bilateral imaging findings are present, reoperation is often "staged" to reduce the chances of major morbidity. The goal of initial parathyroidectomy is durable cure, and the costs of reoperation are higher from every standpoint.[29]

PARATHYROID IMAGING

The variability in parathyroid anatomy together with the inability of imaging tests to reliably exclude multiglandular disease prompted the widely quoted statement of NIH radiologist John L. Doppmann, who taught that "the only localization that a patient needs who has primary hyperparathyroidism is the localization of an experienced surgeon!"[30] However, in the era of minimally invasive parathyroid surgery, preoperative imaging is routinely performed to aid both surgical planning and intraoperative dissection. Identification of abnormal ectopic glands or double adenomata can also provide crucial information to increase the chance of curative surgery. Concomitant evaluation of the thyroid gland for nodules that may require thyroidectomy can help to avoid repeat operations in the neck, which can carry an increased risk of morbidities such as permanent hypoparathyroidism and recurrent laryngeal nerve injury.

A combination of modalities—most often cervical ultrasonography and ^{99m}Tc-sestamibi single-photon emission computed tomography (SPECT)—which blends both anatomic and functional information is typically employed to maximize initial curative outcomes. Computed tomography (CT) and magnetic resonance (MR) have been shown to be useful for localizing abnormal parathyroid glands. Nonetheless ultrasonography, despite being operator-dependent, has emerged as the dominant anatomic imaging modality. Combined SPECT/CT offers another approach combining anatomic and functional imaging, but a determination of the incremental utility of this technique beyond combined ultrasonography and sestamibi SPECT awaits further study. In parathyroid reoperation, combined ultrasonography and sestamibi SPECT is still the first-line preoperative imaging evaluation, with CT and MR used as second line modalities for recurrent or persistent hyperparathyroidism given the increased incidence of ectopic and multiple abnormal glands in these cases. Invasive techniques such as selective venous sampling may be useful in the setting of persistent/recurrent primary hyperparathyroidism when noninvasive techniques fail to localize the offending gland or glands. Imaging can also guide diagnostic and therapeutic interventions such as fine-needle aspiration (FNA) for PTH assay to confirm that a nodule is parathyroid tissue as well as to perform ethanol ablation of hyperfunctioning parathyroid glands.

ULTRASONOGRAPHY
Technique

Cervical sonography should be performed with a high-frequency linear transducer (12–15 MHz) whenever possible, though some patients may require a lower frequency transducer for increased depth penetration (**Fig. 2**). The patient should be supine with the neck slightly hyperextended, with a towel or pillow beneath the shoulders. Longitudinal and transverse images should be obtained from the level of the hyoid bone to the clavicles in the craniocaudal direction and from the carotid arteries laterally to the midline. Inferior parathyroid glands located deep to the clavicles may become visible by having the patient swallow during real-time observation. Limited visualization of the superior mediastinum may be possible with a curved or sector probe. Abnormal glands should be measured in 3 dimensions, and their location should be reported with respect to adjacent anatomic landmarks such as the thyroid gland, trachea, esophagus, and so forth.[31] When

possible, the embryologic origin of the enlarged parathyroid gland should also be stated in the report (eg, inferior but deeply positioned glands are most likely descended superior glands whereas more superficial glands in the inferior neck are inferior glands embryologically), as this can aid the surgeon to explore in the appropriate anatomic compartment when the targeted glands are not readily identified.

Color and power Doppler interrogation of suspected parathyroid glands should be used to evaluate vascularity and to look for a feeding artery. Adequate assessment of lesion vascularity requires attention to optimal color Doppler technique, and includes minimizing the color Doppler region of interest to exclude adjacent large vessels such as the jugular vein and carotid artery, choosing an appropriately low pulse repetition frequency or Doppler scale, and increasing color gain to slightly below the level of excessive noise.

The thyroid gland should also be imaged. The size, location, and sonographic features of any nodules should be documented, as suspicious or indeterminate thyroid nodules should be evaluated prior to cervical exploration for concurrent parathyroid disease in order to minimize the need for reoperative surgery in the neck.

Imaging Findings

The majority of parathyroid adenomas appear as discrete oval nodules that are homogeneously hypoechoic relative to the thyroid gland (**Fig. 3**A–D). Less commonly, lesions may be bilobed or multilobulated, particularly in larger glands. Adenomas are

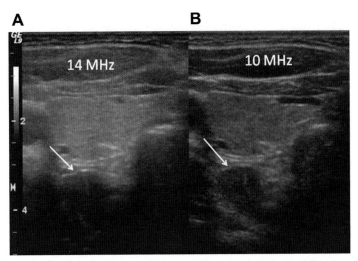

Fig. 2. Transverse sonographic images of a right superior parathyroid adenoma. (*A*) Image obtained with a 14-MHz probe shows diminished acoustic penetration, partially obscuring the enlarged parathyroid gland deep to the thyroid (*arrow*). (*B*) Image obtained with similar orientation using a 10-MHz probe shows better definition of the deeper structures and improves conspicuity of the parathyroid adenoma (*arrow*).

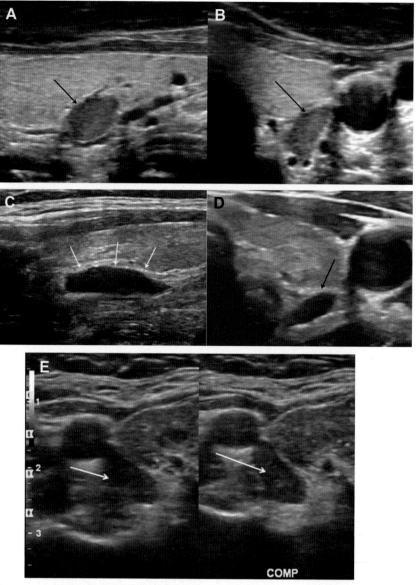

Fig. 3. Typical gray-scale appearance of parathyroid adenomas. (*A, C*) Longitudinal and (*B, D*) transverse sonographic images in two different patients show elongated homogeneously hypoechoic nodules (*black arrows*) deep to the mid-aspect of the left thyroid lobe, a typical sonographic appearance, and location for a superior parathyroid gland. (*C*) Often the echogenic thyroid capsule (*white arrows*) can be identified separating the parathyroid gland from the thyroid. (*E*) Gentle compression over a suspected parathyroid gland can increase the conspicuity of subtle lesions (*arrow*), as a parathyroid adenoma is less compressible than the surrounding soft tissues.

typically discrete from the adjacent thyroid gland, and the echogenic thyroid capsule may be visible separating these structures (see **Fig. 3**C). Parathyroid glands are relatively incompressible compared with their surrounding soft tissue structures, thus graded compression with the ultrasound transducer over suspected lesions or the common

locations of the parathyroid glands may increase the conspicuity of small lesions (see **Fig. 3**E).[32–34]

Normal parathyroid glands are uncommonly seen with ultrasonography, in part due to their small size as well as their isoechogenicity with the thyroid gland (**Fig. 4**). Hyperplastic glands are not consistently visualized because either each

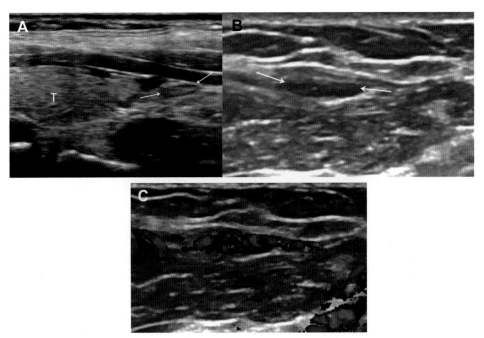

Fig. 4. Pathologically proven normal parathyroid glands. (*A*) 5×3-mm isoechoic nodule (*arrows*) inferior to the left thyroid lobe (T) was subsequently sampled during parathyroid exploration and found to be a normocellular gland. (*B*) Gray-scale and (*C*) color Doppler images of an autotransplanted parathyroid gland into the forearm (*arrows*) showing that the gland is poorly differentiated from surrounding soft tissues other than relative hypervascularity shown with color Doppler interrogation. Normal parathyroid glands are infrequently identified, given their small size and isoechogenicity to surrounding tissues.

individual gland is relatively small or their tissue composition is similar to normal glands (**Fig. 5**).

Color Doppler imaging commonly shows a prominent feeding artery that is typically a branch of the superior or inferior thyroid artery. The artery often courses along the periphery of the gland before penetrating deeper at one of the poles of the gland, leading to what has been described as a vascular arc (**Fig. 6A, B**). Internal vascularity may be visible in larger adenomas and tends to show ramification in the periphery, in contradistinction to typical lymph node vascularity in which a hilar feeding vessel ramifies within the central fatty hilum before coursing peripherally (see **Fig. 6C, D**).[35–37] While not always seen, the identification of a polar feeding vessel has been reported to significantly improve diagnostic accuracy. One prospective study of 98 patients found a polar vessel in 60% of suspected adenomas. Those lesions that showed a feeding vessel were correctly identified 93% of the time, compared with 39% for those lesions where no feeding vessel was identified.[38]

Pitfalls

There are several variants of parathyroid anatomy that can give rise to an atypical imaging appearance (**Fig. 7**). First, cystic degeneration can occur within a parathyroid adenoma in approximately 1% to 2% of cases,[39] giving it a complex cystic morphology, often with a peripheral solid component, or even an entirely cystic appearance (see **Fig. 7A**). Like their solid counterparts, cystic parathyroid adenomas still are found in the typical anatomic locations separate from the thyroid, maintain an elongated oval shape, and may demonstrate a polar feeding vessel with color Doppler flow within the solid components.[40] Small areas of cystic change can be seen within a larger otherwise typical appearing adenoma. Second, although the great majority of parathyroid adenomas are homogeneously hypoechoic relative to the adjacent thyroid gland, larger adenomas can appear more heterogeneous in echogenicity, and can even be hyperechoic. Hyperechogenicity may suggest a parathyroid lipoadenoma—a rare variant of parathyroid adenoma that contains mature adipose tissue within the adenomatous gland (see **Fig. 7B**).[41] Third, the location of certain ectopic parathyroid adenomas may make them impossible to detect using ultrasonography. Mediastinal glands, for example, are obscured by the overlying skeleton and retrotracheal lesions are obscured by air within the trachea. Rarely

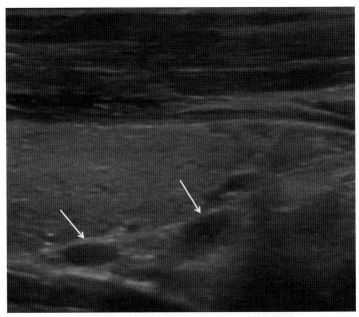

Fig. 5. Parathyroid hyperplasia. Sagittal image of the left lobe showing two small hypoechoic nodules (*arrows*) in the expected location of the parathyroid glands in a patient with chronic renal failure and secondary hyperparathyroidism. A similar finding was identified on the right side (not shown).

(particularly in the setting of previous neck surgery), parathyroid tissue can become disseminated throughout the anterior neck, resulting in a condition known as parathyromatosis. The disseminated nodules of parathyroid tissue may retain tracer at scintigraphy and may appear ultrasonographically as hyperechoic hypervascular cervical nodules. These imaging features may allow for a confident diagnosis in the appropriate clinical setting.[42]

Concurrent thyroid disease can result in several imaging pitfalls as well. Acoustic penetration may be limited in the setting of large multinodular glands, obscuring a parathyroid adenoma positioned deep to the thyroid. In addition, posteriorly positioned and exophytic thyroid nodules can be confused with parathyroid tissue, particularly in cases where the enlarged parathyroid gland is within the thyroid capsule or, more rarely, entirely within the thyroid parenchyma. Color Doppler can be helpful in distinguishing between these entities when an extrathyroidal feeding artery supplying a parathyroid adenoma is identified. Central compartment lymph nodes, which tend to be prominent in the setting of concurrent chronic thyroiditis or thyroid cancer, can also be confused with parathyroid glands (see Fig. 7D). The presence of a prominent fatty hilum and demonstration of hilar vascularity at color Doppler help to distinguish lymph nodes from parathyroid adenomas.

Parathyroid carcinoma is a rare malignancy occurring in fewer than 1% of patients with primary hyperparathyroidism, and can be a challenging diagnosis to make prospectively. Small sonographic series suggest that compared with adenoma, heterogeneity, ill-defined margins, and a taller than wide shape are features suggesting a parathyroid cancer (Fig. 8).[43] Biochemically, parathyroid carcinoma can be associated with markedly elevated serum calcium and PTH levels, but these are by no means always present and in many cases the diagnosis is first made intraoperatively when the surgeon encounters a firm, fibrous, lobulated mass adherent to surrounding structures. When the diagnosis is made preoperatively or intraoperatively, treatment consists of en bloc resection of adherent tissues, including an ipsilateral thyroid lobectomy when appropriate.[44] Given this difference in operative approach, the referring parathyroid surgeon should be urgently alerted when sonographic features suggestive of parathyroid carcinoma are encountered preoperatively.

Effectiveness of Preoperative Parathyroid Localization with Ultrasonography

In recent large series of patients with primary hyperparathyroidism, ultrasound sensitivities for the detection of solitary adenomas ranged from 72% to 89%.[38,45–47] A meta-analysis including 54 studies using ultrasonography for preoperative

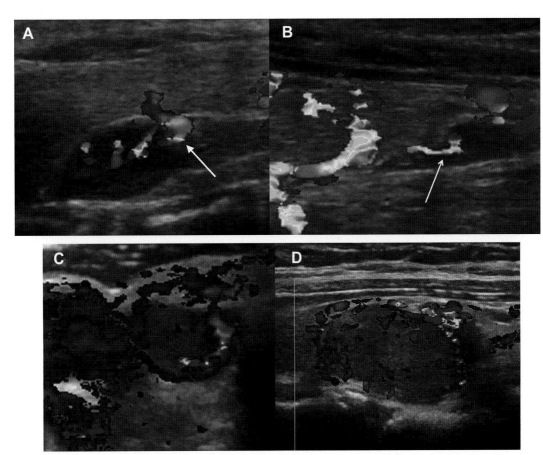

Fig. 6. Color Doppler appearance of parathyroid adenomas. (*A, B*) A prominent feeding vessel (*arrows*), commonly a branch of the inferior thyroidal artery, can commonly be seen feeding a pole of the parathyroid gland. (*C, D*) Feeding vessels may course peripherally before ramifying centrally, in contrast to lymph nodes with vessels feeding the hilum before ramifying peripherally.

parathyroid localization found sensitivities for the detection of solitary adenomas to be 79% (confidence interval [CI] 77–80).[10] In this same meta-analysis, sensitivities for the detection of multiglandular disease were much lower; they were calculated to be 35% for double adenomata and 16% for hyperplasia.[10]

One large prospective study in the surgical literature deserves specific mention, given its unique study design which is unlikely to be replicated given the widespread adoption of focused surgical techniques.[26] The study included 350 patients with primary hyperparathyroidism who underwent preoperative ultrasonography. Initially a focused surgical approach was undertaken based on the ultrasound results, including intraoperative PTH sampling, to resect the abnormal gland or glands and confirm normalization of PTH levels. Then irrespective of these results, a traditional 4-gland exploration was undertaken with pathologic sampling of all 4 parathyroid glands. Given this design, the preoperative imaging findings did not

influence the operation performed, eliminating any selection bias related to imaging findings. Furthermore, the visual evaluation of all parathyroid glands despite a successful focused resection minimized potential false negative imaging results. Using this approach, a preoperative ultrasound scan that suggested a single parathyroid adenoma correctly identified a single abnormal gland at surgery in 74% of patients. Although these results suggest ultrasound sensitivity for the localization of parathyroid adenomas at the lower range of reported values, these findings confirm the utility of ultrasonography in directing focused surgical approaches in the absence of any selection bias that is inherent in retrospective series.

However, even when multiglandular disease is suspected or imaging fails to localize abnormal parathyroid glands, ultrasonography has an important role to play in the management of concurrent thyroid disease. The reported incidence of nodular thyroid disease detected at ultrasonography in patients with concurrent hyperparathyroidism

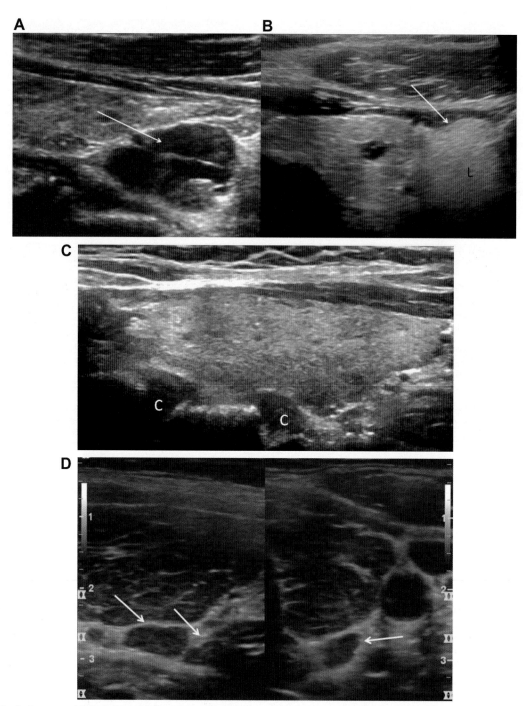

Fig. 7. Sonographic imaging pitfalls. (*A*) Longitudinal sonographic image of a partially cystic inferior parathyroid adenoma (*arrow*). Parathyroid adenomas uncommonly undergo cystic degeneration, resulting in a complex cystic or even entirely cystic morphology. (*B*) Uniformly echogenic nodule (*arrow*) seen lateral to the left thyroid lobe was pathologically proven to be a lipoadenoma (L). (*C*) Hypoechoic nodules deep to the mid and lower poles of the thyroid gland could be mistaken for parathyroid glands, but are shown to be contiguous with the underlying cervical discs (C). (*D*) Longitudinal and transverse views of a heterogeneously hypoechoic thyroid parenchyma with echogenic bands of tissue coursing through it typical for chronic lymphocytic thyroiditis. Prominent central compartment lymph nodes (*arrows*) are commonly seen in this setting, potentially obscuring an underlying parathyroid adenoma.

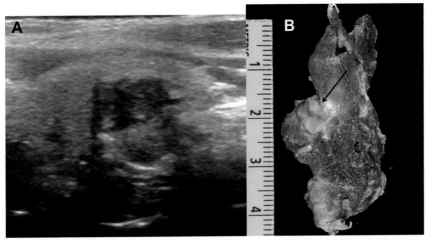

Fig. 8. Parathyroid carcinoma. (*A*) Longitudinal sonographic image of the thyroid shows a heterogeneous nodule with ill-defined borders, which is taller than wide and appears to be entirely intrathyroidal in location. Although sonography is not sensitive for the detection of parathyroid carcinoma, when such features are seen in a suspected parathyroid adenoma the parathyroid surgeon should be alerted, as the appropriate surgical therapy may include en bloc ipsilateral thyroid lobectomy. (*B*) Gross pathologic specimen of the resected thyroid lobe containing an infiltrative and intrathyroidal parathyroid carcinoma (*arrow*).

ranges from 29% to 51% in recent large series.[18–20] The incidence of thyroid malignancy in these same series ranged from 2% to 6%. Preoperative assessment of the thyroid prior to parathyroid exploration spares these patients the need for repeat neck operations and may also avoid unnecessary thyroid surgery. Preoperative thyroid ultrasonography and FNA of indeterminate nodules reduced the need for concomitant thyroid surgery from 30% to 6% in one surgical series.[19]

ULTRASOUND-GUIDED PERCUTANEOUS BIOPSY AND ABLATION

For cases in which sonographic findings are equivocal or discordant with other imaging modalities, ultrasound-guided FNA of a suspected lesion can be performed with an aspirate sent for PTH assay. A parathyroid gland aspirate shows a PTH concentration many orders of magnitude greater than serum concentration. An elevated PTH within the aspirate is highly specific evidence that a lesion is parathyroid in origin and is not a thyroid nodule, lymph node, brown fat, or another lesion that could be confused with a parathyroid gland.[48–50] This technique was 100% specific in one series of 57 sampled lesions, though false-negative results did occur when small glands were sampled.[19] One potential complication of this procedure is the seeding of abnormal parathyroid tissue along the needle tract, resulting in parathyromatosis; however, in one longitudinal study of 81 patients who underwent parathyroid FNA no instance of parathyromatosis was found, with a mean of more than 5 years of follow-up.[51]

PARATHYROID SCINTIGRAPHY
Technique

Technetium-99m sestamibi (^{99m}Tc-sestamibi) is the most commonly used radiotracer for parathyroid scintigraphy. This lipophilic molecule was initially developed as a cardiac imaging agent. It distributes throughout the bloodstream, passively diffuses through cell membranes, and is concentrated within cells with a high concentration of mitochondria, including the myocardium. The normal biodistribution includes the thyroid gland, major salivary glands, heart, and liver. Mild uptake may be seen within the thymus and brown fat. The mitochondrial rich oxyphil cells account for radiotracer uptake within parathyroid tissue, though normal parathyroid glands are typically not detected. Adenomatous and hyperplastic parathyroid tissue show more avid uptake of ^{99m}Tc-sestamibi although initially this activity can be obscured by uptake from the adjacent thyroid gland. Subtraction techniques that use a thyroid agent such as ^{99m}Tc-pertechnitate or ^{123}I coregistered with a ^{99m}Tc-sestamibi image attempt to improve conspicuity of parathyroid tissue by subtracting out the adjacent thyroid uptake.[52,53]

The observation that abnormal parathyroid tissue commonly retains ^{99m}Tc-sestamibi longer than thyroid tissue has led to the widespread use of delayed imaging to improve upon the conspicuity of hyperfunctioning parathyroid tissue. Thus, a commonly used dual-phase single agent protocol includes the intravenous injection of approximately 25 to 30 mCi of ^{99m}Tc-sestamibi followed by early (10–15 minute delay) and delayed (2–3 hours) imaging.[54] Imaging should include the entire neck and chest in order to include potential ectopic parathyroid glands. In patients who have undergone forearm parathyroid autotransplantation (eg, for MEN-1), imaging should also include both forearms. SPECT imaging has been shown to improve detection and localization of hyperfunctioning parathyroid glands as compared with planar imaging, because of an improved ability to discriminate parathyroid tissue uptake from the adjacent thyroid gland.[55–57] Three-dimensional (3-D) SPECT images may be particularly helpful in presurgical planning, and rotating 3-D images are often a useful reference during parathyroid exploration.

Imaging Findings

Detection and localization of abnormal parathyroid tissue depends on both the anatomic location, particularly with respect to the thyroid gland, and the degree of radiotracer uptake and retention. Early-phase uptake of radiotracer within abnormal parathyroid tissue is typically similar to that of the thyroid gland but can also be hyperintense relative to the thyroid gland. In cases where uptake within the parathyroid tissue is isointense to the thyroid on the early images, lesion detection depends on the observation of a focus of activity separate from the thyroid gland, or a bulge or asymmetry of the thyroid contour in cases where the parathyroid tissue is contiguous with the thyroid gland.[58] Differential washout of radiotracer between the parathyroid and thyroid tissue, with retention of contrast within the parathyroid tissue, can increase the conspicuity of parathyroid lesions on the delayed images (see **Fig. 8**A). Correlation with extrathyroidal uptake or thyroid gland asymmetries seen on the early-phase images can improve diagnostic confidence. However, the degree of radiotracer retention within abnormal parathyroid tissue is variable and can show rapid washout in which early-phase uptake is not detectable on the delayed imaging (see **Fig. 8**B).[55,58] Thus, while a focus of extrathyroidal delayed-phase radiotracer uptake has a high probability of representing abnormal parathyroid tissue in a patient with hyperparathyroidism, the lack of radiotracer retention within a lesion detected in the early

phase should not be used as evidence to dismiss such a finding.

Pitfalls

Common causes of false-positive studies include ^{99m}Tc-sestamibi uptake within a thyroid adenoma, a multinodular goiter, lymph node, or even in ectopic thyroid tissue (**Fig. 9**A, B). Even when uptake is clearly shown to be positioned within the thyroid gland, abnormal parathyroid tissue cannot be excluded on the basis of the scintigraphic imaging alone, as rarely a parathyroid adenoma can be intrathyroidal.[59,60] In these cases, correlation with cervical ultrasonography may better characterize such lesions as thyroid or parathyroid in origin. The most common cause of false-positive sestamibi uptake is within a thyroid nodule; follicular adenomas and carcinomas, colloid nodules, and Hürthle cell lesions may all selectively take up tracer (see **Fig. 9**).[61] Multiple case reports describe an array of other potential conditions that may lead to false-positive sestamibi studies including metastases from a variety of tumors, uptake within remnant thymus, brown fat, and reactive lymph nodes (see **Fig. 9**C).[62–66] Physiologic uptake within normal structures such as the submandibular glands can also confound an accurate diagnosis in the setting of ectopic parathyroid glands positioned high within the anterior neck. Activity within the adjacent submandibular gland has reportedly obscured ectopic parathyroid glands, while asymmetric submandibular gland uptake can lead to a false-positive diagnosis of an ectopic parathyroid gland.[67,68]

False-negative studies can occur with early washout of ^{99m}Tc-sestamibi from abnormal parathyroid tissue as already described (**Fig. 10**B). In these cases, lesion detection relies on the ability to discriminate early parathyroid uptake from the adjacent thyroid gland. Particularly in instances where no abnormal uptake is identified on the delayed images, any asymmetry or contour bulge detected on the early images should be reported both to alert the surgeon to the potential for an abnormal parathyroid gland in these locations and to focus attention on these areas during cervical sonography. False-negative studies are more common in the setting of parathyroid hyperplasia as well as double adenomata[24,47,69]; this has been postulated to be a consequence of the decreased volume of parathyroid tissue in the individual glands of multiglandular disease. Several factors may also contribute to the decreased sensitivity of sestamibi SPECT for the detection of double adenomas, including differential uptake and retention of radiotracer within the abnormal

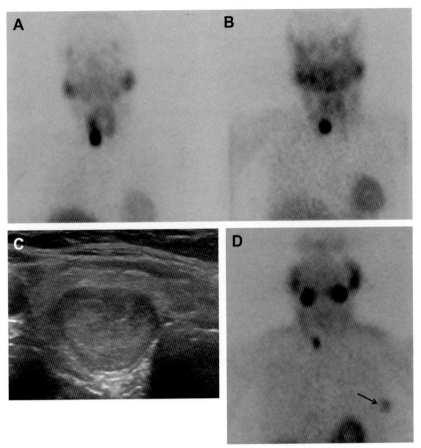

Fig. 9. False-positive sestamibi SPECT. (*A*) Early sestamibi SPECT image showing intense radiotracer in the right neck, which persists on the delayed (*B*) image, a typical appearance for a parathyroid adenoma. Correlation with sonography (*C*) reveals a solid isoechoic thyroid nodule found to be a Hürthle cell lesion at resection. (*D*) Delayed sestamibi SPECT image in a separate patient, which shows retention of radiotracer in the inferior right neck consistent with a parathyroid adenoma but also with a focus of retained activity in the left breast (*arrow*), which was subsequently found to be a breast carcinoma.

gland or confusion of multifocal uptake for activity within a multinodular goiter.[60,61]

Effectiveness of Sestamibi Scintigraphy for Preoperative Parathyroid Localization

Recent series using preoperative ^{99m}Tc-sestamibi SPECT in the setting of primary hyperparathyroidism report sensitivities for the detection of solitary adenomas that range from 68% to 95%; this range is similar to that reported for sonography alone.[26,70–72] The meta-analysis of Ruda and colleagues[10] included 96 studies using sestamibi scintigraphy in the setting of primary hyperparathyroidism, and calculated a sensitivity of 88% (CI 87–89) for detection of solitary adenomas. On the other hand, the sensitivities for the detection of multiglandular disease were relatively low;

sensitivities were calculated to be 44% (CI 41–48) for hyperplasia and 30% (CI 2–62) for double adenomata.

COMBINED IMAGING APPROACH FOR PRIMARY HYPERPARATHYROIDISM

Preoperative parathyroid localization with a combination of the functional data of scintigraphy combined with anatomic information of sonography more accurately predicts the presence and location of solitary adenomas than either technique alone.[10,26,45,73] Suspected lesions within the neck seen with sestamibi can be further localized anatomically with ultrasonography, and pitfalls including sestamibi uptake within thyroid nodules and early washout from parathyroid adenomas can be avoided by correlation with

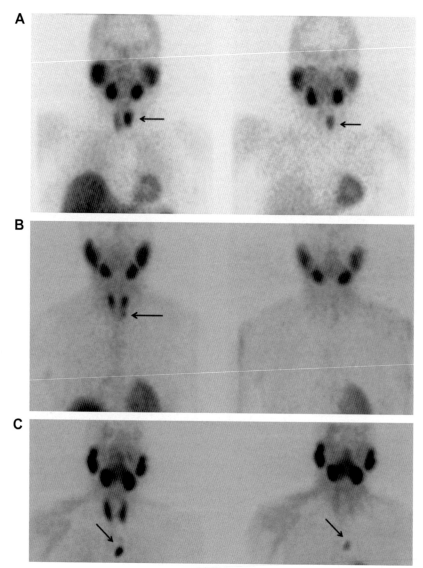

Fig. 10. Sestamibi SPECT of parathyroid adenoma. (*A*) Early (*left*) and delayed (*right*) 3-D sestamibi SPECT images show early focal uptake overlying the midpole of the left thyroid lobe that persists on delayed imaging (*arrows*), a typical appearance for a parathyroid adenoma. (*B*) A focus of radiotracer uptake (*arrow*) inferior to the lower pole of the left lobe does not clearly persist on delayed imaging, an example of early washout from a left inferior parathyroid adenoma. (*C*) Both early (*left*) and delayed (*right*) images show intense radiotracer uptake within the mediastinum (*arrows*), indicating an ectopic mediastinal parathyroid adenoma.

ultrasound images. Several of the largest series report combined sensitivities of scintigraphy and ultrasonography ranging from 74% to 95% compared with 74% to 80% for ultrasonography alone and 68% to 87% for scintigraphy alone.[26,45,73] Using this combined approach to guide focused parathyroid resections, cure rates are greater than 95% and are very similar to the high cure rates of traditional bilateral parathyroid exploration. A recent survey of surgeons confirms the widespread use of this combined approach, with 62% of surgeons routinely obtaining preoperative sestamibi and cervical ultrasound studies compared with 2% performing ultrasonography alone and 26% obtaining only sestamibi imaging.[2] Scintigraphy also has a clear advantage over ultrasonography in the detection of the rare ectopic gland within the mediastinum (see **Fig. 10**C).

The combined imaging approach is not sufficiently accurate for the detection of multiglandular disease to facilitate a focused operative approach in many cases. Although there is incremental improvement in the detection of multiglandular disease when both techniques are combined, one study found that multiglandular disease was only correctly predicted 30% of the time, whereas for 30% of patients subsequently found to have multiglandular disease preoperative imaging studies only identified a single adenoma.[74] Similarly, a study of double adenomata observed a sensitivity of 60% when both techniques were used together.[69] Thus even when imaging studies appear concordant for a single adenoma, surgeons cannot rely solely on imaging to exclude the presence of multiglandular disease. This caveat highlights the importance of both surgical experience and the use of intraoperative PTH assay to achieve cure when a selective surgical approach is used.

COMPUTED TOMOGRAPHY

Contrast-enhanced CT (CECT) can be used to detect abnormal parathyroid glands. Lesion conspicuity is increased by the intense enhancement of the lesions. The small size of most parathyroid adenomas relative to the field of view of CT can make further characterization difficult, but an avidly enhancing soft tissue nodule in a characteristic location in a patient with primary hyperparathyroidism should raise the index of suspicion (**Fig. 11**). Sensitivities of CECT for the detection of a single parathyroid adenoma range from 46% to 87%.[75] As with sestamibi SPECT, one advantage of CT is the ability to image the entire neck and mediastinum with a single modality that evaluates all potential locations of ectopic glands. Despite this presumed advantage, studies that have combined sonography and CT for preoperative localization purposes show only

a small improvement in sensitivity over ultrasonography alone. This finding is not unexpected, given the rarity of ectopic mediastinal parathyroid adenomas (approximately 1 per 1000).[76–78] Thus, CECT is typically reserved for localization in patients requiring parathyroid reoperation as well as for confirmation of ectopic glands identified by parathyroid scintigraphy.

COMBINED SPECT/CT

SPECT/CT scanning offers the ability to coregister functional scintigraphic data with anatomic imaging, with an aim toward improving lesion detection and more precise anatomic localization. The protocol for ^{99m}Tc-sestamibi SPECT imaging is the same, but additional CT acquisitions are obtained following both the early and delayed SPECT images. The image quality of the CT examination is inferior to that of a diagnostic neck CT performed on a dedicated multidetector CT scanner because of the low tube current and long acquisition times (approximately 10 minutes). These technical limitations preclude the use of intravenous contrast, but CT still provides additional anatomic detail helpful in lesion localization. SPECT and CT images can be viewed separately and be coregistered to form fused images (**Fig. 12**). CT data can also be used for attenuation correction of the SPECT images. Imaging pitfalls unique to SPECT/CT include patient motion leading to misregistration of the SPECT and CT images, as well as attenuation correction artifacts that could result from surgical clips or densely calcified structures such as thyroid nodules and lymph nodes.

Initial reports using SPECT/CT confirm that the addition of CT imaging improves the anatomic localization of SPECT abnormalities, particularly in patients with ectopic glands or distorted anatomy. Reported sensitivities range from 88%

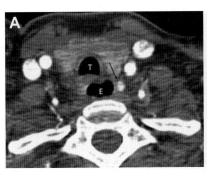
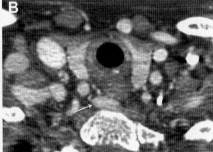

Fig. 11. Contrast-enhanced CT (CECT) of parathyroid adenomas. (*A*) Axial CECT image shows a small but briskly enhancing parathyroid adenoma (*arrow*) deep to the mid-left thyroid lobe. T, trachea; E, esophagus. (*B*) Axial CECT of a retroesophageal parathyroid adenoma (*arrow*), a location typically obscured with cervical sonography.

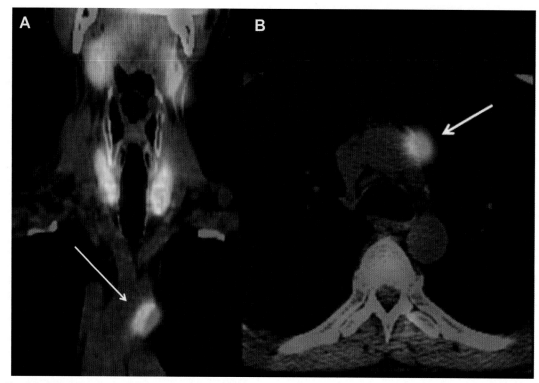

Fig. 12. SPECT/CT. Coronal (*A*) and axial (*B*) fused SPECT/CT images show an ectopic mediastinal parathyroid adenoma (*arrows*) clearly localized to the prevascular space.

to 93%.[79–87] Several earlier reports also suggested that improved detection of single normotopic parathyroid adenoma by the addition of CT may be minimal, but the ability to more precisely localize detected lesions improves.[80,81,83] More recent reports suggest that the incremental benefit of SPECT/CT over SPECT alone may be greater in patients with multinodular goiter or multiglandular disease.[85,87] The incremental utility of SPECT/CT over the commonly used combined imaging approach of ultrasonography and sestamibi SPECT has not been determined. Further study will be required before consensus is reached on the appropriate role of SPECT/CT in routine preoperative imaging prior to initial parathyroid surgery.

MAGNETIC RESONANCE

Cervical MR imaging provides similar sensitivity to other imaging techniques for the detection of normotopic parathyroid adenoma.[88,89] As with CT, the limited availability and increased cost of MR relative to cervical ultrasonography has decreased its clinical utility. The authors tend to use MR (and CT) at their institution solely in patients with an imaging-occult source of persistent or recurrent hyperparathyroidism.

MR imaging of the anterior neck is generally performed from the skull base through the sternal notch, often using an anterior surface coil. T1-weighted and T2-weighted fast spin-echo sequences are obtained in at least 2 imaging planes. Gadolinium-enhanced T1-weighted images can increase the sensitivity for detection of parathyroid adenomas, particularly in cases in which the T1 and T2 characteristics are not typical.

The MR signal characteristics of parathyroid tissue vary depending on the histology of the gland.[90] Most commonly, parathyroid adenomas are T2 hyperintense and T1 iso- to hypointense relative to skeletal muscle (**Fig. 13**). However, subacute hemorrhage into parathyroid parenchyma can result in T1 hyperintensity. Fibrosis and chronic hemorrhage can diminish the T2 signal and cause lesions to appear isointense or hypointense. Contrast enhancement can improve detection of abnormal parathyroid tissue in instances where the MR signal characteristics are not typical, but may not increase the sensitivity for the typical cases in which lesions are T2 hyperintense.[89]

With MR, the most significant pitfall lies in the differentiation of parathyroid adenomas from cervical lymph nodes, as both entities have similar signal characteristics. As with CT and

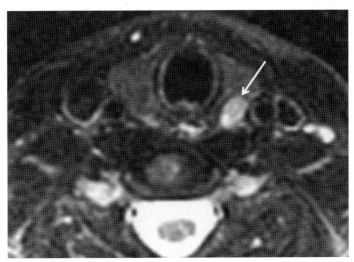

Fig. 13. MR of parathyroid adenoma. T2-weighted axial image of the neck at the level of the mid-thyroid gland shows a typical T2-hyperintense superior parathyroid adenoma (*arrow*).

ultrasonography, an accurate MR diagnosis depends on clinical context and a knowledge of the typical locations and morphology of enlarged parathyroid glands.

VENOUS SAMPLING

Most cases of primary hyperparathyroidism are cured (>95%) with selective parathyroid exploration guided by preoperative localization studies or bilateral 4-gland exploration. However, for the small group of patients with recurrent or persistent hyperparathyroidism in whom additional imaging fails to identify the abnormal parathyroid tissue, venous sampling is an additional technique shown to be effective in localization.[91,92] The principle of the technique involves the collection of venous blood samples from a catheter positioned in multiple veins within the neck and mediastinum. Measurement of PTH concentrations within the samples should reveal a gradient emanating from the vein closest to the abnormal parathyroid gland; such a gradient focuses the area for reexploration. By the same principle, intraoperative internal jugular venous sampling with rapid PTH assay has been used by some endocrine surgeons to help lateralize an abnormal parathyroid gland during surgery.[93,94]

SUMMARY

Radiologists interpreting parathyroid imaging studies should be familiar with the anatomy, embryology, and pathophysiology of the parathyroid glands, and should understand the role that imaging may play for patient management. The goal is to identify and localize any and all abnormal parathyroid tissue to provide the surgeon with the necessary information with which to plan the operative approach in minimally invasive parathyroidectomy. A combined imaging approach that includes both anatomic and functional studies, most commonly cervical ultrasonography and sestamibi SPECT, is currently used by the majority of surgeons for preoperative localization in the setting of initial surgery for primary hyperparathyroidism. Such an approach is sufficient in the large majority of cases. Negative imaging does not obviate initial parathyroid exploration but it does predict a higher likelihood of multiglandular disease. Other imaging modalities such as CT, MR, and selective venous sampling are not routinely used in the preoperative setting but have a role in the evaluation of persistent or recurrent hyperparathyroidism requiring reoperation. The utility of SPECT/CT for parathyroid localization has been demonstrated in initial studies, but the appropriate routine use in primary hyperparathyroidism awaits further research.

REFERENCES

1. Lew JI, Solorzano CC. Surgical management of primary hyperparathyroidism: state of the art. Surg Clin North Am 2009;89(5):1205–25.
2. Greene AB, Butler RS, McIntyre S, et al. National trends in parathyroid surgery from 1998 to 2008: a decade of change. J Am Coll Surg 2009;209(3): 332–43.

3. Grant CS, Thompson G, Farley D, et al. Primary hyperparathyroidism surgical management since the introduction of minimally invasive parathyroidectomy: Mayo Clinic experience. Arch Surg 2005; 140(5):472–8 [discussion: 478–9].

4. Udelsman R. Six hundred fifty-six consecutive explorations for primary hyperparathyroidism. Ann Surg 2002;235(5):665–70 [discussion: 670–2].

5. Udelsman R, Donovan PI, Sokoll LJ. One hundred consecutive minimally invasive parathyroid explorations. Ann Surg 2000;232(3):331–9.

6. Burkey SH, Snyder WH 3rd, Nwariaku F, et al. Directed parathyroidectomy: feasibility and performance in 100 consecutive patients with primary hyperparathyroidism. Arch Surg 2003;138(6):604–8 [discussion: 608–9].

7. Akerstrom G, Malmaeus J, Bergstrom R. Surgical anatomy of human parathyroid glands. Surgery 1984;95(1):14–21.

8. Wang C. The anatomic basis of parathyroid surgery. Ann Surg 1976;183(3):271–5.

9. Grimelius L, Bondeson L. Histopathological diagnosis of parathyroid diseases. Pathol Res Pract 1995;191(4):353–65.

10. Ruda JM, Hollenbeak CS, Stack BC Jr. A systematic review of the diagnosis and treatment of primary hyperparathyroidism from 1995 to 2003. Otolaryngol Head Neck Surg 2005;132(3):359–72.

11. Yip L, Ogilvie JB, Challinor SM, et al. Identification of multiple endocrine neoplasia type 1 in patients with apparent sporadic primary hyperparathyroidism. Surgery 2008;144(6):1002–6 [discussion: 1006–7].

12. Fraser WD. Hyperparathyroidism. Lancet 2009; 374(9684):145–58.

13. Udelsman R, Pasieka JL, Sturgeon C, et al. Surgery for asymptomatic primary hyperparathyroidism: proceedings of the Third International Workshop. J Clin Endocrinol Metab 2009;94(2):366–72.

14. Bilezikian JP, Potts JT Jr, Fuleihan Gel H, et al. Summary statement from a workshop on asymptomatic primary hyperparathyroidism: a perspective for the 21st century. J Clin Endocrinol Metab 2002; 87(12):5353–61.

15. Pitt SC, Sippel RS, Chen H. Secondary and tertiary hyperparathyroidism, state of the art surgical management. Surg Clin North Am 2009;89(5):1227–39.

16. Schamp S, Dunser E, Schuster H, et al. Ultrasound-guided percutaneous ethanol ablation of parathyroid hyperplasia: preliminary experience in patients on chronic dialysis. Ultraschall Med 2004;25(2):131–6.

17. Cintin C, Karstrup S, Ladefoged SD, et al. Tertiary hyperparathyroidism treated by ultrasonically guided percutaneous fine-needle ethanol injection. Nephron 1994;68(2):217–20.

18. Morita SY, Somervell H, Umbricht CB, et al. Evaluation for concomitant thyroid nodules and primary hyperparathyroidism in patients undergoing parathyroidectomy or thyroidectomy. Surgery 2008; 144(6):862–6 [discussion: 866–8].

19. Milas M, Mensah A, Alghoul M, et al. The impact of office neck ultrasonography on reducing unnecessary thyroid surgery in patients undergoing parathyroidectomy. Thyroid 2005;15(9):1055–9.

20. Adler JT, Chen H, Schaefer S, et al. Does routine use of ultrasound result in additional thyroid procedures in patients with primary hyperparathyroidism? J Am Coll Surg 2010;211(4):536–9.

21. Sosa JA, Powe NR, Levine MA, et al. Profile of a clinical practice: thresholds for surgery and surgical outcomes for patients with primary hyperparathyroidism: a national survey of endocrine surgeons. J Clin Endocrinol Metab 1998;83(8):2658–65.

22. Bergenfelz A, Lindblom P, Tibblin S, et al. Unilateral versus bilateral neck exploration for primary hyperparathyroidism: a prospective randomized controlled trial. Ann Surg 2002;236(5):543–51.

23. Baliski C, Stewart J, Anderson D, et al. Selective unilateral parathyroid exploration: an effective treatment for primary hyperparathyroidism. Am J Surg 2005;189(5):596–600.

24. Yip L, Pryma DA, Yim JH, et al. Can a lightbulb sestamibi SPECT accurately predict single-gland disease in sporadic primary hyperparathyroidism? World J Surg 2008;32(5):784–92 [discussion: 793–4].

25. Carty SE, Worsey J, Virji MA, et al. Concise parathyroidectomy: the impact of preoperative SPECT ^{99m}Tc sestamibi scanning and intraoperative quick parathormone assay. Surgery 1997;122(6):1107–14 [discussion: 1114–6].

26. Siperstein A, Berber E, Mackey R, et al. Prospective evaluation of sestamibi scan, ultrasonography, and rapid PTH to predict the success of limited exploration for sporadic primary hyperparathyroidism. Surgery 2004;136(4):872–80.

27. Dralle H, Lorenz K, Nguyen-Thanh P. Minimally invasive video-assisted parathyroidectomy–selective approach to localized single gland adenoma. Langenbecks Arch Surg 1999;384(6):556–62.

28. Henry JF, Defechereux T, Gramatica L, et al. Minimally invasive videoscopic parathyroidectomy by lateral approach. Langenbecks Arch Surg 1999; 384(3):298–301.

29. Doherty GM, Weber B, Norton JA. Cost of unsuccessful surgery for primary hyperparathyroidism. Surgery 1994;116(6):954–7 [discussion: 957–8].

30. Brennan MF. Lessons learned. Ann Surg Oncol 2006;13(10):1322–8.

31. American Institute of Ultrasound in Medicine. AIUM Practice Guideline for the performance of thyroid and parathyroid ultrasound examination. J Ultrasound Med 2003;22(10):1126–30.

32. Reading CC, Charboneau JW, James EM, et al. High-resolution parathyroid sonography. AJR Am J Roentgenol 1982;139(3):539–46.

33. Kamaya A, Quon A, Jeffrey RB. Sonography of the abnormal parathyroid gland. Ultrasound Q 2006; 22(4):253–62.

34. Simeone JF, Mueller PR, Ferrucci JT Jr, et al. High-resolution real-time sonography of the parathyroid. Radiology 1981;141(3):745–51.

35. Wolf RJ, Cronan JJ, Monchik JM. Color Doppler sonography: an adjunctive technique in assessment of parathyroid adenomas. J Ultrasound Med 1994; 13(4):303–8.

36. Lane MJ, Desser TS, Weigel RJ, et al. Use of color and power Doppler sonography to identify feeding arteries associated with parathyroid adenomas. AJR Am J Roentgenol 1998;171(3):819–23.

37. Reeder SB, Desser TS, Weigel RJ, et al. Sonography in primary hyperparathyroidism: review with emphasis on scanning technique. J Ultrasound Med 2002;21(5):539–52 [quiz: 553–4].

38. Rickes S, Sitzy J, Neye H, et al. High-resolution ultrasound in combination with colour-Doppler sonography for preoperative localization of parathyroid adenomas in patients with primary hyperparathyroidism. Ultraschall Med 2003;24(2):85–9.

39. McCoy KL, Yim JH, Zuckerbraun BS, et al. Cystic parathyroid lesions: functional and nonfunctional parathyroid cysts. Arch Surg 2009;144(1):52–6 [discussion: 56].

40. Johnson NA, Yip L, Tublin ME. Cystic parathyroid adenoma: sonographic features and correlation with 99mTc-sestamibi SPECT findings. AJR Am J Roentgenol 2010;195(6):1385–90.

41. Turner WJ, Baergen RN, Pellitteri PK, et al. Parathyroid lipoadenoma: case report and review of the literature. Otolaryngol Head Neck Surg 1996;114(2): 313–6.

42. Tublin ME, Yim JH, Carty SE. Recurrent hyperparathyroidism secondary to parathyromatosis: clinical and imaging findings. J Ultrasound Med 2007; 26(6):847–51.

43. Hara H, Igarashi A, Yano Y, et al. Ultrasonographic features of parathyroid carcinoma. Endocr J 2001; 48(2):213–7.

44. Dudney WC, Bodenner D, Stack BC Jr. Parathyroid carcinoma. Otolaryngol Clin North Am 2010;43(2): 441–53, xi.

45. Solorzano CC, Carneiro-Pla DM, Irvin GL. Surgeon-performed ultrasonography as the initial and only localizing study in sporadic primary hyperparathyroidism. J Am Coll Surg 2006;202(1):18–24.

46. Haber RS, Kim CK, Inabnet WB. Ultrasonography for preoperative localization of enlarged parathyroid glands in primary hyperparathyroidism: comparison with (99m)technetium sestamibi scintigraphy. Clin Endocrinol 2002;57(2):241–9.

47. Tublin ME, Pryma DA, Yim JH, et al. Localization of parathyroid adenomas by sonography and technetium Tc 99m sestamibi single-photon emission

computed tomography before minimally invasive parathyroidectomy: are both studies really needed? J Ultrasound Med 2009;28(2):183–90.

48. Gooding GA, Clark OH, Stark DD, et al. Parathyroid aspiration biopsy under ultrasound guidance in the postoperative hyperparathyroid patient. Radiology 1985;155(1):193–6.

49. Sacks BA, Pallotta JA, Cole A, et al. Diagnosis of parathyroid adenomas: efficacy of measuring para-thormone levels in needle aspirates of cervical masses. AJR Am J Roentgenol 1994;163(5):1223–6.

50. Stephen AE, Milas M, Garner CN, et al. Use of surgeon-performed office ultrasound and parathyroid fine needle aspiration for complex parathyroid localization. Surgery 2005;138(6):1143–50 [discussion: 1150–1].

51. Kendrick ML, Charboneau JW, Curlee KJ, et al. Risk of parathyromatosis after fine-needle aspiration. Am Surg 2001;67(3):290–3 [discussion: 293–4].

52. Neumann DR, Esselstyn CB Jr, Go RT, et al. Comparison of double-phase ^{99m}Tc-sestamibi with ^{123}I-^{99m}Tc-sestamibi subtraction SPECT in hyperparathyroidism. AJR Am J Roentgenol 1997;169(6): 1671–4.

53. Bergenfelz A, Tennvall J, Valdermarsson S, et al. Sestamibi versus thallium subtraction scintigraphy in parathyroid localization: a prospective comparative study in patients with predominantly mild primary hyperparathyroidism. Surgery 1997;121(6): 601–5.

54. Taillefer R, Boucher Y, Potvin C, et al. Detection and localization of parathyroid adenomas in patients with hyperparathyroidism using a single radionuclide imaging procedure with technetium-99m-sestamibi (double-phase study). J Nucl Med 1992;33(10): 1801–7.

55. Lorberboym M, Minski I, Macadziob S, et al. Incremental diagnostic value of preoperative ^{99m}Tc-MIBI SPECT in patients with a parathyroid adenoma. J Nucl Med 2003;44(6):904–8.

56. Spanu A, Falchi A, Manca A, et al. The usefulness of neck pinhole SPECT as a complementary tool to planar scintigraphy in primary and secondary hyperparathyroidism. J Nucl Med 2004;45(1):40–8.

57. Slater A, Gleeson FV. Increased sensitivity and confidence of SPECT over planar imaging in dual-phase sestamibi for parathyroid adenoma detection. Clin Nucl Med 2005;30(1):1–3.

58. Bajoghli M, Muthukrishnan A, Mountz JM. Posterior bulge sign for parathyroid adenoma on Tc-99m MIBI SPECT. Clin Nucl Med 2006;31(8):470–1.

59. Yusim A, Aspelund G, Ahrens W, et al. Intrathyroidal parathyroid adenoma. Thyroid 2006;16(6):619–20.

60. McIntyre RC Jr, Eisenach JH, Pearlman NW, et al. Intrathyroidal parathyroid glands can be a cause of failed cervical exploration for hyperparathyroidism. Am J Surg 1997;174(6):750–3 [discussion: 753–4].

61. McBiles M, Lambert AT, Cote MG, et al. Sestamibi parathyroid imaging. Semin Nucl Med 1995;25(3): 221–34.

62. Wong KK, Brown RK, Avram AM. Potential false positive Tc-99m sestamibi parathyroid study due to uptake in brown adipose tissue. Clin Nucl Med 2008;33(5):346–8.

63. Taillefer R, Robidoux A, Lambert R, et al. Technetium-99m-sestamibi prone scintimammography to detect primary breast cancer and axillary lymph node involvement. J Nucl Med 1995;36(10):1758–65.

64. Yen TC, Tzen KY, Lee CM, et al. Squamous cell carcinoma of the lung mimicking an ectopic mediastinal parathyroid adenoma demonstrated by Tc-99m sestamibi in a hypercalcemic patient. Clin Nucl Med 1999;24(11):895–6.

65. Mudun A, Kocak M, Unal S, et al. Tc-99m MIBI accumulation in remnant thymus. A cause of false-positive interpretation in parathyroid imaging. Clin Nucl Med 1995;20(4):379–80.

66. Leslie WD, Riese KT, Mohamed C. Sestamibi retention in reactive lymph node hyperplasia: a cause of false-positive parathyroid localization. Clin Nucl Med 2000;25(3):216–7.

67. Dam HQ, Intenzo CM, Kairys JC. Supernumerary parathyroid tissue hidden by high uptake in the submandibular gland. Clin Nucl Med 2002;27(12): 893–4.

68. Campeau RJ, Reuther WL, Wayne J. False-positive Tc-99m sestamibi examination for parathyroid adenoma in a case of asymmetrical salivary gland enlargement. Clin Nucl Med 1999;24(9):723–4.

69. Haciyanli M, Lal G, Morita E, et al. Accuracy of preoperative localization studies and intraoperative parathyroid hormone assay in patients with primary hyperparathyroidism and double adenoma. J Am Coll Surg 2003;197(5):739–46.

70. Civelek A, Ozalp E, Donovan P, et al. Prospective evaluation of delayed technetium-99m sestamibi SPECT scintigraphy for preoperative localization of primary hyperparathyroidism. Surgery 2002;131(2): 149–57.

71. Moka D. Technetium 99m-MIBI-SPECT: a highly sensitive diagnostic tool for localization of parathyroid adenomas. Surgery 2000;128(1):29–35.

72. Nichols KJ, Tomas MB, Tronco GG, et al. Preoperative parathyroid scintigraphic lesion localization: accuracy of various types of readings. Radiology 2008;248(1):221–32.

73. Lumachi F, Zucchetta P, Marzola MC, et al. Advantages of combined technetium-99m-sestamibi scintigraphy and high-resolution ultrasonography in parathyroid localization: comparative study in 91 patients with primary hyperparathyroidism. Eur J Endocrinol 2000;143(6):755–60.

74. Sugg SL, Krzywda EA, Demeure MJ, et al. Detection of multiple gland primary hyperparathyroidism in the era of minimally invasive parathyroidectomy. Surgery 2004;136(6):1303–9.

75. Gotway MB, Higgins CB. MR imaging of the thyroid and parathyroid glands. Magn Reson Imaging Clin N Am 2000;8(1):163–82, ix.

76. van Dalen A, Smit CP, van Vroonhoven TJ, et al. Minimally invasive surgery for solitary parathyroid adenomas in patients with primary hyperparathyroidism: role of US with supplemental CT. Radiology 2001;220(3):631–9.

77. Spieth ME, Gough J, Kasner DL. Role of US with supplemental CT for localization of parathyroid adenomas. Radiology 2002;223(3):878–9 [author reply: 879].

78. Gross ND, Weissman JL, Veenker E, et al. The diagnostic utility of computed tomography for preoperative localization in surgery for hyperparathyroidism. Laryngoscope 2004;114(2):227–31.

79. Clark PB, Perrier ND, Morton KA. Detection of an intrathymic parathyroid adenoma using single-photon emission CT 99mTc sestamibi scintigraphy and CT. AJR Am J Roentgenol 2005;184(Suppl 3):S16–8.

80. Krausz Y, Bettman L, Guralnik L, et al. Technetium-99m-MIBI SPECT/CT in primary hyperparathyroidism. World J Surg 2006;30(1):76–83.

81. Gayed IW, Kim EE, Broussard WF, et al. The value of 99mTc-sestamibi SPECT/CT over conventional SPECT in the evaluation of parathyroid adenomas or hyperplasia. J Nucl Med 2005;46(2):248–52.

82. Papathanassiou D, Flament JB, Pochart JM, et al. SPECT/CT in localization of parathyroid adenoma or hyperplasia in patients with previous neck surgery. Clin Nucl Med 2008;33(6):394–7.

83. Prommegger R, Wimmer G, Profanter C, et al. Virtual neck exploration. Ann Surg 2009;250(5):761–5.

84. Wimmer G, Bale R, Kovacs P, et al. Virtual neck exploration in patients with hyperparathyroidism and former cervical operations. Langenbecks Arch Surg 2008;393(5):687–92.

85. Pata G, Casella C, Besuzio S, et al. Clinical appraisal of 99mTechnetium-sestamibi SPECT/CT compared to conventional SPECT in patients with primary hyperparathyroidism and concomitant nodular goiter. Thyroid 2010;20(10):1121–7.

86. Roach PJ, Schembri GP, Ho Shon IA, et al. SPECT/CT imaging using a spiral CT scanner for anatomical localization: impact on diagnostic accuracy and reporter confidence in clinical practice. Nucl Med Commun 2006;27(12):977–87.

87. Wimmer G, Profanter C, Kovacs P, et al. CT-MIBI-SPECT image fusion predicts multiglandular disease in hyperparathyroidism. Langenbecks Arch Surg 2010;395(1):73–80.

88. McDermott VG, Fernandez RJ, Meakem TJ 3rd, et al. Preoperative MR imaging in hyperparathyroidism: results and factors affecting parathyroid detection. AJR Am J Roentgenol 1996;166(3):705–10.

89. Lopez Hanninen E, Vogl TJ, Steinmuller T, et al. Preoperative contrast-enhanced MRI of the parathyroid glands in hyperparathyroidism. Invest Radiol 2000;35(7):426–30.

90. Gotway MB, Reddy GP, Webb WR, et al. Comparison between MR imaging and ^{99m}Tc MIBI scintigraphy in the evaluation of recurrent of persistent hyperparathyroidism. Radiology 2001;218(3):783–90.

91. Reidel M, Schilling T, Graf S, et al. Localization of hyperfunctioning parathyroid glands by selective venous sampling in reoperation for primary or secondary hyperparathyroidism. Surgery 2006; 140(6):907–13.

92. Ogilvie CM, Brown PL, Matson M, et al. Selective parathyroid venous sampling in patients with complicated hyperparathyroidism. Eur J Endocrinol 2006;155(6):813–21.

93. Ito F, Sippel R, Lederman J, et al. The utility of intraoperative bilateral internal jugular venous sampling with rapid parathyroid hormone testing. Ann Surg 2007;245(6):959–63.

94. Carneiro-Pla D. Effectiveness of "office"-based, ultrasound-guided differential jugular venous sampling (DJVS) of parathormone in patients with primary hyperparathyroidism. Surgery 2009;146(6): 1014–20.

Adrenal Imaging: From Addison to Algorithms

Giles W.L. Boland, MD

KEYWORDS

- Adrenal lesion • Hyperfunctioning • Computed tomography
- Characterization • Algorithm

Despite their small size, pathologic condition of the adrenal glands is often far from insignificant. Hyperfunctioning disease with excessive hormonal function has long been recognized to be potentially fatal,[1] metastatic disease often alters the staging and prognosis of the primary disease, infiltrative and infectious diseases (relatively common in the developing world) can lead to prolonged morbidity, and primary adrenal malignancies left untreated are usually fatal. Despite these facts, most adrenal masses are innocuous. The challenge for any physician is to sort out which masses can be safely ignored and which cannot. Fortunately, novel and innovative modern imaging techniques have transformed the investigation of adrenal disease and have consequently placed radiologists center stage in adrenal mass detection and characterization. No longer is it simply sufficient for a modern day imager to state that there is an adrenal mass on cross-sectional imaging; for most patients, the imager should be able to differentiate between those lesions that can safely be left alone and those that may potentially do harm. In fact, it is a central role of contemporary imagers to guide referring physicians and patients toward the correct diagnosis, with a specificity that obviates invasive tissue sampling. It is therefore vital that any imaging department develop the knowledge and expertise to differentiate such lesions. Whereas the adrenal imaging algorithm may at first glance appear complex and perhaps confusing, the imaging skills required are, in fact, relatively simple. It behooves imagers, therefore, to become familiar with this algorithm if they are to realize their full value in adrenal lesion diagnosis and characterization. This article, therefore, outlines the range of possible abnormalities encountered in the adrenal gland, the imaging modalities and specialized techniques used to detect and characterize them, the principles based on which these techniques are used, and finally a working imaging algorithm that can be readily used in daily practice. We have come a long way since Addison[1] first published in 1855 that a disease of the adrenal glands can cause a particular bronzing of the skin.

ADRENAL PATHOLOGY

Adrenal masses can be variously classified, but the simplest approach is to divide them into benign or malignant and functioning or nonfunctioning.[2] Functioning, hormone-producing adrenal masses have challenged even the most savvy of diagnostic clinicians throughout the ages because of the myriad and often-subtle presenting symptoms and signs that they produce (the details of which are outside the scope of this article). Even today, it is probably a minor coup for a diagnostician to identify, especially if early, a hyperfunctioning adrenal tumor, thereby preventing the patient from prolonged morbidity and sometimes death. The syndrome these tumors produce depends on which cells are hyperfunctioning and therefore whether they arise from the cortex or medulla.[2] Famous, almost iconic, clinicians have their names eponymously associated to the various syndromes and diseases, including Cushing, Conn, and of course, Addison, amongst others. Most hyperfunctioning tumors are relatively rare, although

Department of Radiology, Massachusetts General Hospital, Harvard Medical School, White Building 270C, 55 Fruit Street, Boston, MA 02114, USA
E-mail address: gboland@partners.org

Radiol Clin N Am 49 (2011) 511–528
doi:10.1016/j.rcl.2011.02.010

there is some new evidence that hyperaldosteron-ism (Conn disease) may be more common than once thought and might account for up to 10% of hypertension.[3] The true frequency of identification of these tumors on imaging, like that of most other adrenal masses, is unknown, but is generally thought to be between 5% and 10% of identified adrenal masses.[2] Most are also benign, although some malignant lesions, particularly the aggressive ones, can produce excessive hormones, sometimes prolifically (**Tables 1** and **2**). These aggressive tumors are even rarer than benign hyperfunctioning tumors, and early diagnosis is often impossible. Thus, patients may present when the adrenal mass is already relatively large.[2]

Nonfunctioning benign tumors are the most commonly encountered lesion in the general population and at imaging, are seen in approximately 5% of all abdominal computed tomographic (CT) imaging. The prevalence of these adrenal lesions at CT increases to approximately 7% to 8% in the elderly (see **Table 1**).[2,4] Almost all lesions are cortical adenomas for which no treatment or follow-up, once characterized, is needed. As will be seen, however, many, at least at first presentation, cannot initially be differentiated from other, more sinister, lesions. However, depending on the clinical context (ie, the patient has no history of malignancy), it can be strongly inferred that the lesion is indeed benign, so much so that it could be argued that additional imaging is not required. However, even though the a priori chance of an incidentally detected mass is a benign adrenocortical adenoma in the appropriate clinical setting, most imagers recommend additional tests to solidify the diagnosis. Other nonfunctioning benign lesions (see **Table 1**) are rare and may only be ultimately diagnosed by tissue diagnosis, but this is generally not required

because a simple diagnosis of benignity should suffice. Infectious and infiltrative causes are rare in the West but should definitely be considered in the developing world (see **Tables 1** and **2**).

Perhaps, imagers have become critical to the detection and characterization of adrenal masses because malignant, mainly metastatic, adrenal disease is not uncommon, particularly in older patients, given the increased prevalence of malignancy in the elderly. In fact, some studies suggest that microscopic adrenal metastases are seen in up to 27% of patients with an extra-adrenal malignancy.[5] More notable to most imagers is the frequency with which macroscopic metastases to the adrenal gland are identified—approximately 50% in most series.[4] It should come as no surprise, therefore, that the presence of a known underlying extra-adrenal malignancy completely alters the approach to characterizing these lesions. While the a priori chance of a lesion being metastatic in a patient without a known primary malignancy is close to nil,[4,6] this certainly cannot be said for patients with an extra-adrenal malignancy. The presence of an adrenal metastasis can have profound prognostic implications for the patient, and oncologic therapy is guided by such a finding. Imagers must thus be confident in their diagnoses and appropriately direct further characterization if a diagnosis is not possible by imaging, It clearly serves no purpose to any party in the clinical care process (least of all the patient) if an imager diagnoses the adrenal lesion to be benign when in fact it is metastatic. The patient will very likely undergo unnecessary prolonged aggressive treatment in an attempt to cure, when cure is often not possible. Conversely, diagnosing a metastasis when the lesion is in fact benign can deny the patient a chance for cure. Therefore, it is less critical for the imager to characterize adrenal

Table 1
Type, frequency, and growth rate of benign adrenal masses

Type	Frequency Amongst All Adrenal Masses	Growth Rate
Adenoma	Common, approximately 50%–80% Nonfunctioning in the majority	Stable or very slow
Myelolipoma	5%–10%	Stable to slow
Pheochromocytoma (90% benign)	5% (figure likely less in clinical practice)	Slow
Hematoma	1%	Rapid
Cyst	1%	Usually stable
Ganglioneuroma	Very rare	Variable, slow to rapid
Hemangioma	Very rare	Usually slow
Granulomatous	Rare outside Asia	Variable, slow to intermediate

Table 2
Type, frequency, and growth rate of malignant adrenal masses

Type	Frequency	Growth Rate
Metastasis	No Cancer: uncommon; known cancer: common (up to 50%)	Variable, slow to rapid
Lymphoma	Primary rare, metastatic more common	Variable, slow to rapid
Carcinoma	Rare, <5%	Variable, usually slow
Pheochromocytoma (10% malignant)	5% (figure likely less in clinical practice)	Slow
Neuroblastoma	Very rare, more common in children	Variable, slow to rapid

lesions with great sensitivity than with very high specificity to avoid the scenario described earlier.

This scenario should be a rare event because most lesions can be confidently diagnosed into the correct category. Correct characterization depends on multiple factors including clinical history and age (as has been discussed), the modality selected, and the technique and protocol used. Imaging can now exploit various physiologic principles to achieve this goal, and each is described in detail.

IMAGING PRINCIPLES IN ADRENAL MASS CHARACTERIZATION
Macroscopic Features

Whereas some masses can be readily diagnosed by specific macroscopic features, most cannot, at least at first presentation. Most masses when detected, irrespective of their cause, are relatively small and generally look alike (**Figs. 1** and **2**). Therefore, imagers are strongly advised to not conclude based on the macroscopic features alone. That being said, there are a few lesions that can be confidently diagnosed by simple macroscopic features alone. The benign myelolipoma, as its name suggests, often (but not always) has visible fat that can be readily identified on cross-sectional imaging techniques, although the amount of fat does vary (**Fig. 3**). Should macroscopic fat be seen, the lesion is effectively always a myelolipoma, and no further imaging is required. Smooth-walled water density lesions are consistent with adrenal cysts (**Fig. 4**), but not all low-density lesions are cysts. Necrotic metastases can look cystic, even though they are usually not water-density cysts (**Fig. 5**). Large, especially if irregular, lesions offer a strong clue that they are

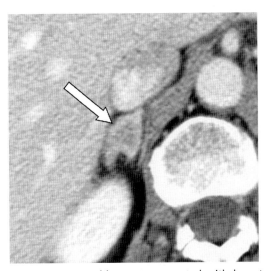

Fig. 1. A 53-year-old woman presented with breast cancer. A contrast-enhanced CT demonstrates a 1.9-cm right adrenal mass (*arrow*), which cannot be characterized by this test alone. It was subsequently demonstrated to be a metastasis at follow-up imaging.

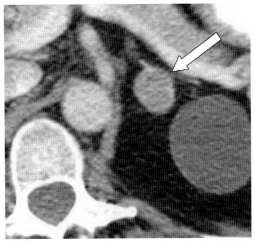

Fig. 2. A 77-year-old man presented with bladder cancer. Contrast-enhanced CT demonstrates a 2-cm left adrenal mass (*arrow*). This cannot be characterized by visual analysis, but follow-up imaging at 8 months demonstrated lesion stability, consistent with a benign adenoma.

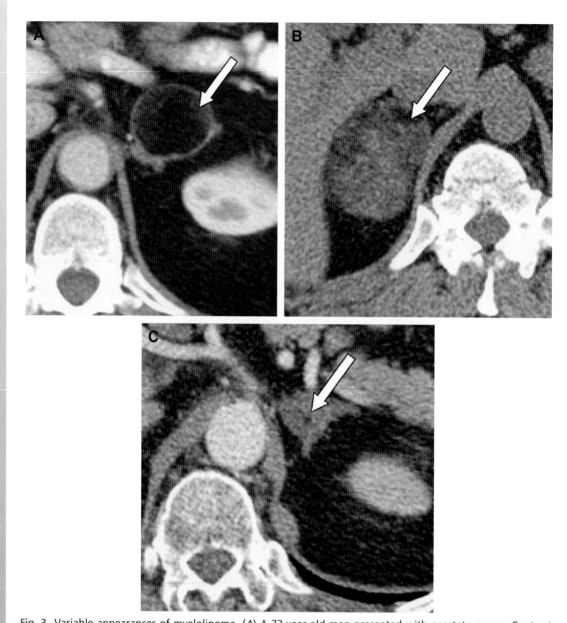

Fig. 3. Variable appearances of myelolipoma. (*A*) A 72-year-old man presented with prostate cancer. Contrast-enhanced CT demonstrates a uniformly fatty mass in the left adrenal gland (*arrow*) consistent with myelolipoma. (*B*) A 54-year-old woman presented with abdominal pain. A contrast-enhanced CT demonstrates a 5.2-cm heterogeneous right adrenal mass with fat elements (*arrow*), consistent with myelolipoma. (*C*) A 63-year-old man presented with bladder cancer. A contrast-enhanced CT demonstrates a 1.9-cm left adrenal lesion with a small punctuate region of fat (*arrow*), sufficient to make a diagnosis of myelolipoma.

malignant. One study documented that more than 70% of lesions greater than 4 cm in diameter are malignant and that this percentage increases even further with even larger masses.[7] Occasionally, a benign cortical adenoma or myelolipoma (especially if it has hemorrhaged) may measure more than 4 cm, but malignancy should be definitively excluded before confidently characterizing the disease as benign. In a patient presenting with a larger lesion without any known history of malignancy, adrenal cortical carcinoma (ACC) should be excluded before proceeding because these lesions are often indolent and present late (**Fig. 6**).[2] Most large lesions, however, are ultimately diagnosed as metastatic disease. Necrosis is almost unique to malignancy (see **Figs. 5** and **6**).

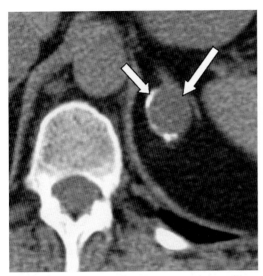

Fig. 4. A 53-year-old woman presented with endometrial cancer. A noncontrast CT demonstrates a 1.7-cm left adrenal mass (*long arrow*) with rim calcification (*short arrow*). Density values measured 3 HU, consistent with an adrenal cyst.

Adrenal calcification can be seen in malignant ACC, granulomatous disease, and sometimes in the wall of benign cysts (see **Fig. 4**).

Serial Imaging

The adage that the "old film" is the imager's best friend still holds just true. Woe is the imager who fails to compare current studies with any relevant prior available cross-sectional image. Indeed, prior images are so crucial to correct adrenal lesion characterization that if cross-sectional imaging has been performed at an outside institution (and a diagnosis is not possible based on current studies), the imager should recommend to the patient or referring physician that they obtain a copy with the final word on the definitive diagnosis/management withheld until those images obtained at the outside institution are available. Benign lesions rarely enlarge on serial imaging, and if they do, they enlarge only very slowly.[4] Therefore, if sufficient time has elapsed between one cross-sectional study and the next (usually, by wide consensus, considered to be 6 months)[4] and the lesion is stable (irrespective of the underlying history), the lesion can confidently be assumed to be benign (**Fig. 7**). The converse usually holds up—if a lesion grows, it is almost always malignant (**Fig. 8**).[4] There is, however, a caveat; adrenal hemorrhage will rapidly enlarge the adrenal gland (**Fig. 9**), whether in a preexisting normal adrenal or in the one with an underlying pathologic condition (ie, myelolipoma that have a propensity to bleed). Imagers are sometimes confused when an adrenal mass actually becomes smaller on serial imaging. This change usually results from a benign hemorrhagic mass or from a malignancy treated with chemotherapy. This pattern may be most dramatic with adrenal lymphoma (**Fig. 10**).

Unfortunately, serial imaging is not always available, particularly in patients without a history of malignancy. This presents a different problem—how to characterize a mass without the aid of the imagers "best friend." Fortunately, there are several imaging principles and techniques that can now be recruited to trump this conundrum,

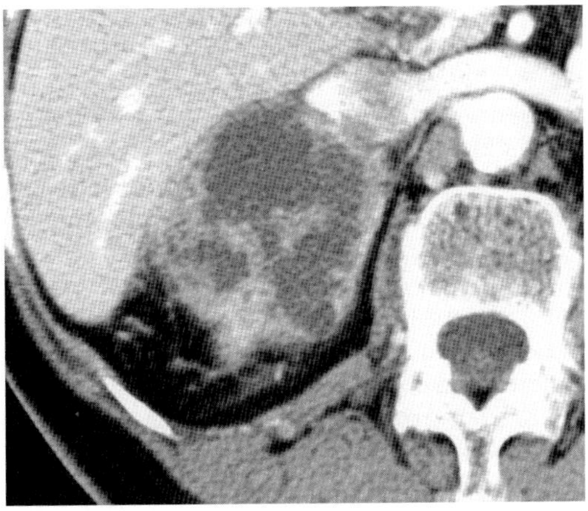

Fig. 5. A 71-year-old woman presented with lung cancer. A contrast-enhanced CT demonstrates a 7.1-cm heterogeneous and necrotic right adrenal confirmed to be metastatic when compared with prior imaging.

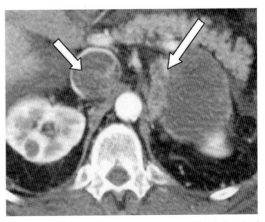

Fig. 6. A 54-year-old man presented with abdominal pain and an ACC. A contrast-enhanced CT demonstrates an 8.2-cm heterogeneous left adrenal mass with peripheral vascular enhancement (*long arrow*). The inferior vena cava is expanded because of tumor invasion (*short arrow*).

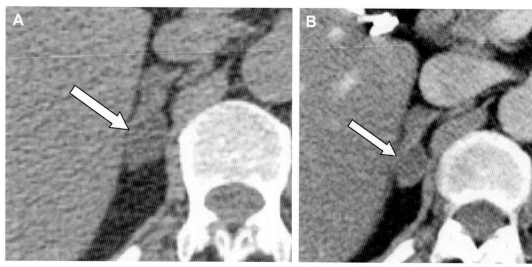

Fig. 7. A 53-year-old woman was investigated for renal stone disease. (*A*) A noncontrast CT performed in 2010 demonstrates a 1.8-cm right adrenal mass (*arrow*). (*B*) A contrast-enhanced CT from 2006 confirms that the lesion is stable and consistent with a benign adenoma (*arrow*).

including lipid-sensitive imaging, physiologic perfusional washout protocols, and metabolic imaging. Each is discussed in turn.

Lipid-Sensitive Imaging

It was serendipitously noted in the late 1980's that a surprising number of benign adrenal cortical adenomas demonstrated low density on CT, whereas malignant lesions did not (Peter Hahn, personal communication, 1995). They then went on to formally test their hypothesis, which confirmed their suspicion, and published their finding in a seminal article almost a generation ago. Lee and colleagues[8] documented that many benign adenomas indeed demonstrate a significantly lower density than malignant lesions on non-contrast CT (NCCT) images. They reported that no lesions that have attenuation less than 0 Hounsfield units (HU) were malignant and that all of these lesions were benign adenomas. It was subsequently demonstrated by Korobkin and colleagues[9] that this phenomenon was predicated on the intracellular lipid concentration of the lesion, with many cortical adenomas demonstrating abundant fat and almost all malignant lesions devoid of such fat. Most low-density lesions are therefore deemed lipid rich, and malignant lesions are deemed lipid poor. Multiple other reports have now validated these initial findings by Boland and colleagues,[10] and a pooled-analysis of 10 NCCT reports evaluating this phenomenon confirmed it as a firmly established tool with which to differentiate benign form malignant diseases. This study, by varying the threshold up or down the density scale, documented a range of sensitivities and specificities for the test to accurately characterize a lesion as a benign adenoma. The investigators chose 10 HU as the optimal threshold, giving sufficient sensitivity (71%) for the test to be relevant and specificity (98%) for the test to be sufficiently accurate. It should be noted that the test is not 100% specific, potentially undermining the usefulness of the adrenal imager. However, there are often other clues that can lead the imager to suspect with variable degrees of certainty that the lesion is, in fact, not a benign adenoma, but rather something more sinister. Perhaps, prior imaging is available or macroscopic features that suggest malignancy (discussed previously) are present. The reason for the less-than-perfect specificity is that an occasional malignant lesion demonstrates a density of less than 10 HU.[4] In clinical practice, however, this is very uncommon, unless the imager has included necrotic areas within the region of interest (ROI). A further mistake, sometimes made by inexperienced adrenal imagers, is incorrect ROI placement, either because they have included a portion of surrounding retroperitoneal fat within the ROI, or more commonly because they have chosen an ROI that is too small, thereby including too few pixels to represent the lesion density average. In any anatomic structure, there are variable pixel densities, and one can usually make a lesion appear lipid rich or poor simply by moving a small ROI (one of a few pixels) around the lesion (**Fig. 11**).

Other lipid-sensitive techniques, aside from NCCT, can also be used to detect the intracytoplasmic fat found in many adrenal adenomas. Fat-sensitive MR imaging techniques have been

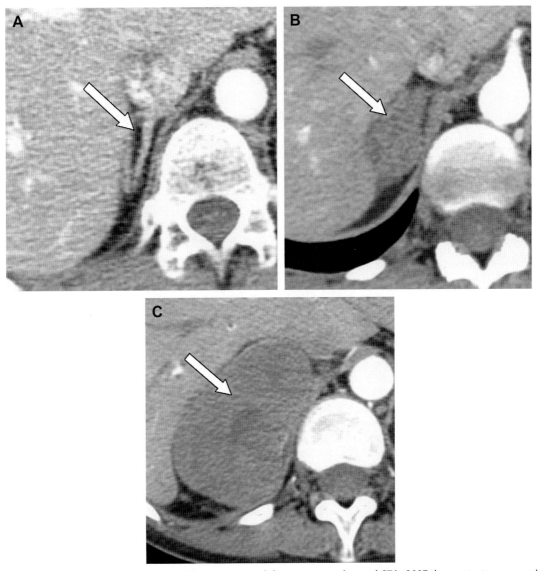

Fig. 8. A 45-year-old man presented with colon cancer. (*A*) A contrast-enhanced CT in 2007 demonstrates a normal right adrenal gland (*arrow*). (*B*) A follow-up CT in 2008 demonstrates a new mass in the right adrenal (*arrow*), consistent with metastatic disease. (*C*) A further follow-up CT in 2009 demonstrates enlargement of the right adrenal metastasis (*arrow*).

demonstrated to be effective tools with which to characterize adrenal lesions. The premise is really no different to that of NCCT. If one can detect sufficient intracellular fat within the lesion (not macroscopic as seen in myelolipoma), the lesion can confidently be assumed to be benign. Although there are differing fat suppression MR imaging techniques, the commonest used, mainly because of its speed, availability, and ease of use, is chemical shift imaging (CSI). This technique has been used almost as long as NCCT and has stood the test of time, although there is some controversy as to whether NCCT or chemical shift (CS) MR

imaging is a better test. Some investigators state that CS MRI is superior to CT, perhaps because it is more sensitive in detecting intracellular fat.[11,12] Other investigators have challenged this notion and have stated that MR imaging might be useful under certain criteria.[13,14] As can be inferred from the discussion on lipid-sensitive NCCT imaging, up to one-third of benign adenomas do not contain sufficient intracellular fat for their density to measure less than 10 HU on NCCT. These lipid-poor lesions, therefore, mimic malignant lesions, which are almost always lipid-poor.[4,15] NCCT is therefore unhelpful to characterize this group of

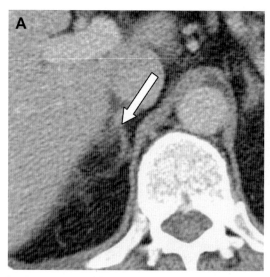
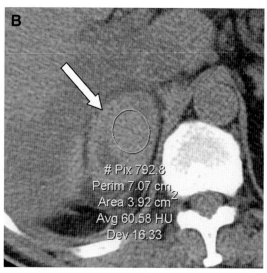

Fig. 9. A 71-year-old man presented with leukemia. (*A*) Contrast-enhanced CT performed to evaluate for liver abscess, demonstrates a normal right adrenal (*arrow*). (*B*) Noncontrast CT performed 3 days later, again to evaluate for liver abscess, demonstrates a new 4.8-cm hyperdense mass (61 HU) (*arrow*), consistent with an acute adrenal hematoma.

adenomas, and this technique can only determine them to be indeterminate (along with most malignant lesions). Some investigators have proposed that it is in this group of benign lesions that CS MR imaging can be more effective than NCCT because it may be more sensitive at detecting lipid.[13] In practice, these findings have not entered mainstream practice, so it is left to the imager to decide which modality to use. Given that CS MR imaging offers little advantage over NCCT, most investigators prefer NCCT, but others, perhaps being more familiar with MR imaging techniques continue to recommend CS MR imaging to differentiate lipid-rich benign disease from lipid-poor indeterminate malignant and some benign lesions. MR imaging offers no radiation exposure to the patient, so is perhaps preferred to CT, particularly for younger patients, but MR imaging is less available, more expensive, and for some individuals, uncomfortable.

The premise behind the CS MR imaging technique is based on a complicated physical phenomenon, really only fully understood though complex mathematical formulas that are

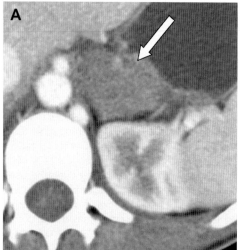
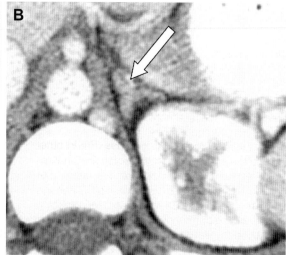

Fig. 10. A 23-year-old woman presented with lymphoma. (*A*) Contrast-enhanced CT demonstrates a 4-cm left adrenal lesion (*arrow*) in a patient with known lymphoma. (*B*) A subsequent contrast-enhanced CT 4 years later demonstrates a normal adrenal gland (*arrow*), consistent with a curative response.

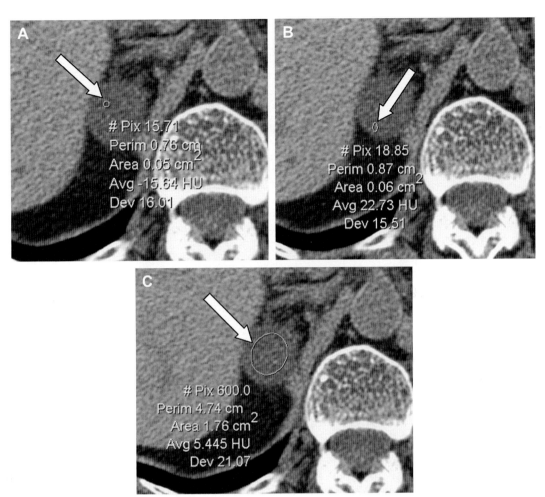

Fig. 11. An 82-year-old woman presented with lung cancer. (*A*) An ROI that is too small (*arrow*) yields a density in the right adrenal gland of −15 HU. (*B*) Again, the ROI is too small (*arrow*), yielding a density of 23 HU, which would be consistent with a lipid-poor indeterminate lesion. (*C*) Correct ROI measurement (*arrow*) yields a density of 5 HU, consistent with a lipid-rich adrenal adenoma.

incomprehensible to most.[16] However, the general concept is that each MR imaging voxel contains a variable proportion of fat and water protons.[15] These protons can be manipulated to precess (rotate) at different frequencies such that at predetermined times (in milliseconds), the amplitude of the different fat and water signals in the MR detectors varies.[15] At precisely the right time, these protons will be precessing in-phase (IP); in other words, their signals summate to produce a large-amplitude signal in the detector. At another predetermined time, their signals will be opposed causing signal drop-off in the detectors. Being aligned is analogous to the proton signals being IP, and being on opposite sides of the track, to out of phase (OOP). If there are equal concentrations of fat and water protons in the voxel, these 2 signals cancel each other out, hence the term signal drop-off. This physical phenomenon can

be portrayed on the MR image as a bright signal in the adrenal gland on IP images but a darker signal on OOP images (**Fig. 12**). It has been demonstrated that qualitative evaluation of this drop-off on the MR image is sufficient to diagnose a lipid-rich adenoma,[17] but some investigators prefer to use a quantitative method to demonstrate the fractional signal drop-off from the IP image to the OOP image. A signal drop-off of 16.5% is generally considered to indicate a lipid-rich adenoma.[18] In practice, even in centers with subspecialty MR imaging expertise, the quantitative method is often not used. One caveat to relying on qualitative analysis alone is that sometimes a steatotic liver also demonstrates signal drop-off on OOP images, so the imager can be fooled into thinking that there is no signal drop-off in a lipid-rich adjacent right adrenal adenoma.[4,17] The spleen (or muscle) should

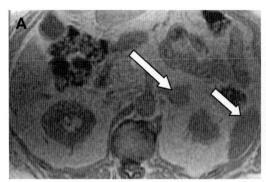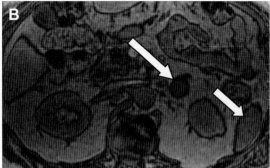

Fig. 12. An 82-year-old woman presented with colon cancer. (*A*) An IP gradient echo (GRE) MR imaging demonstrating a 2-cm left adrenal lesion (*long arrow*) with signal intensity similar to the spleen (*short arrow*). (*B*) OOP GRE MR imaging demonstrates signal drop-off in the left adrenal gland (*long arrow*) when compared with the spleen (*short arrow*), consistent with a lipid-rich adenoma.

therefore be used as the internal control when attempting to determine any qualitative signal drop-off.[17] Lipid-poor lesions (most malignancies and a few adenomas), on the other hand, demonstrate no signal drop-off, being devoid of fat protons to cancel out the water protons on OOP images (**Fig. 13**). Given that the most signal drop-off that can be encountered is when there are equal fat and water protons within a voxel, voxels with pure fat (ie, seen in most myelolipomas) may not demonstrate any signal drop-off at all.[4]

Although lipid-sensitive imaging is a useful tool when characterizing adrenal lesions, it usually cannot differentiate benign lipid-poor lesions form malignant ones. Assuming there is no prior imaging to help make a definitive diagnosis, other imaging tests are needed to characterize this subset. Furthermore, most patients, particularly those with an underlying malignancy, are usually imaged with contrast-enhanced CT (CECT) rather than with NCCT. Use of CECT renders the test useless because both adenomas and malignant lesions enhance to a variable and often the same degree after the administration of intravenous (IV) contrast material.[19] Unless one were to perform an NCCT at a separate setting (which is to be discussed as part of the adrenal CT protocol), a different test is needed.

Physiologic CT Washout Test

This test relies on a principle completely different from that of lipid-sensitive imaging. It was noticed on MR imaging in the late 1980's by Krestin and colleagues[20] that benign and malignant adrenal lesions behave differently after the injection of MR contrast agents. After the injected IV contrast medium had circulated into the adrenal gland, it rapidly washed-out in benign lesions. On the other

hand, contrast was retained for relatively longer periods in malignant adrenal lesions. No one has been able to reproduce this MR imaging phenomenon, but Korobkin and colleagues,[21] a few years later, noticed that the same phenomenon occurs on CECT. The CT washout test, as it came to be known, has been replicated by other investigators and has, in fact, been demonstrated to be a more accurate test than lipid-sensitive techniques.[19,22–25] Why malignant lesions retain injected IV contrast longer than benign lesions is not known. It has been speculated that the slow washout in malignant lesions is because of diffusion of contrast through porous malignant microvasculature into the extravascular space. Contrast rapidly washes out from benign adrenal lesions because it stays intravascular, within intact capillaries.[4] Whatever the reason, the CT washout test is now routinely used as one of the standard imaging tests to characterize most adrenal disease. Furthermore, most lipid-poor benign lesions (up to 30% of adenomas) also washout faster than malignant lesions, although perhaps not as avidly as lipid-rich adenomas.[22] The test therefore can characterize almost all adenomatous diseases (whether lipid-rich or poor) with accuracy rates close to 100%.

In practice, a washout fraction represents the density of the adrenal gland on dynamic CECT (approximately 70-second scan delay after the injection of IV contrast) compared with its density on a delayed image (usually 15 minutes later). To calculate the percentage washout, the formula given in **Table 3** is used.

An absolute washout can be calculated if the NCCT density is known; a relative washout is calculated if the NCCT density is unavailable. In practice, the relative percentage washout (RPW) has been demonstrated to be just as accurate as

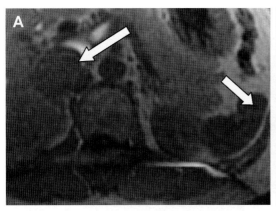
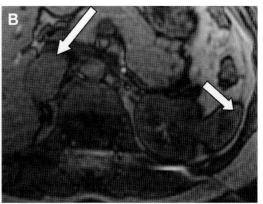

Fig. 13. A 49-year-old woman presented with lung cancer and right adrenal metastasis confirmed from serial imaging. (A) An IP GRE MR imaging sequence demonstrates a 3.8-cm right adrenal mass (*long arrow*). It is slightly hyperintense compared with the spleen (*small arrow*). (B) An OOP GRE sequence demonstrates no signal drop-off in the right adrenal (*long arrow*) when compared with the spleen (*small arrow*) consistent with a lipid-poor indeterminate lesion.

the absolute percentage washout (APW). Korobkin and colleagues[21] proposed that an RPW of greater than 40% (or >60% for APW) is consistent with benign adenomatous disease (**Fig. 14**), whereas lesions that washout less than 40% are nonadenomatous and usually malignant (**Fig. 15**).

Although the washout formula is relatively simple, it is often not remembered, even by most subspecialty imagers. In practice, most imagers now input the term adrenal washout formula into a Web search engine, which offers numerous Web sites in which the density values can be inserted into the on-screen formula and the RPW and APW calculated. Although an NCCT is not essential for this test, it is recommended. Assuming an adrenal lesion is detected on a CECT scan (as it mostly will be), the patient is asked to return for a dedicated adrenal CT protocol. This protocol starts with an NCCT, and diligent imagers will abort the rest of the test if the lesion density is less than 10 HU because a benign adenoma has been diagnosed. This abortion avoids further radiation (the test should

be limited to the region of the adrenal glands anyway), time, and the slight risk of a reaction to IV contrast material. If the density is greater than 10 HU, CT washouts are performed and the RPW and APW calculated. It is better to use the washout test with an online calculator than to advise the patient to return for either a more invasive or expensive test (such as positron emission tomography [PET]/CT).

METABOLIC IMAGING

It has been long known that pheochromocytoma can be readily diagnosed with the use of metaiodobenzylguanidine (MIBG). MIBG has almost 100% specificity, but variable sensitivity, for the diagnosis of pheochromocytomas.[26,27] Occasionally octreotide, a somatostatin analogue can be helpful, but it is only 30% sensitive.[28] More recently, however, there has been a proliferation in the installed base and use of PET/CT to evaluate a range of malignant diseases, usually to determine the metastatic disease burden of the primary disease. PET was first demonstrated in the early 1990's to be highly accurate in differentiating benign from malignant disease, and multiple other reports have now confirmed these initial findings.[29–37] One meta-analysis documented that PET alone has approximately 97% sensitivity and 91% specificity for differentiating benign from malignant adrenal disease.[38] The premise, no different to PET imaging malignancy elsewhere, is that malignant cells are glucose avid due to their high metabolic rate because they rapidly divide and grow.[32] The physics of how a PET scanner works is beyond the scope of this article, but, in short, a glucose analogue, 18F-fluoro-deoxyglucose (^{18}F FDG) is

Table 3	
Washout formulas for characterizing both lipid-rich and lipid-poor adenomas	
Absolute % Washout Benign if >60%	[Dynamic enhanced (HU)−Delayed (HU)]/ [Dynamic enhanced (HU)−Unenhanced (HU)]
Relative % Washout Benign if >40%	[Dynamic enhanced (HU)−Delayed (HU)]/ Dynamic enhanced (HU)

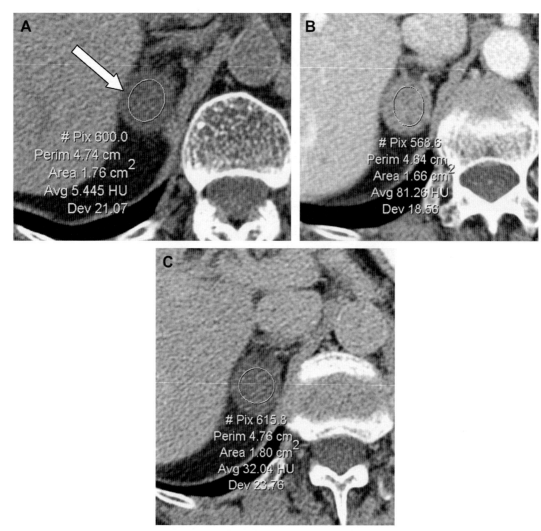

Fig. 14. An 82-year-old woman presented with lung cancer. (*A*) An NCCT demonstrates a 2.2-cm right adrenal mass (*arrow*) with density measurements of 5 HU. This is consistent with an adrenal adenoma. Imaging could be stopped here. (*B*) Dynamic CECT demonstrates that the right adrenal gland enhances to 82 HU. (*C*) Delayed CECT demonstrates a density value of 32 HU and an RPW of 61%, consistent with benign disease.

injected intravenously, which (as most glucose is) is rapidly and preferentially absorbed by malignant cells. However, whereas phosphorylated glucose (part of the glycolytic pathway) can rapidly exit the cell, ^{18}F FDG cannot and steadily accumulates within the malignant cells. The emitted positrons, originating from the accumulated foci of ^{18}F FDG within malignant cells, are captured by the PET detectors and depicted on a PET image as increased signal intensity indicating malignant disease. Like other malignant disease, adrenal metastases from the primary disease can be readily detected by PET, although lesions less than 1 cm are often difficult to detect because of their size and insufficient accumulation of the radiotracer.[30] However, PET can sometimes detect very early

forms of adrenal disease (**Fig. 16**) well before there is any appreciable macroscopic change. The intensity of the visualized uptake varies depending on the type of metastasis and its histologic grade, but most metastases can be detected this way. Most investigators simply evaluate the images qualitatively, but some reports suggest that the standardized uptake value or the standardized uptake ratio (a quantitative value of the adrenal signal compared with the liver) is effective.[4]

Most malignant lesions are highly ^{18}F FDG avid (**Fig. 17**), but some lesions can demonstrate mild ^{18}F FDG avidity (**Fig. 18**). Some benign lesions also demonstrate mild FDG avidity (up to 10%) and should not, therefore, be confused with malignant disease (**Fig. 19**). It is therefore recommended

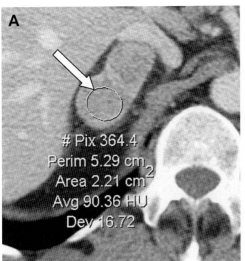 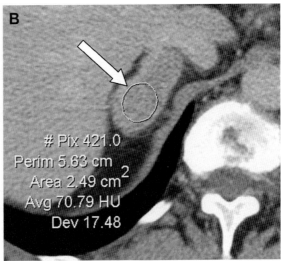

Fig. 15. A 64-year-old woman presented with colon cancer. (*A*) A dynamic CECT demonstrates a 5.2-cm right adrenal mass (*arrow*). Densitometry yields a density value of 90 HU. (*B*) Delayed CECT yields an adrenal mass density of 71 HU with a calculated RPW of 21% (*arrow*), consistent with metastatic disease.

that lesions demonstrating mild FDG avidity should be considered indeterminate unless other features are present (large irregular lesion, or new lesion compared with prior imaging).[4] Only extremely rarely will a benign lesion demonstrate marked FDG uptake, so under almost all circumstances, marked uptake, particularly in a patient with a known malignancy, should be considered a marker for malignant disease.

Given that PET imaging is now frequently combined with CT imaging (CT/PET), the combined modalities should, at least in theory, offer advantages over the modalities alone when attempting to characterize adrenal masses. Theoretically, CT/PET might combine all 4 adrenal imaging principles into 1 patient visit: the CT component might assess the gross appearance of the lesion, its lipid content, and washout kinetics, whereas PET might assess metabolic activity. In practice, PET/CT

imagers use a variety of CT techniques as part of the PET/CT. Ideally, a CECT should be performed as part of the PET/CT (CECT is well known to be far more sensitive for vdetecting and characterizing malignant disease compared with NCCT), but often it is not. Either an NCCT or possibly only a low-dose attenuation correction CT is performed. At least with a standard-dose NCCT, macroscopic and lipid-sensitive assessments can be used, but it has been demonstrated that the adrenal attenuation (measured in Hounsfield units) is too variable (the signal to noise is too low) on low-dose attenuation correction CT's and the images are often grainy, so macroscopic features are difficult to evaluate.[39] In theory, a contrast-enhanced washout CT could also be performed if one knew a priori that an adrenal lesion existed. One investigator did combine adrenal PET/CT findings with CT washout tests performed at a different time with perfect

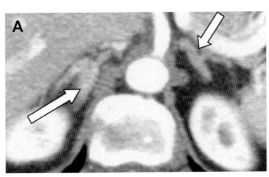 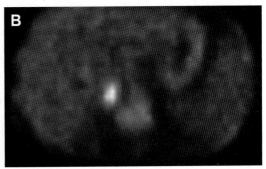

Fig. 16. A 71-year-old woman presented with breast cancer. (*A*) A CECT scan demonstrates a normal left adrenal gland (*short arrow*) and a slightly thickened right adrenal gland (*long arrow*). (*B*) ¹⁸F FDG-PET demonstrates marked FDG uptake in the right adrenal gland. This was confirmed as metastasis by surgical removal.

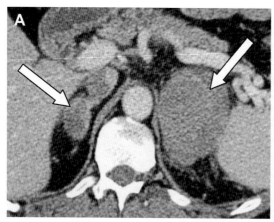
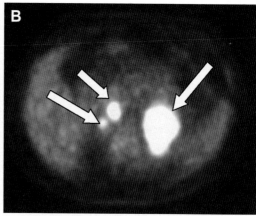

Fig. 17. A 53-year-old man presented with colon cancer. (*A*) A CECT from PET/CT demonstrates bilateral adrenal metastases because the lesions were enlarged since prior imaging (*arrows*). (*B*) ^{18}F FDG-PET as part of the same examination demonstrates marked uptake in both adrenal glands (*long arrows*) consistent with metastatic disease. A further area of uptake (*short arrow*) corresponds to a metastatic lymph node, identified on a different slice on the CT.

accuracy[32] but the complicated logistics involved have prevented the adoption of this technique in clinical practice.

SPECIFIC ADRENAL MASSES

Adrenal myelolipoma cyst, hemorrhage, infections, and hyperfunctioning cortical adenomas have already been discussed. Three specific conditions warrant further discussion.

PHEOCHROMOCYTOMA

This rare catecholamine-secreting tumor still fascinates imagers and referring physicians alike because of its subtle clinical manifestations and because detection can be life saving. Up to 10%

of tumors are detected incidentally at imaging, and 10% are also bilateral or extra-adrenal in location (along the paraganglionic sympathetic nervous system) or malignant.[40] The imaging features of this tumor can be highly characteristic. Typically, these lesions can be markedly bright on T2-weighted MR imaging (**Fig. 20**), but this sign is not very specific.[41] They avidly enhance after administration of IV contrast media, and washout characteristics typically follow malignant lesion characteristics, regardless of whether the pheochromocytoma is malignant or benign,[25] although sometimes they show the opposite, with washout values consistent with benign disease. Occasionally, these tumors demonstrate low attenuation on NCCT or poor enhancement after administration of IV contrast media, and even macroscopic

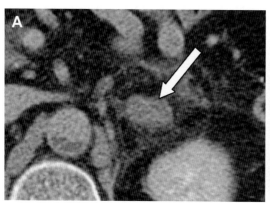
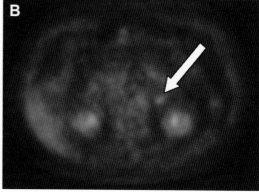

Fig. 18. A 68-year-old man had lung cancer and a left adrenal metastasis. (*A*) CECT from a PET/CT demonstrates a 2.3-cm left adrenal mass (*arrow*). (*B*) PET imaging during the same examination demonstrates mild ^{18}F FDG avidity (*arrow*). By PET alone, this lesion is indeterminate because some benign lesions are mildly PET avid.

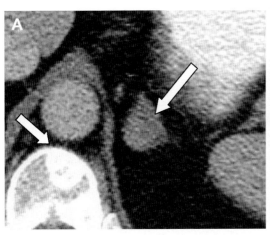
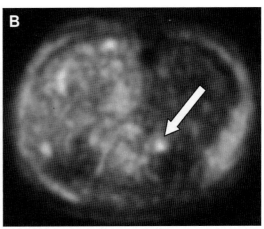

Fig. 19. A 74-year-old woman presented with breast cancer. (*A*) CECT as part of a PET/CT demonstrates a 2-cm left adrenal adenoma (*long arrow*), proved at percutaneous biopsy. An incidental bone metastasis in noted in the thoracic vertebral body (*short arrow*). (*B*) PET as part of the same examination demonstrates mild ^{18}F FDG uptake in the left adrenal gland (*arrow*). At PET alone, this lesion is indeterminate because some metastases also demonstrate mild ^{18}F FDG uptake.

fat has been identified on rare occasions.[41] As discussed, MIBG imaging has consistently demonstrated high accuracy for detecting both adrenal and extra-adrenal pheochromocytomas, but its use is decreasing with the adoption of PET, which often demonstrates increased FDG activity.[42]

ACC

This very rare, potentially fatal, primary tumor of the adrenal gland is the endocrinologist's nemesis.[2] To detect a small adrenal lesion on cross-sectional imaging in a patient, only to

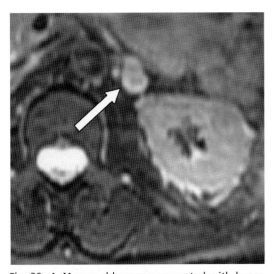

Fig. 20. A 41-year-old woman presented with hypertension. An axial T2 fast spin echo with fat saturation demonstrates a 1.8-cm hyperintense left adrenal mass (*arrow*). These characteristics are suggestive, but not diagnostic, of pheochromocytoma.

assume it benign (because the patient has an otherwise unremarkable history) can very rarely lead to catastrophic error for the patient. Some ACC's grow so slowly (or so it is thought) that even 6-month serial imaging may lead the imager to mistake that the lesion is benign because of no appreciable change in lesion size over this time frame. It is just because of this risk, albeit very rare, that some endocrinologists are uncomfortable performing single 6-month follow-up CT in a patient thought to harbor a benign adrenal adenoma. The formal endocrinologic recommendation for any patient without any suspicious underlying history and an incidentally detected adrenal lesion is for 6-month, 1-year, 2-year, and 3-year follow-up cross-sectional imagings to finally confirm lesion stability and rule out an ACC.[2] To many imagers, and probably referring physicians, this recommendation seems excessive, particularly given the rarity of AAC. Furthermore, considering that approximately 60 million CT's are performed annually in the United States (several million of which will be chest and abdominal CT's), a large number (likely hundreds of thousands) of incidental adrenal lesions will be detected, which in all likelihood will be benign a priori.[43] To perform 4 follow-up CT's in each of these patients will induce not only a significant radiation burden to a large proportion of the population but also incur an appreciable cost to the overall health system. In practice, most imagers therefore recommend a single 6-month follow-up CT for patients in whom an adrenal mass is incidentally detected. Alternatively, an adrenal protocol CT can be performed within a short time interval, which should put the issue to rest and avoid any further follow-up at all, reassuring to both the patient and referring physician. Either recommendation (6-month follow-up imaging or adrenal protocol CT) is, however, appropriate, and the recommendation will partly depend on the local physician, patient, and imaging preferences. However, that the chance that an incidentally detected lesion in this group of patients is malignant is close to nil.[4,6]

However, if there is any growth on serial imaging or there are features on an adrenal protocol CT that do not suggest benign disease, further short-term follow-up is probably warranted to exclude AAC or perhaps another nonadenomatous lesion (ie, an incidental adrenal metastasis in a patient not known to harbor an underlying extra-adrenal malignancy) (see **Tables 1** and **2**). The next step may involve percutaneous biopsy, or sometimes PET or PET/CT.

DIFFERENTIATION BETWEEN BENIGN ADENOMAS AND METASTASES

In practice, differentiation between benign adenomas and metastases will be the commonest clinical conundrum facing imagers. Most are small when detected, appear similar, but have vastly different implications for disease management. It has been discussed earlier that if the patient has no history of an extra-adrenal malignancy, the lesion is almost always benign and either an adrenal protocol or a 6-month serial CT is performed to confirm the diagnosis (assuming there is no prior cross-sectional image to confirm lesion stability) (see **Fig. 7**). If there is any prior imaging available and the lesion has grown, particularly in a patient with an oncologic history, then the chance that the lesion is metastatic is very high and should be assumed to be as such until proven otherwise (see **Fig. 8**). No further investigation is usually required, but if there is no prior imaging or there is a need to further confirm the diagnosis, an adrenal protocol CT, PET (or PET/CT), or ultimately percutaneous biopsy can be performed.

AN IMAGING ALGORITHM TO CHARACTERIZE ADRENAL LESIONS DETECTED AT IMAGING

Considering adrenal lesions are often detected at imaging, and most busy imaging practices will likely see at least 1 lesion daily, it behooves the imager to be familiar with an algorithm for definitive lesion diagnosis. With the array of imaging options available as discussed earlier, it should be possible for almost all lesions to be characterized without the need for invasive tests. The suggested algorithm is as follows:

1. Adrenal lesion is detected at imaging (usually CT).
2. Consider endocrine hormonal testing to rule out hyperfunctioning disease, especially in a patient without a known extra-adrenal malignancy. This consideration will depend on local endocrinologic practices. Although rare, pheochromocytoma is a possibility.
3. What is the age of the patient (adenomas are more likely in younger patients, malignant lesions become more common in the elderly)?
4. Does the patient have an underlying history of malignancy (metastasis are much more common)?
5. Does the patient have prior cross-sectional imaging (stability consistent with benign disease, growth usually represents malignancy)?
6. Are there characteristic imaging features (cyst, myelolipoma, hemorrhage, necrosis, large size)?
7. Has an NCCT been performed (is the lesion lipid-rich, consistent with benign disease)? CS MR imaging is an acceptable alternative.
8. If CECT is performed, recommend CT washout tests (6-month follow-up CT in the nononcologic patient is acceptable).
9. Does the lesion conform to benign or malignant disease at CT washouts?
10. Most lesions will now be characterized.
11. Some indeterminate lesions (conflicting macroscopic, lipid-sensitive, or perfusional washout test results) may benefit from ^{18}F FDG-PET or percutaneous biopsy.

NEWER DEVELOPMENTS

Several studies have demonstrated poor results with diffusion-weighted MR imaging for differentiating benign from malignant adrenal disease.[44,45] Such results are disappointing considering the success of using apparent diffusion coefficient maps elsewhere.[44] At this time, this MR imaging application is not recommended.

MR spectroscopy on the other hand, has demonstrated more promise.[46] The details of this technique are outside the scope of this article, and its use is likely reserved for a few specialized centers. However, threshold values of 1.2 for choline-creatine ratio and 0.38 for the choline-lipid ratio have generally yielded high sensitivity and specificity (>90% each) for adenomas (and pheochromocytomas) to be distinguished from AAC and metastases. A lipid-creatine ratio of 2.1 demonstrated lower sensitivity (45%) but perfect specificity. Furthermore, adenomas and metastases could be differentiated from pheochromocytomas and AAC's using a 4.0 to 4.3 ppm/creatine ratio greater than 1.5 and by comparing choline-creatine ratio with 4.0 to 4.3 ppm/creatine ratios. It remains to be seen whether these initial results are confirmed by other reports and whether it use has any advantage over the already established, more conventional, techniques.

Considering more conventional techniques, a recent report has challenged the notion that the adrenal CT washout protocol can be performed with a 10-minute, rather than a 15-minute delayed CECT.[47] In 2000, a report by Pena and colleagues[19] recommended this shorter interval as accurate as the longer protocol, thereby aiding busy CT workflows. However, a larger study, revisiting the 10-minute protocol, demonstrated suboptimal sensitivity (approximately 70%) for the 10-minute delayed imaging to differentiate adenomatous from nonadenomatous disease compared with the greater than 90% sensitivity as published for 15-minute delayed protocols.[4] The investigators therefore recommended that the 10-minute delayed protocol be abandoned and all CT washout tests be performed using the 15-minute delay protocol. This recommendation seems prudent, considering this was a large study and no other investigator has recommended the 10-minute delayed technique.

SUMMARY

Adrenal lesions are commonly detected at cross-sectional imaging. Numerous reports have now confirmed that imaging alone can characterize almost all masses into benign adenomatous disease or nonadenomatous (usually metastatic) lesions. Diagnostic percutaneous biopsy is rarely necessary and should be reserved for the few remaining indeterminate lesions (or because some patients require a tissue diagnosis to enter a specific investigational clinical trial). Imagers should therefore be familiar with the principles and techniques that underpin the ability of imaging to characterize most lesions. Ignorance of these techniques fails to deliver the necessary imaging value to referrers and patients alike.

REFERENCES

1. Addison T. On the constitutional and local effects of disease of the suprarenal capsule. In: Highley S, editor. A collection of the published writings of the late Thomas Addison MD. London: Taylor and Francis; 1855.
2. Young WF Jr. The incidentally discovered adrenal mass. N Engl J Med 2007;356:601–10.
3. Rayner B. Primary aldosteronism and aldosterone-associated hypertension. J Clin Pathol 2008;61: 825–31.
4. Boland GW, Blake MA, Hahn PF. Incidental adrenal lesions: principles, techniques, and algorithms for imaging characterization. Radiology 2008;249:756–75.
5. Abrams HL, Spiro B, Goldstein N. Metastases in carcinoma: analysis of 1000 autopsy cases. Cancer 1950;3:74–85.
6. Song J, Chaudhry FS, Mayo-Smith WW. The incidental adrenal mass on CT: prevalence of adrenal disease in 1,049 consecutive adrenal masses in patients with no known malignancy. Am J Roentgenol 2008;190:1163–8.
7. Mannsman G, Lau J, Balk E, et al. The clinically inapparent adrenal mass: update in diagnosis and treatment. Endocr Rev 2004;25:309–40.
8. Lee MJ, Hahn PF, Papanicolou N, et al. Benign and malignant adrenal masses: CT distinction with attenuation coefficients, size, and observer analysis. Radiology 1991;179:415–8.
9. Korobkin M, Giordano TJ, Brodeur FJ, et al. Adrenal adenomas: relationship between histologic lipid and CT and MR findings. Radiology 1996;200:743–7.
10. Boland GW, Lee MJ, Gazelle GS, et al. Characterization of adrenal masses using unenhanced CT: analysis of the CT literature. Am J Roentgenol 1998;171:201–4.
11. Mitchell DG, Crovello M, Matteucci T, et al. Benign adrenocortical masses: diagnosis with chemical shift MR imaging. Radiology 1992;185:345–51.
12. Reinig JW, Stutley JE, Leonhurdt CM, et al. Differentiation of adrenal masses with MR imaging: comparison of techniques. Radiology 1994;192:41–6.
13. Haider MA, Ghai S, Jhaveri K, et al. Chemical shift MR imaging of hyperattenuating (>10 HU) adrenal masses: does it still have a role? Radiology 2004;231:711–6.
14. Israel GM, Korobkin M, Wang C, et al. Comparison of unenhanced CT and chemical shift MRI in evaluating lipid-rich adrenal adenomas. Am J Roentgenol 2004;183:215–9.
15. Mayo-Smith WW, Boland GW, Noto RB, et al. State-of-the-art adrenal imaging. Radiographics 2001;21: 995–1012.
16. Twieg DB. The k-trajectory formulation of the NMR imaging process with applications in analysis and synthesis of imaging methods. Med Phys 1983; 10(5):610–21.
17. Mayo-Smith WW, Lee MJ, McNicholas MM, et al. Characterization of adrenal masses (<5 cm) by use of chemical shift MR imaging: observer performance versus quantitative measures. Am J Roentgenol 1995;165:91–5.
18. Fujiyoshi F, Nakajo M, Kukukura Y, et al. Characterization of adrenal tumors by chemical shift fast-low angle shot MR imaging: comparison of four methods of quantitative evaluation. Am J Roentgenol 2003; 180:1649–57.

19. Pena CS, Boland GW, Hahn PF, et al. Characterization of indeterminate (lipid-poor) adrenal masses: use of washout characteristics at contrast-enhanced CT. Radiology 2000;217:798–802.

20. Krestin GP, Steinbrich W, Friedmann G. Adrenal masses: evaluation with fast gradient-echo MR imaging and Gd-DTPA-enhanced dynamic studies. Radiology 1989;171:675–80.

21. Korobkin M, Brodeur FJ, Francis IR, et al. CT time-attenuation washout curves of adrenal adenomas and nonadenomas. Am J Roentgenol 1998;170:747–52.

22. Caoili EM, Korobkin M, Francis IR, et al. Delayed enhanced CT of lipid-poor adrenal adenomas. Am J Roentgenol 2000;175:1411–5.

23. Blake MA, Kalra MK, Sweeney AT, et al. Distinguishing benign from malignant adrenal masses: multidetector row CT protocol with 10-minute delay. Radiology 2006;238:578–85.

24. Caoili EM, Korobkin M, Francis IR, et al. Adrenal masses: characterization with combined unenhanced and delayed enhanced CT. Radiology 2002;222:629–33.

25. Szolar DH, Korobkin M, Reittner P, et al. Adrenocortical carcinomas and adrenal pheochromocytomas: mass and enhancement loss evaluation at delayed contrast-enhanced CT. Radiology 2005;234:479–85.

26. Maurea S, Klain M, Mainolfi C, et al. The diagnostic role of radionuclide imaging in evaluation of patients with nonhypersecreting adrenal masses. J Nucl Med 2001;42:884–92.

27. Tenenbaum F, Lumbroso J, Schlumberger M, et al. Comparison of radiolabeled octreotide and metaiodobenzylguanidine (MIBG) scintigraphy in malignant pheochromocytoma. J Nucl Med 1995;36:1–6.

28. Van der Harst E, de Herder WW, Bruining HA, et al. [(123)I] metaiodobenzylguanidine and [(111)In] octreotide uptake in benign and malignant pheochromocytomas. J Clin Endocrinol Metab 2001;86:685–93.

29. Boland GW, Goldberg MA, Lee MJ, et al. Indeterminate adrenal mass in patients with cancer: evaluation at PET with 2-[F-18]-fluoro-2-deoxy-D-glucose. Radiology 1995;194:131–4.

30. Elaini AB, Shetty SK, Chapman VM, et al. Improved detection and characterization of adrenal disease with PET-CT. Radiographics 2007;27:755–67.

31. Metser U, Miller E, Lerman H, et al. ^{18}F-FDG PET/CT in the evaluation of adrenal masses. J Nucl Med 2005;47:32–7.

32. Blake MA, Slattery JMA, Kalra K, et al. Adrenal lesions: characterization with fused PET/CT image in patients with proved or suspected malignancy—initial experience. Radiology 2006;238:970–7.

33. Jana S, Zhang T, Milstein DM, et al. FDG-PET and CT characterization of adrenal lesions in cancer patients. Eur J Nucl Med Mol Imaging 2006;33:29–35.

34. Han SJ, Kim TS, Jeon SW, et al. Analysis of adrenal masses by ^{18}F-FDG positron emission tomography scanning. Int J Clin Pract 2007;61:802–9.

35. Park BK, Kim CK, Kim B, et al. Comparison of delayed enhanced CT and 18F-FDG PET/CT in the evaluation of adrenal masses in oncology patients. J Comput Assist Tomogr 2007;31:550–6.

36. Caoili EM, Korobkin M, Brown RKJ, et al. Differentiating adrenal adenomas from nonadenomas using 18F-FDG PET/CT: quantitative and qualitative evaluation. Acad Radiol 2007;14:468–75.

37. Boland GWL, Blake MA, Holalkere N, et al. PET/CT for the characterization of adrenal masses in patients with cancer: qualitative versus quantitative accuracy in 150 consecutive patients. Am J Roentgenol 2009;192:956–62.

38. Jagtiani M, Boland GW, Blake MA, et al. Characterization of adrenal lesions using 18F-FDG PET: an analysis of the PET literature. Presented at the 94th Scientific Assembly and Annual Meeting, Radiological Society of North America. Chicago, November 30–December 5, 2008.

39. Boland GW. Adrenal adenoma attenuation values: comparison of low dose (Attenuation Correction) PET/CT versus Normal Dose CT. Presented at the 95th Scientific Assembly and Annual Meeting, Radiological Society of North America. Chicago, November 28 to December 3, 2009.

40. Francis IR, Korobkin M. Pheochromocytoma. Radiol Clin North Am 1996;34:1101–12.

41. Blake MA, Kalra MK, Maher MM, et al. Pheochromocytoma: an imaging chameleon. Radiographics 2004;24:S87–9.

42. Shulkin BL, Thompson NW, Shapiro B, et al. Pheochromocytomas: imaging with 2-[fluorine-18]fluoro-2-deoxy-D-glucose PET. Radiology 1999;212:35–41.

43. Brenner DJ, Eric J, Hall EJ. Computed tomography—an increasing source of radiation exposure. N Engl J Med 2007;357:2277–84.

44. Tsushima Y, Takahashi-Taketomi A, Endo K. Diagnostic utility of diffusion-weighted MR imaging and apparent diffusion coefficient value for the diagnosis of adrenal tumors. J Magn Reson Imaging 2009;29:112–7.

45. Miller FH, Wang Y, McCarthy RJ, et al. Utility of diffusion-weighted MRI in characterization of adrenal lesions. Am J Roentgenol 2010;194:459; [web]W179–85.

46. Faria JF, Goldman SM, Szejnfeld J, et al. Adrenal masses: characterization with in vivo proton MR spectroscopy–initial experience. Radiology 2007;245:788–97.

47. Sangwiaya MJ, Boland GW, Cronin CG, et al. Incidental adrenal lesions: accuracy of characterization with contrast-enhanced washout multidetector CT—10-minute delayed imaging protocol revisited in a large patient cohort. Radiology 2010;256:504–10.

Imaging of Neuroendocrine Tumors

Matthew T. Heller, MD[a],*, Amar B. Shah, MD[b]

KEYWORDS

• Neuroendocrine • Tumor • Carcinoid • Imaging

IMAGING OVERVIEW OF NEUROENDOCRINE TUMORS

Neuroendocrine tumors (NETs) were first described by Langhans[1] and Lubarsch[2] in the late nineteenth century. These tumors are commonly referred to as carcinoids because of their early description as *karzinoide* (carcinoma-like) in the early twentieth century by Oberndorfer.[3] This term referred to the less-aggressive biological behavior of carcinoids compared with the more common gastrointestinal carcinomas. Less than a decade later, it was shown that carcinoids harbor silver salt–reducing granules, which established the notion that these tumors were derived from the enteroendocrine (Kulchitsky) cells of the small intestine.[4] The nomenclature and classification of carcinoids have undergone several revisions since the initial descriptions. An early classification scheme described by Williams and Sandler[5] was based on the differences in clinico-pathologic features of carcinoids because of their anatomic location and embryologic origin. This classification scheme has proved to be useful because carcinoid tumors have unique clinical, imaging, and pathologic features based on their location. However, because this classification scheme did not adequately address the behavior of carcinoid tumors, the World Health Organization (WHO) classified the NETs into 3 groups: well-differentiated NETs, well-differentiated neuroendocrine carcinomas, and poorly differentiated endocrine carcinomas.[6] Well-differentiated NETs are regarded as having low or unknown malignant potential and are commonly referred to as carcinoids. Well-differentiated neuroendocrine carcinomas are low-grade neoplasms and often referred to as malignant carcinoids. Poorly differentiated neuroendocrine carcinomas are high-grade neoplasms and are considered to be small cell neoplasms. The WHO classification addresses the clinicobiological heterogeneity of NETs and takes into account the tumor size, vascular invasion, mitotic activity, histologic differentiation, hormonal activity, and presence of metastases and organ invasion. However, although the biological behavior of carcinoids varies by location and cell type, all carcinoids are considered to have some malignant potential.[7] Therefore, in this article the term carcinoid is used interchangeably with well-differentiated NETs having malignant potential; poorly differentiated endocrine carcinomas are designated separately.

NETs are a diverse group of related neoplasms that originate from various types of endocrine cells found throughout the neuroendocrine system. Most NETs occur in the gastrointestinal tract (67%) and tracheobronchial structures (25%).[8] Of gastrointestinal tract carcinoids, 42% occur in the small intestine, 27% in the rectum, 24% in the appendix, and 9% in the stomach.[8] NETs arise from endocrine cells in the mucosa and submucosa derived from the neural crest, neuroectoderm, and endoderm. The term neuroendocrine reflects the

The authors have nothing to disclose.

[a] Division of Abdominal Imaging, Department of Radiology, University of Pittsburgh Medical Center, 200 Lothrop Street, Suite 4895 PUH S. Tower, Pittsburgh, PA 15213, USA

[b] Division of Body Imaging, Department of Radiology, New York Medical College, 100 Woods Road, Macy Pavilion SW 257, Valhalla, NY 10595, USA

* Corresponding author.

E-mail address: hellermt@upmc.edu

antigens that are common to both tumors and nerve cells and the ability of these tumors to synthesize, store, and secrete messenger chemicals such as neuropeptides and amines.[9] NETs of the gastrointestinal tract, pancreas, and bile ducts are rare; most neoplasms of these organ systems are adenocarcinomas. NETs comprise only approximately 1.5% of all gastrointestinal and pancreatic neoplasms, with an estimated of 1 to 2 new cases reported per 100,000 persons per year. The average age at diagnosis is 61 years.[10,11] Most NETs occur sporadically but a small percentage are associated with complex familial syndromes such as multiple endocrine neoplasia type 1 (MEN-1), von Hippel-Lindau (vHL) disease, and neurofibromatosis 1 (NF-1).

Thoracic NETs

Bronchial carcinoids are rare pulmonary neoplasms, comprising approximately 1% to 2% of all lung tumors.[12] The tumors have variable clinical behavior and histologic differentiation ranging from indolent low-grade neoplasms to high-grade small cell carcinomas. Unlike most bronchogenic carcinomas, typical bronchial carcinoids affect men and women almost equally and manifest at an earlier age.[13] Approximately half of the patients with bronchial carcinoids are symptomatic because of the central location of the tumor; common symptoms include cough, recurrent infection, and hemoptysis.[14] Hormonal manifestations of bronchial carcinoids are rare; only 2% of patients have Cushing syndrome, whereas less than 5% have carcinoid syndrome. The carcinoid syndrome is usually because of liver metastases and is extremely rare in cases of isolated bronchial carcinoids and is discussed later.[15]

The imaging findings of bronchial carcinoids are protean because of their site of origin and degree of histologic differentiation. A common radiographic and computed tomographic (CT) finding is a well-circumscribed slightly lobulated hilar mass (**Fig. 1**); occasionally, carcinoids present as

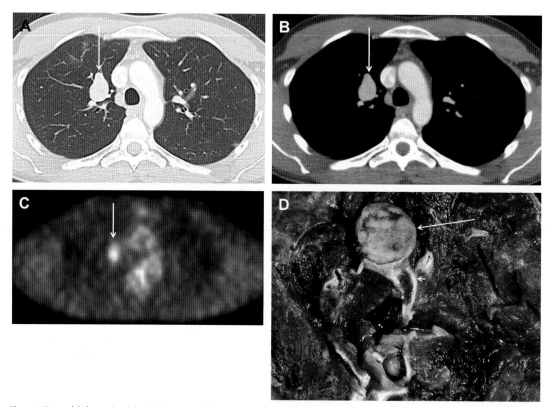

Fig. 1. Bronchial carcinoid. A 35-year-old man presented with recurrent hemoptysis. (*A*) Contrast material–enhanced chest CT displayed in lung windows shows a well-marginated nodule (*arrow*) in the orifice of the anterior segmental bronchus of the right upper lobe. (*B*) Contrast material–enhanced chest CT displayed in soft tissue windows shows homogeneous enhancement of the right upper lobe nodule (*arrow*). (*C*) Positron emission tomographic image shows moderate fludeoxyglucose avidity in the right upper lobe nodule (*arrow*). (*D*) Gross pathology specimen shows the round tumor (*long arrow*) at the orifice of the anterior segmental bronchus (*short arrow*) of the right upper lobe. (*Courtesy of* Carl. R. Fuhrman, MD, Pittsburgh, PA.)

peripheral subpleural nodules, usually with well-marginated borders. Carcinoids can occasionally be entirely endoluminal, although most have an endoluminal and an extrabronchial (parenchymal) component with variable degrees of invasion of the bronchial wall, cartilaginous rings, and lung parenchyma.[16] Central carcinoids, and those with a large endoluminal component, can result in bronchial occlusion and postobstructive atelectasis, inflammation, and mucoid impaction (**Fig. 2**). Central bronchial carcinoids are typically larger than peripheral lesions. Whereas typical and atypical carcinoids have similar imaging features, atypical carcinoids, tumors with more aggressive features such as increased mitotic activity and increased nuclear pleomorphism, are usually larger than typical indolent carcinoids.[16] The more aggressive atypical carcinoids are more likely to invade the adjacent structures (lungs, vessels, and lymphatics), metastasize, and exhibit necrosis and hemorrhage.[17] Metastases occur in approximately 15% of bronchial carcinoids.[18] Additional CT findings of bronchial carcinoids include variable tumor calcification and enhancement; however, not all bronchial carcinoids show contrast material enhancement and the degree of enhancement alone cannot be used to differentiate a carcinoid from bronchogenic carcinoma.[19] At MR imaging, carcinoids show high signal intensity on both T1- and T2-weighted imaging.

Carcinoids are also rare primary malignancies of the thymus. These tumors typically manifest in the fifth decade and are 3 times more common in men. Thymic carcinoids are usually more aggressive than bronchial carcinoids and symptoms are commonly because of mass effect on, or invasion of, mediastinal structures.[20] Thymic carcinoids are hormonally active in approximately 50% of patients, with Cushing syndrome affecting up to 40% of the affected patients.[21] In addition, up to 25% of patients with thymic carcinoids have MEN-1. Most thymic NETs are considered to be atypical carcinoids and have histologic features resembling bronchial carcinoids. As such, thymic carcinoids are commonly large heterogeneous masses that show local invasion or metastases in up to 30% of patients at the time of diagnosis.[21]

At radiography, the most common finding is a contour abnormality of the anterior mediastinum. CT and MR imaging typically show a large heterogeneously enhancing mass with variable degrees of invasion of adjacent mediastinal structures (**Fig. 3**). Distant metastases typically involve the lung, pleura, and brain.

GASTROINTESTINAL SITE-SPECIFIC FEATURES
Stomach

Gastric carcinoids comprise 8.7% of all gastrointestinal NETs and 1.8% of gastric malignancies.[8] Most gastric carcinoids are derived from the enterochromaffin-like (ECL) cell; 3 types of gastric ECL cell carcinoids have been described. Type 1 carcinoids account for up to 80% of cases and are associated with autoimmune chronic atrophic gastritis.[22] These tumors are usually clinically silent and incidentally discovered at endoscopy as numerous submucosal lesions of the gastric fundus and body that typically measure less than 2 cm in diameter. However, limited metastases to regional nodes have been reported in 5% of cases.[23] Type II gastric carcinoids account for 6% of gastric endocrine tumors. They are also usually multifocal and small (<2 cm); however,

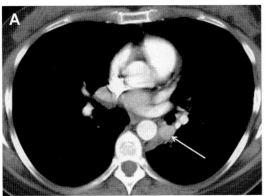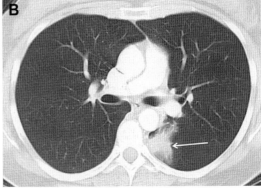

Fig. 2. Bronchial carcinoid. A 42-year-old woman presented with persistent cough. (*A*) Contrast material–enhanced chest CT displayed in soft tissue windows shows a well-marginated enhancing lesion (*arrow*) in the superior segmental bronchus of the left lower lobe. (*B*) Contrast material–enhanced chest CT displayed in lung windows shows postobstructive atelectasis (*arrow*) and volume loss in the superior segment of the left lower lobe. (*Courtesy of* Carl. R. Fuhrman, MD, Pittsburgh, PA.)

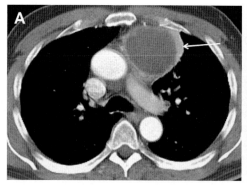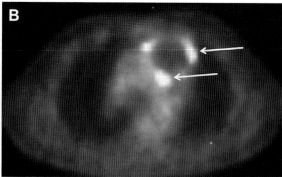

Fig. 3. Thymic carcinoid. A 61-year-old man was found to have a mediastinal mass during cardiac evaluation for chest discomfort. (*A*) Contrast material–enhanced chest CT displayed in soft tissue windows shows a 7-cm anterior mediastinal mass. The mass has central necrosis and enhancing solid components (*arrow*) along the periphery. (*B*) Positron emission tomographic image shows foci of fluorodeoxyglucose (FDG) avidity (*arrows*) corresponding to the peripheral solid components and lack of FDG avidity in the central necrotic portion of the mass. (*Courtesy of* Carl. R. Fuhrman, MD, Pittsburgh, PA.)

metastases occur in 10% to 30% of cases.[23] Type II gastric carcinoids are associated with Zollinger-Ellison syndrome (ZES) in the setting of MEN-1; approximately one-third of patients with these syndromes develop a type II carcinoid, whereas less than 1% of patients with sporadic ZES develop a gastric NET.[24] Type III gastric NETs are sporadic and usually occur in the body and fundus of the stomach. Compared with the other types of gastric NETs, these tumors are usually solitary, larger (>2 cm), and more likely to show vascular invasion; patients typically present with signs and symptoms of an aggressive mass and have no endocrine manifestations. At the time of diagnosis, metastases are present in up to 70% of well-differentiated tumors and up to nearly 100% of poorly differentiated tumors.[23]

The imaging findings of gastric NETs are variable and reflect the histologic differentiation and classification of the tumor. Because most gastric NETs are of types I and II, their sizes and imaging/endoscopic appearances cannot be reliably differentiated from those of the more common small submucosal tumors and polyps encountered in polyposis syndromes. Thin collimation CT can show a focal mural mass with variable contrast enhancement, although the small size of many tumors renders them undetectable by CT.[25] With double-contrast barium examinations, a small submucosal mass can be depicted, whereas larger carcinoids may show surface ulcerations manifesting as irregular collections of contrast or air on the ulcer crater surface. For less-differentiated gastric carcinoids, the imaging findings begin to parallel the more common gastric adenocarcinomas. CT findings may include a large ulcerated mass with associated perigastric adenopathy and liver metastases. Such findings are nonspecific, and differential considerations include gastrointestinal stromal tumor, adenocarcinoma, and lymphoma. Some poorly differentiated gastric NETs can be infiltrative and scirrhous; CT findings can be limited to wall thickening or luminal distortion because of the infiltrative nature of the primary tumor. These types of tumors may be underestimated at CT unless an intraluminal fungating or polypoid component is present. Barium examinations of the larger, less-differentiated tumors can show ulcerations, poor gastric distensibility, annular or focal luminal distortion, and a fungating mass projecting into the lumen. Although exceedingly rare, NETs of the esophagus are typically located distally and can potentially extend to the gastric cardia.[26] However, these tumors are typically depicted as small ulcerative or polypoid masses at esophagography and endoscopy.

Small Intestine

Carcinoids of the duodenum are rare, accounting for 2% to 3% of all gastrointestinal NETs.[8] Gastrin cell tumors are the most common type of duodenal NETs; one-third of these are functional gastrinomas that cause abdominal pain, gastric ulceration, bleeding, and diarrhea associated with ZES. Most sporadic gastrinomas are solitary and 85% occur in the gastrinoma triangle, defined superiorly by the junction of the cystic and common bile ducts, inferiorly by the junction of the second to third portions of the duodenum, and medially by the junction of the neck and body of the pancreas. Gastrinomas associated with ZES and MEN-1 are typically multiple, subcentimeter, and located in the wall of the proximal duodenum; in patients with MEN-1, up to 90%

develop multiple gastrinomas. Less common types of duodenal NETs include D cell (somatostatin producing) tumors, nonfunctioning tumors, poorly differentiated ampullary carcinomas, and gangliocytic paragangliomas. Duodenal somatostatinomas occur exclusively in the periampullary region and are associated with NF-1; up to 50% of patients with D cell carcinoids have NF-1. Clinically, systemic effects of elevated somatostatin levels are rare; however, if large, the tumor may cause local obstruction and pancreatitis.

Duodenal carcinoids can be difficult to detect at CT because of their size and location; most carcinoids are 1 to 2 cm in diameter. Approximately 50% of duodenal carcinoids manifest as intraluminal polypoid masses, whereas 40% are intramural (Fig. 4).[27] At contrast-enhanced CT, carcinoids often show brisk arterial phase enhancement with loss of enhancement on delayed phase imaging; this enhancement pattern can be used to differentiate carcinoids from other periampullary tumors (such as adenomas and adenocarcinomas) which do not typically show arterial enhancement. Use of a negative oral contrast agent, such as water or ultralow-dose barium suspension, can aid in the detection of small hypervascular mural and intraluminal lesions at CT. Barium examinations show a well-defined intraluminal polypoid mass or an intramural mass with focal ulceration.[27]

Gastrointestinal NETs are most commonly found in the distal ileum, and ileal NETs account for up to 30% of all cases.[27,28] These tumors arise from enterochromaffin (EC) cells in the distal ileum. Whereas these tumors commonly produce serotonin, the clinical presentation is usually indolent and nonspecific. Patients commonly present with vague pain, bleeding, or intermittent partial bowel obstruction. Only approximately 10% of patients present with classic carcinoid syndrome that occurs when nondegraded vasoactive metabolites enter the systemic circulation.[29] The syndrome is most commonly encountered in patients with ileal carcinoids, hepatic metastases, or retroperitoneal metastases. Clinically, the syndrome consists of

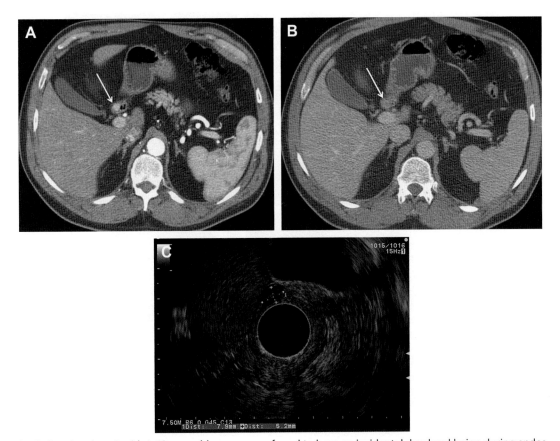

Fig. 4. Duodenal carcinoid. A 58-year-old woman was found to have an incidental duodenal lesion during endoscopy for dyspepsia. (A) Contrast material–enhanced CT shows a briskly enhancing round lesion (arrow) in the lumen of the proximal duodenum during the arterial phase. (B) Contrast material–enhanced CT shows that the lesion (arrow) becomes isoattenuating to the adjacent duodenum on the portal venous phase. (C) Image from corresponding endoscopic ultrasonography shows the well-marginated solid lesion.

cutaneous flushing, sweating, bronchospasm, abdominal pain, diarrhea, and fibrosis of right-sided heart valves.

Radiographic localization of enteric NETs can be challenging because of their small size coupled with bowel underdistension and tortuosity; in addition, ileal NETs can be multifocal in up to 40% of cases. At small bowel follow-through, typical carcinoids are usually shown as small, smooth, polypoid, mucosal and submucosal lesions in the distal ileum (Fig. 5A, B). The tumor can cause ulceration of the overlying mucosa. Ulceration results in a barium-filled crater overlying the primary lesion. At contrast-enhanced CT or MR imaging, the primary carcinoid can manifest as a focal, enhancing, intramural nodule that may protrude into the lumen; this may serve as a lead point for intussusception in some cases. The primary carcinoid can also infiltrate the bowel wall and cause submucosal fibrosis; this is manifested at CT as asymmetric or annular mural

thickening and at small bowel follow-through as a fixed distorted segment of small bowel. Advanced tumoral infiltration and fibrosis can result in an abrupt turn or kinking of the small bowel referred to as the hairpin turn. At the time of diagnosis, ileal NETs would have typically traversed the muscularis propria, infiltrated the adjacent mesentery, and metastasized to regional nodes; in addition, up to 20% of patients have hepatic metastases during diagnosis.[28] The regional infiltration of tumor and release of serotonin commonly results in a desmoplastic reaction in the mesentery; typical imaging findings including a stellate soft tissue mass, which is commonly calcified; adjacent bowel wall kinking/retraction; and bowel obstruction (see Fig. 5C, D). Adjacent mesenteric vessels can thicken and develop multifocal stenoses because of the substances released from the tumor; this elastic vascular sclerosis can eventually lead to vascular occlusions and bowel ischemia.[30] Advanced

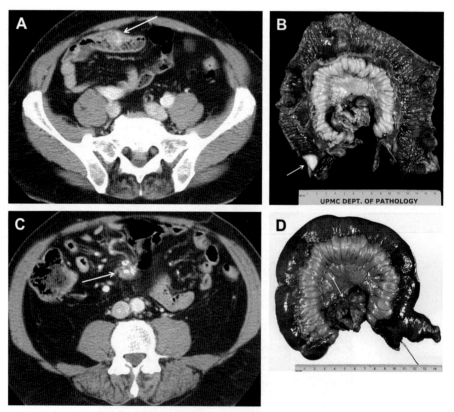

Fig. 5. Well-differentiated multifocal NET of the ileum. A 64-year-old man presented with nonspecific abdominal pain and underwent CT examination. (A) Contrast material–enhanced CT shows a submucosal lesion (arrow) in the distal ileum. A total of 4 ileal NETs were found at pathology, but only 1 was apparent at CT. (B) Gross specimen of a segment of the ileum shows a submucosal NET (arrow). (C) More superiorly, there is a central mesenteric metastasis (arrow) with stippled calcification resulting in tethering of the adjacent mesentery and bowel segments. (D) Gross specimen shows the mesenteric metastasis (arrow) distorting the adjacent fat and tethering the small bowel.

mesenteric disease may progress to miliary peritoneal implants and caking. Hepatic metastases are generally hypervascular and show strong arterial phase enhancement with subsequent washout on later phases of imaging (**Fig. 6**). Differential considerations for small bowel carcinoids include primary adenocarcinoma, lymphoma, gastrointestinal stromal tumors, and metastases from melanoma, breast, and lung carcinomas. Occasionally, Crohn disease and ischemic changes may simulate the bowel changes and mesenteric metastases caused by ileal carcinoid.

Gastrointestinal carcinoids are associated with other tumors, especially when the carcinoid is located in the small bowel[8]; in this population, 29% of patients harbor synchronous or metachronous malignancies (commonly adenocarcinoma).[31]

Appendix

Appendiceal carcinoids are most commonly derived from EC cells and produce serotonin. These tumors have the best prognosis of all gastrointestinal tract NETs because of their indolent biological behavior and early symptom onset with subsequent appendectomy. Most of (70%) these tumors affect the more distal appendix and are discovered incidentally in appendectomy specimens.[32] These tumors rarely penetrate the appendiceal wall and usually do not infiltrate the mesoappendix or metastasize; however, the goblet cell carcinoid is a more aggressive variant that is more closely related to adenocarcinoma.

The relative paucity of reported imaging features of appendiceal carcinoids reflects their small size, confinement, and benign behavior. Secondary findings of periappendiceal inflammation because of the tumor obstructing a portion of the lumen are typically the initial manifestations. Rarely, a focal soft tissue mass or circumferential wall thickening may be shown.[32]

Colon and Rectum

Colonic NETs are rare EC cell–derived tumors. They typically present as large ulcerating masses.

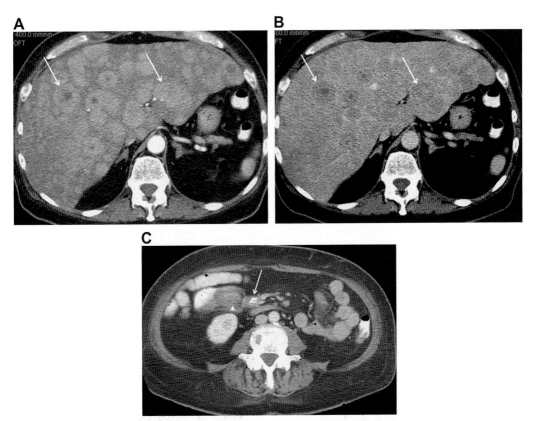

Fig. 6. Metastatic ileal carcinoid. A 66-year-old man presented with tachycardia, flushing, diarrhea, and dyspnea, consistent with carcinoid syndrome. (*A*) Contrast material–enhanced CT during the arterial phase shows innumerable hypervascular metastases (*arrows*) throughout the liver. (*B*) Contrast material–enhanced CT during the portal venous phase shows hypoattenuation of the lesions (*arrows*) due to washout of the contrast material. (*C*) More inferiorly, a partially calcified mesenteric metastasis (*long arrow*) is adjacent to a segment of thickened tethered distal ileum (*arrowhead*); this was the site of the primary carcinoid.

Weight loss and pain are the typical symptoms; carcinoid syndrome from metastatic disease is a less-common presentation. Most of these tumors are poorly differentiated carcinomas and have already metastasized at the time of diagnosis. In contrast, rectal NETs are derived from enteroendocrine cells and account for up to 27% of all gastrointestinal NETs and 1% of all rectal cancers. Compared with colonic carcinoids, rectal carcinoids are typically small (<1 cm) and asymptomatic. They have a better prognosis because most of these tumors are confined to the rectal wall[28]; if a rectal carcinoid does metastasize, symptoms of carcinoid syndrome are usually absent.

There are relatively few reports in the literature describing the imaging features of colorectal carcinoids. Colonic carcinoids are commonly large ulcerating masses in the ascending colon and are indistinguishable from large polypoid adenomas or adenocarcinomas; the tumors may have regions of low attenuating necrosis at CT and may cause colocolonic intussusception; rarely, the tumors may be annular and infiltrative.[7] Rectal carcinoids are usually not apparent at CT because of their small size and submucosal location; transrectal ultrasonography (US) can be used to assess the depth of invasion.[33]

Rare Locations

Carcinoids have been infrequently reported in the esophagus, Meckel diverticulum, enteric duplication cysts, and biliary system, but these are all exceedingly rare locations of carcinoids and difficult to identify radiographically.[7]

PANCREAS

Pancreatic NETs are a rare diverse group of related neoplasms that have variable hormone production and secretion. The first report of a pancreatic NET was published in 1902 by Nicholls.[34] He described a tumor originating from pancreatic islet cells. This relatively recent description of pancreatic NETs may be because of their rarity; they are estimated to occur in approximately 1 in 100,000 people, although some autopsy series have reported the incidence to be as high as 1.5%.[35] Pancreatic exocrine tumors are overwhelmingly more common because adenocarcinoma is diagnosed approximately 125 times more often than pancreatic NETs.[36] Although less common and typically less aggressive than pancreatic adenocarcinoma, pancreatic NETs metastasize to the liver more commonly than all tumors except colon cancer. The most common cause of death from pancreatic NET is hepatic failure.[37,38]

Historically, several investigators have suggested that these tumors derive from the amine precursor uptake and decarboxylation cells; the general term apudomas includes pancreatic NETs (previously commonly referred to as islet cell tumors), carcinoids, pheochromocytomas, and medullary thyroid cancers.[39] Other evidence indicates that pancreatic NETs may originate from the multipotential cells of the pancreatic ductal epithelium. Despite the debate over their cause, the various types of pancreatic NETs often overlap in their clinical features, imaging characteristics, treatment options, and prognosis[40]; however, these tumors also have key clinical and imaging distinctions.

The most basic groups of pancreatic NETs are functioning and nonfunctioning tumors. A functioning tumor produces a typical clinically evident syndrome. The moniker for functioning tumors most commonly refers to the hormone produced. Insulinoma and gastrinoma are the common types of functioning tumors, whereas somatostatinoma, VIPoma (vasoactive intestinal peptide), glucagonoma, and adrenocorticotropic hormone–producing tumor are much less common. Conversely, nonfunctioning tumors are often clinically silent and unnamed. Nonfunctioning pancreatic NETs may not be clinically apparent because of insufficient hormone production, lack of secretion of produced hormone, or lack of end-organ physiologic effect of the produced hormone. Nonfunctioning pancreatic NETs are reported in 30% to 40% of all patients with pancreatic NETs.[41] Although clinically silent and functioning tumors cannot be reliably distinguished histologically, functioning islet cell tumors usually manifest earlier because of unique signs and symptoms associated with the endocrine syndrome and nonfunctioning tumors more commonly present with locally advanced or metastatic disease.

While most pancreatic NETs occur sporadically, some are associated with inherited genetic syndromes. The most common syndrome associated with pancreatic NETs is MEN-1. This syndrome is most commonly characterized by tumors of the pituitary gland, parathyroid glands, and NETs of the pancreas. Less commonly, patients develop carcinoid, adrenal, thyroid, and ovarian tumors. MEN-1 follows an autosomal dominant pattern of inheritance and has been associated with mutations on chromosome 11.[42] Less commonly, pancreatic NETs are associated with vHL disease; this syndrome also follows autosomal dominant inheritance and is caused by a mutation on chromosome 3. vHL is characterized by cerebellar and retinal hemangioblastomas and tumors and cysts of the pancreas, kidney, and epididymis. Approximately 14% of patients with vHL have pancreatic NETs and more than half of the patients have multiple tumors; the majority of these tumors are nonfunctional.

Cross-Sectional Imaging Findings

Imaging has evolved to play a pivotal role in both diagnosis and postoperative surveillance for pancreatic NETs. Various studies have shown the importance of preoperative imaging in reducing the operative time and risk of pancreatic injury.[43,44] The imaging and surgical pathologic characteristics of pancreatic NETs are a direct result of the functioning versus nonfunctioning status of the tumor. Because functioning tumors usually produce symptoms and syndromes earlier, they are detected and resected earlier; this results

in discovery and treatment of typically small (commonly 1–2 cm) homogeneous tumors. Typically, such tumors are not metastatic and are not locally invasive at the time of diagnosis. On the other hand, nonfunctioning NETs are typically larger (several centimeters) and heterogeneous; as such, they commonly contain areas of irregular calcification, necrosis, and cystic changes. Local invasion, vascular invasion, and distant metastatic disease are typically observed (**Fig. 7**).[45]

Role of CT in Pancreatic NETs

The primary imaging modality for pancreatic disease in most radiology departments is CT. Its widespread availability, speed, and spatial resolution make CT a reproducible, well-tolerated, noninvasive examination. The development of dose-modulating scanners has been effective in

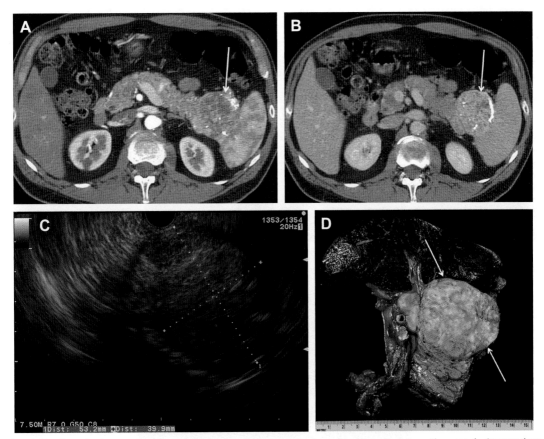

Fig. 7. Nonfunctioning pancreatic NET. A 61-year-old man was found to have a pancreatic mass during workup for nephrolithiasis. (*A*) Contrast material–enhanced chest CT during the pancreatic parenchymal phase shows heterogeneous enhancement of a large mass (*arrow*) in the pancreatic tail. There are scattered calcifications in the mass. (*B*) Contrast material–enhanced chest CT during the portal venous phase shows more homogeneous enhancement of the pancreatic mass (*arrow*). (*C*) Image from endoscopic ultrasonography shows a solid hypoechoic mass (*graticules*) in the pancreatic tail. Fine-needle aspiration was consistent with well-differentiated NET. (*D*) Gross pathology specimen following distal pancreatectomy and splenectomy shows the round fleshy tumor (*arrows*) arising in the pancreatic tail and abutting the splenic hilum.

reducing radiation exposure. Because pancreatic NETs are often hypervascular, performing an arterial phase leads to improved detection of these tumors.[46] Therefore, the typical protocol for CT of the pancreas is a triphasic examination consisting of an initial noncontrast phase followed by arterial and portal venous phases. Peak arterial enhancement can be determined by the use of bolus timing software. The images are usually acquired at 2.5 mm collimation using helical technique. A negative contrast agent, such as water, is the preferred oral contrast because it may aid in depicting small hypervascular tumors adjacent to the duodenal wall. Postoperative follow-up examinations should also be performed with the triphasic technique to provide the most sensitive evaluation for small hypervascular liver metastases.

Although pancreatic NETs are often hypervascular, their imaging characteristics somewhat depend on their size. Some subcentimeter tumors may be detectable only in the arterial phase, whereas larger tumors may be best identified in

the parenchymal phase. Therefore, performing CT in both the arterial and parenchymal phases improves detection of pancreatic NETs (**Fig. 8**).[46] The sensitivity of detection of pancreatic NETs is variable and directly related to their size. Occasionally, pancreatic NETs present as cystic lesions at CT and MR imaging (**Fig. 9**); differential considerations include pancreatic cysts, pseudocysts, and mucinous cystic neoplasms. Evaluation with endoscopic ultrasonography (EUS) and fine-needle aspiration (FNA) allow for better characterization.

Role of MR Imaging in Pancreatic NETs

The lack of ionizing radiation and exquisite soft tissue contrast resolution of MR imaging have made it an increasingly important modality in the evaluation of pancreatic NETs.[47] Refinement of protocols and application of parallel imaging have decreased the scan time for MR imaging. The typical protocol for MR imaging of the

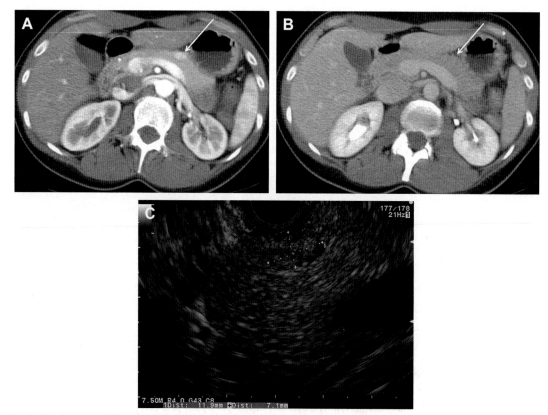

Fig. 8. Insulinoma. A 36-year-old woman presented with persistent hypoglycemia and underwent CT protocol for evaluation of pancreas. (*A*) Contrast material–enhanced chest CT during the pancreatic parenchymal phase shows an ovoid hypervascular lesion (*arrow*) in the distal pancreatic body. (*B*) Contrast material–enhanced chest CT during the portal venous phase shows the lesion is inconspicuous because of its isoattenuation to background pancreas (*arrow* shows expected location of lesion). (*C*) Image from endoscopic ultrasonography shows the iso-echoic, well-marginated, ovoid lesion (graticules).

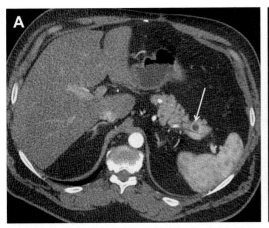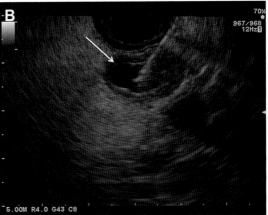

Fig. 9. Cystic NET of the pancreas. A 53-year-old man presented with back pain, and a pancreatic lesion was found at CT. (*A*) Contrast material–enhanced CT during the arterial phase shows a well-marginated near-water attenuation lesion (*arrow*) with a thin rim of peripheral enhancement in the pancreatic tail. (*B*) Image from endoscopic ultrasonography shows the cystic lesion and needle entering the lesion (*arrow*) during fine-needle aspiration; the aspirate was consistent with NET, and the patient subsequently underwent distal pancreatectomy.

pancreas includes a combination of T1- and T2-weighted sequences and dynamic precontrast and postcontrast volumetric T1-weighted sequences with fat saturation. The postcontrast sequences should include an arterial and more delayed phases of imaging to allow detection of small hypervascular lesions. Studies have shown an overall sensitivity and specificity of 80% and 100%, respectively.[48] The typical MR findings include a hypervascular lesion showing low T1 signal and intermediate T2 signal intensities; larger necrotic tumors may show heterogeneous signal and enhancement.

Role of US in Pancreatic NETs

Transabdominal US plays a limited role in the detection and follow-up of pancreatic NETs because the pancreas is rarely able to be insonated in its entirety because of artifact from the overlying bowel. However, EUS has evolved to play a major role in the workup of pancreatic lesions. EUS performed at experienced centers usually allows complete evaluation of the gland; the close apposition of the probe to the lesion results in a higher-resolution image compared with that obtained by transabdominal US and allows for performance of FNA at the time of the scan. Intraoperative US plays a pivotal role in localizing small NETs as discussed in detail in the following sections.

TUMOR-SPECIFIC FEATURES
Insulinoma

Insulinoma is the most common type of functional pancreatic NET with a reported incidence of 4

cases per 1 million people per year.[49,50] Typically, insulinoma is clinically suspected in a patient with persistent, symptomatic, and episodic hypoglycemia. The diagnosis may often be delayed because insulinoma is an overall unusual cause of hypoglycemia. However, the hypoglycemia due to insulinoma typically occurs during a fasting state or after exercise and allows differentiation from the more common postprandial or reactive hypoglycemia. In fact, Whipple described a triad in 1935 in an attempt to better identify patients with insulinoma more accurately; the triad consists of signs and symptoms of hypoglycemia after fasting or exercise, blood glucose levels less than 45 mg/dL when symptomatic, and symptoms relieved by intravenous or oral glucose. Neuroglycopenic symptoms are common and include dizziness, amnesia, confusion, personality changes, and seizure; it is not uncommon for patients with insulinoma to be initially diagnosed with a neurologic disorder. Cardiovascular symptoms are less common and include tachycardia, chest pain, and diaphoresis.[51] The average duration of symptoms before diagnosis is 18 months.[50] The relative rarity and subtle presentation of these tumors makes diagnosis difficult and underscores the importance of a well-performed cross-sectional imaging study.

The first operative procedure for insulinoma was performed in 1926.[52] Approximately 95% of tumors are benign when diagnosed[53]; in one series of 224 patients with insulinoma, 87% had solitary benign tumors, 7% had multiple benign tumors, and 6% had malignant tumors.[54] The overall 5-year survival rate is 97%.[53] The incidence of MEN-1 in patients diagnosed with insulinoma is approximately 8%; patients with MEN-1 are more likely to have multiple tumors compared with patients with sporadic insulinomas.[54]

The overwhelming majority of insulinomas are found in the pancreas, with only 3% found in the peripancreatic tissues.[55] Insulinomas are equally distributed throughout the pancreas and 10% are multifocal. In these cases, MEN-1 should be considered, even though only 10% of patients with hyperinsulinism will have MEN-1.[56] Most insulinomas are small; 66% of these tumors measure less than 1.5 cm, whereas more than 90% measure less than 2 cm.[57] Only approximately 10% of insulinomas are malignant. When metastases do occur, the most common sites are the peripancreatic lymph nodes and the liver.

Preoperative imaging of patients with suspected or biochemically confirmed insulinoma is crucial in surgical planning. A National Institutes of Health (NIH) study of 25 patients with insulinomas reported that the sensitivities for the commonly performed preoperative tests are as follows: 88% for arterial stimulation with venous sampling, 68% for percutaneous transhepatic portal venous sampling, 43% for MR imaging, 36% for arteriography, 17% for CT, and 9% for transabdominal US.[58] Despite the variable sensitivity of these examinations, preoperative protocol for CT or MR imaging of the pancreas with dynamic postcontrast sequences is usually performed at most institutions. Although 97% of insulinomas are located in the pancreas, preoperative localization by imaging aids in surgical planning and patient education by allowing the surgeon to determine whether a Whipple procedure, a distal pancreatectomy/splenectomy, a central pancreatectomy, or an enucleation have to be undertaken. If the tumor is large, CT and MR imaging allow evaluation of adjacent structures. Most importantly, preoperative cross-sectional imaging may detect lymph node and hepatic metastases and may obviate an unnecessary surgery.

The success of localization has been greatly improved since the introduction of intraoperative US. Studies have shown that intraoperative US can identify 75% to 90% of nonpalpable insulinomas.[59] Moreover, intraoperative US aids in determining the relationship between the splenic artery and vein, superior mesenteric vessels, common bile duct, and pancreatic duct. Although the overall sensitivity of intraoperative palpation (75%–90%) is similar to that of intraoperative US, palpating tumors in the body and tail of the pancreas is easier than in the head and uncinate process. In addition, the combination of intraoperative palpation and intraoperative US results in the sensitivity approaching 100%.[60] Therefore, most centers now perform the preoperative protocol for CT or MR imaging of the pancreas and intraoperative US in the evaluation for insulinoma.

Gastrinoma

Gastrinoma is the second most common type of pancreatic NET after insulinoma.[61] Gastrinoma results in hypersecretion of gastrin, which causes gastric acid hypersecretion. The combination of duodenal-jejunal ulceration, gastric acid hypersecretion, and a neoplasm of the endocrine pancreas constitutes the ZES.[62] More than 90% of patients with gastrinomas have peptic ulcer disease[63]; because of the large volume of gastric acid secretion, common initial complaints include diarrhea and abdominal pain. Diagnosis of gastrinoma begins with an elevated serum gastrin level. The secretin stimulation test can differentiate between patients with ZES and other causes of hypergastrinemia.[64] The tumor is typically diagnosed in the sixth to eighth decades and is almost twice as common in men.[37] Up to 35% of gastrinomas are associated with MEN-1 (**Fig. 10**).[65] During diagnosis, more than 50% of patients have hepatic metastases.[66]

Approximately 60% of gastrinomas are located in the pancreas, whereas 30% are located in the duodenum.[55,67,68] The anatomic region between the junction of the pancreatic body and neck, the junction of the second and third portions of the duodenum, and the junction of the cystic duct and common bile duct constitutes the gastrinoma triangle. Up to 90% of gastrinomas are found in this triangle (**Figs. 11** and **12**).[69] CT and MR imaging can show enhancing tumors in the pancreas; however, the presence of a large percentage of gastrinomas in the duodenal wall results in decreased sensitivity. Somatostatin receptor scintigraphy (SRS) has been proved to be useful for localization of these small duodenal tumors; the sensitivity of planar SRS has been reported as 58%. Sensitivity is increased with the addition of single-photon emission computed tomography (**Fig. 13**).[70,71] EUS is a useful compliment to SRS. The sensitivity of EUS for duodenal gastrinomas as small as 2 mm has been reported to be between 82% and 93%.[68,72]

Glucagonoma

The classic clinical presentation of glucagonoma is referred to as the 4D syndrome. The syndrome consists of diabetes, dermatitis, deep venous thrombosis, and depression. The dermatitis component consists of a rash that develops erythematous plaques on the face, abdomen, groin, and lower extremities; the plaques coalesce and the borders become blistered and

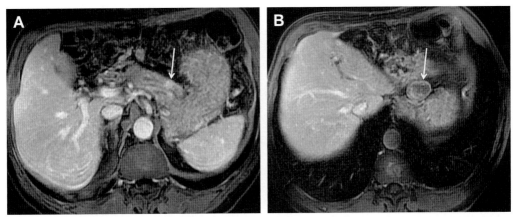

Fig. 10. Gastrinoma in the setting of MEN-1. A 70-year-old man with MEN-1 was found to have a pancreatic lesion, gastrohepatic ligament adenopathy, and a persistently elevated gastrin level. (*A*) Contrast material–enhanced T1-weighted MR imaging with fat suppression shows a subcentimeter hypervascular lesion (*arrow*) in the pancreatic body, consistent with gastrinoma. (*B*) More superiorly, an enlarged metastatic node (*arrow*) along the gastrohepatic ligament enhances heterogeneously.

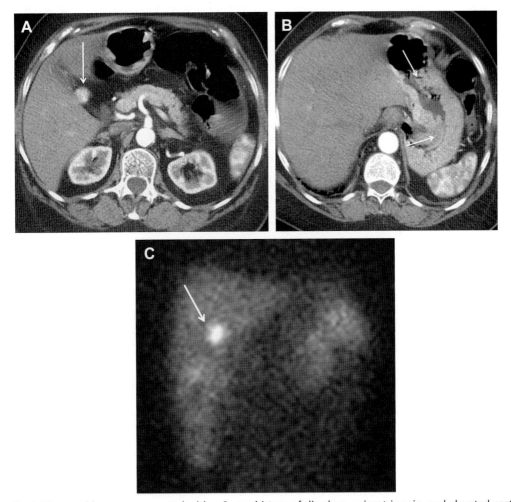

Fig. 11. A 70-year-old woman presented with a 6-year history of diarrhea, epigastric pain, and elevated gastrin level. (*A*) Contrast material–enhanced CT during the arterial phase shows a briskly enhancing lesion in the gallbladder fossa (*arrow*). (*B*) More superior section during CT shows thickened gastric folds (*arrows*) due to hypergastrinemia. (*C*) Coronal image from octreotide scan shows focal intense uptake (*arrow*) in the gallbladder fossa corresponding to the lesion on CT.

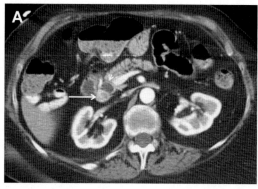
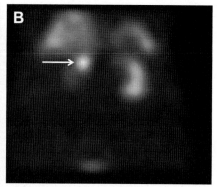

Fig. 12. A 71-year-old woman presented with persistent diarrhea and elevated gastrin levels after endoscopic removal of a duodenal gastrinoma. (*A*) Contrast material–enhanced CT shows a round enhancing lesion (*arrow*) adjacent to the distal common bile duct (*arrowhead*) and anterior to the kidney. (*B*) Coronal image from octreotide scan shows intense focal uptake (*arrow*) inferior to the liver and just anterior to the kidney, corresponding to the lesion on CT. (*Courtesy of* Nathan Johnson, MD, Pittsburgh, PA.)

encrusted.[73] The rash is referred to as necrolytic migratory erythema. Diabetes occurs in 75% to 95% of patients, and deep venous thrombosis occurs in up to 30% of patients.[74,75] Patients usually present in the fifth decade of life, and there is an equal gender distribution. Diagnosis can be made by a combination of classic symptoms and an elevated serum glucagon level.

Glucagonomas are usually greater than 4 cm at the time of initial imaging presentation. The tumors are almost always found in the pancreatic body and tail.[76] Hepatic metastases have been reported in more than 50% of patients at the time of diagnosis[77]; metastases can also occur in the adrenals, lymph nodes, bones, and lungs. Tumor size is correlated to the chance of malignancy; tumors greater than 5 cm in diameter have a 60% to 80% chance of being malignant.[54] CT

is the preferred imaging modality, and the typical imaging findings include a large heterogeneously enhancing mass in the pancreatic body and tail. If the tumor is not identified by CT, EUS has been proved to be effective, yielding a sensitivity of 82% and a specificity of 95%.[68]

Somatostatinoma

Somatostatin is a peptide that usually functions in a paracrine role by inhibiting secretion of insulin, gastrin, gastric acid, and cholecystokinin (CCK)-mediated pancreatic enzymes. Although often discovered incidentally, the classic presentation is diabetes due to somatostatin's inhibitory effect on insulin secretion, cholelithiasis due to inhibition of CCK and gallbladder contractility, and steatorrhea due to inhibition of pancreatic enzyme and

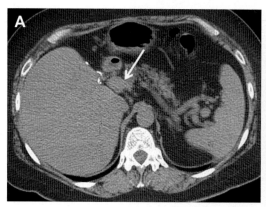
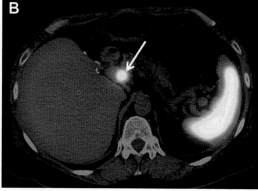

Fig. 13. Metastatic NET. A 55-year-old woman underwent surveillance CT after left hepatic lobectomy for metastatic NET. (*A*) Noncontrast CT shows a potential ill-defined soft tissue lesion (*arrow*), which was inseparable from the main portal vein. (*B*) Fused image from single-photon emission computed tomography-CT after injection of octreotide shows focal intense uptake (*arrow*) corresponding to the nodule on CT, consistent with a metastasis. There is physiologic uptake in the liver and spleen. (*Courtesy of* Judith Joyce, MD and Ashok Muthukrishnan, MD, Pittsburgh, PA.)

bicarbonate secretion.[78–80] The condition is diagnosed by an elevated fasting somatostatin level. Surgery is the only curative treatment; surgical debulking of metastatic disease may decrease symptoms of diarrhea and steatorrhea.[81] Duodenal somatostatinomas have a better prognosis than extraduodenal tumors.[82]

At imaging, most somatostatinomas are large heterogeneous tumors; 56% to 70% occur in the pancreas, and of these, 66% occur in the pancreatic head. Most extrahepatic somatostatinomas are located in the duodenum, ampulla, or small bowel; duodenal tumors are associated with NF-1.[83]

VIPoma

VIPoma is a rare tumor, usually occurring in adults in the fourth to sixth decade; the frequency is estimated to be approximately 1 in 10,000,000 per year.[84] VIPoma is caused by hypersecretion of vasoactive intestinal peptide. This amino acid peptide binds to receptors in the intestinal lumen to stimulate the secretion of sodium, chloride, potassium, and water into the lumen while increasing bowel motility. These actions lead to secretory diarrhea, hypokalemia, and dehydration. This clinical scenario is referred to as the Verner-Morrison syndrome[85]; it is also referred to as the WDHA syndrome, consisting of watery diarrhea, hypokalemia, and achlorhydria. Additional clinical manifestations include flushing, hypercalcemia, and hyperglycemia.[86] In addition to the clinical findings, diagnosis is made by stool analysis and a fasting plasma vasoactive intestinal polypeptide level. Definitive cure can be accomplished by surgery. In the setting of metastatic disease, aggressive debulking complements medical management of residual disease. Octreotide, a long-acting somatostatin analogue, can stop the diarrhea and allow easier correction of the metabolic derangements.

At imaging at initial presentation, most VIPomas are typically solitary and larger than 3 cm. Approximately 90% of VIPomas are located in the pancreas, with 75% of these found in the pancreatic tail. Less commonly, these tumors have been reported to arise in the colon, bronchus, adrenals, liver, and sympathetic ganglia.[55,84] In 60% to 80% of cases, VIPomas are metastatic when they are initially diagnosed.[87] CT or MR imaging shows a large heterogeneous tumor typically located in the pancreatic tail. Less commonly, somatostatin receptor scintigraphy can also be used for localization.

Nonfunctioning Pancreatic NETs

Many pancreatic NETs are not associated with a syndrome related to hormone hypersecretion and are therefore considered nonfunctioning. However, the tumors may secrete high levels of hormones that produce no symptoms; common hormones include pancreatic polypeptide, neurotensin, and calcitonin. Alternatively, the nonfunctioning tumors may produce minute amounts of biologically active hormones or inactive forms of hormones. Regardless, the nonfunctioning moniker of these pancreatic NETs stems from the lack of association with a hormonal symptom complex. The incidence of nonfunctioning pancreatic NETs has been reported to be as high as 48%.[41,88]

Because of the lack of clinical findings, nonfunctioning NETs present later than their functioning counterparts. Therefore, nonfunctioning pancreatic NETs are typically large at the time of resection, averaging a diameter of 4 cm compared with 1.9 cm for other types of pancreatic NETs.[88,89] The initial patient presentation is usually because of the size of the tumor; common clinical presentations include abdominal pain, weight loss, or jaundice, with abdominal pain being the most common symptom.[88] Although there is some controversy as to whether patients with nonfunctioning tumors have a worse prognosis than patients with functioning tumors,[90–92] nonfunctioning tumors are more commonly metastatic at the time of diagnosis compared with functioning tumors (60%–80% vs 25%).[53,88,93] The presence of metastases is a key finding in the evaluation of patients with pancreatic NETs and is best diagnosed with contrast-enhanced CT or MR imaging. The presence of metastases significantly affects survival: the 3-year survival for patients without liver metastases was 82% compared with 56% for patients with hepatic involvement.[94] At imaging, nonfunctioning NETs are shown as large heterogeneously enhancing pancreatic masses at CT and MR imaging (**Fig. 14**). Metastases are often found in the liver or by direct invasion of surrounding organs such as the spleen, stomach, and duodenum. However, the imaging features are nonspecific and differential considerations include pancreatic adenocarcinoma, metastases, and lymphoma.

Overview of Nuclear Medicine in NETs

Peptide receptor scintigraphy was shown to be of clinical utility for tumor localization through the successful in vivo demonstration of scintigraphic activity utilizing radioiodinated tyr-3-octeotide to bind to tumors that give positive test results for somatostatin receptor.[95,96] This development using an agent labeled with iodine 123 (^{123}I) (tyr-3-somatostatin 201–995, a synthetic

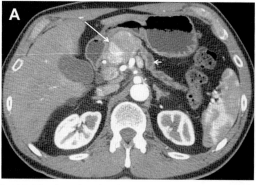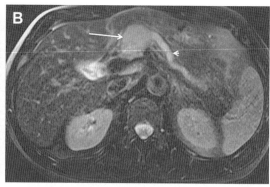

Fig. 14. Nonfunctional pancreatic NET. A 56-year-old man underwent surveillance CT for previously resected prostate cancer, and an incidental pancreatic mass was found. (A) Contrast material–enhanced CT during the pancreatic parenchyma phase shows a heterogeneously enhancing hypervascular lesion (arrow) in the pancreatic body, associated upstream pancreatic ductal dilatation (arrowhead), and parenchymal atrophy. (B) T2-weighted MR imaging shows high signal intensity in the pancreatic mass (arrow) and the dilated upstream pancreatic duct (arrowhead).

derivative of somatostatin) lead to the successful commercial development of 2 agents diethylene triamine pentaacetic acid (DTPA) labeled with indium 111 (^{111}In-DTPA) and ^{123}I-meta-iodobenzylguanidine (^{123}I-MIBG).[97] Of these 2 agents, ^{111}In-DTPA octreotide scintigraphy is most commonly used in clinical practice for evaluating gastrointestinal NETs.

Subsequent research identified alternative agents to ^{111}In-DTPA octreotide scintigraphy. The 2 most notable agents are technetium Tc 99m–labeled EDDA/HYNIC-TOC and gallium 68–labeled DOTA-Tyr3 (^{68}Ga-DOTA-Tyr3), which are used for conventional scintigraphy and positron emission tomography (PET), respectively.[98] However, neither of these compounds is commonly used in clinical practice at medical centers in the United States. The following sections focus on ^{111}In-DTPA octreotide scintigraphy, the most commonly used agent, and PET, a growing area of clinical interest.

Octreoscan

^{111}In-DTPA octreotide (Octreoscan) is the most commercially available and commonly used agent for somatostatin-based radionuclide receptor imaging (SRI) (Fig. 15).[99] Technetium Tc 99m-depreotide and [^{111}In-DOTA] lanreotide have been developed for SRI; however, they are not ideally suited for imaging abdominal NETs, primarily because of the their diminished sensitivity compared with ^{111}In-DTPA octreotide.[99,100]

Somatostatin receptors have been identified in vitro in a large number of human neoplasias.[99] There is a high incidence and density of somatostatin receptors, particularly in gastrointestinal NETs and other nongastrointestinal malignancies such as pituitary adenoma, meningioma, neuroblastoma, pheochromocytoma, paraganglioma,

medullary thyroid cancer, and small cell lung carcinoma.[101] Although other tumors, such as lymphoma, breast cancer, renal cell cancer, hepatocellular cancer, prostate cancer, sarcoma, and gastric cancer, can express somatostatin receptors, the somatostatin receptor subtype-2 is expressed in low amounts, and consequently, the activity is not shown in these malignancies.[99]

SRI has a high sensitivity for detecting gastrointestinal pancreatic NETs, particularly, gastrinomas, nonfunctioning NETs, and functioning endocrine pancreatic tumors except insulinomas and carcinoids. However, SRI has intermediate sensitivity for insulinomas.[70,99,102]

False-positive results using Octreoscan have been reported in up to 12% of all studies.[70] However, this result has been most commonly due to radiation pneumonitis, accessory spleen, focal collection of stools, surgical scar tissue, gallbladder uptake, nodular goiter, ventral hernia, bacterial pneumonia, respiratory tract infections, common cold (nasal uptake), cerebrovascular accident, concomitant granulomatous disease, diffuse breast uptake, adrenal uptake, urine contamination, and concomitant second primary tumor.[103]

PET

PET has recently emerged as an additional method to stage gastrointestinal NETs, because of improved spatial resolution and its ability to evaluate organs that have high background uptake with conventional SRS.[98,104] ^{68}Ga-DOTA-Tyr[3]-octreotide, rather than fludeoxyglucose F18 (^{18}F-FDG), has been used as a radiotracer for evaluating NETs, secondary to ^{18}F-FDG's low sensitivity for detecting tumors with slow growth and malignant potential.[98,105]

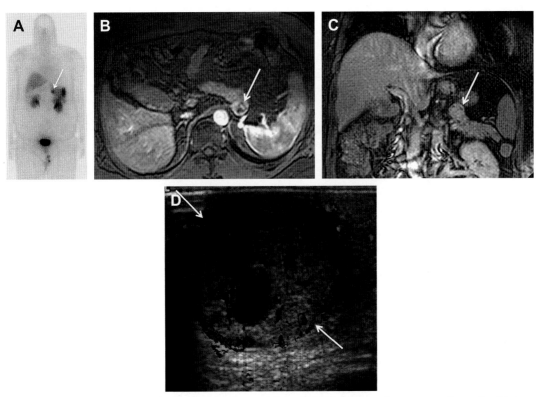

Fig. 15. Pancreatic NET. (*A*) Whole body planar image 4 hours after injection of octreoscan shows focal intense uptake (*arrow*) in the left upper quadrant, concerning for a NET. The remainder of the activity was physiologic. (*B*) Axial and (*C*) coronal postcontrast T1-weighted images with fat suppression show the corresponding hypervascular lesion (*arrows*) arising from the pancreatic body. (*D*) Intraoperative US shows heterogeneous color flow in a predominantly solid lesion (*arrow*) in the pancreatic tail. Pathology confirmed a well-differentiated NET.

However, ^{68}Ga-DOTA-Tyr^3-octreotide has improved diagnostic accuracy compared with conventional SRS, particularly with regard to osseous metastasis. However, visceral metastases, particularly involving the liver, remain best evaluated by CT secondary to radiotracer accumulation.[106]

SUMMARY

NETs constitute a large group of diverse neoplasms with a wide spectrum of clinical, imaging, and pathologic findings. Imaging diagnosis of NETs can be challenging, and several complementary imaging modalities may be needed during the diagnostic workup. Accurate interpretation of the imaging findings is important to facilitate diagnosis and contribute to patient management.

REFERENCES

1. Langhans T. Uber einen drusenpolyp im ileum. Virchows Arch Pathol Anat Physiol Klin Med 1867; 38:559–60 [in German].

2. Lubarsch O. Ueber den primaren krebs des ileum nebst bemerkungen uber das gleichzeitige vorkommen von krebs and tuberculose. Virchows Arch Pathol Anat Physiol Klin Med 1888;111:280–317 [in German].

3. Oberndorfer S. Karzinoide tumoren des dunndarms. Frankf Z Pathol 1907;1:426–32 [in German].

4. Gosset A, Masson P. Tumeurs endocrines de l'appendice. Presse Med 1914;2:237–40 [in French].

5. Williams ED, Sandler M. The classification of carcinoid tumours. Lancet 1963;1(7275):238–9.

6. Solcia E, Klöppel G, Sobin LH, et al. Histologic typing of endocrine tumours. Paper presented at WHO international histologic classification of tumours. Berlin, February 3, 2000.

7. Levy AD, Sobin LH. From the archives of the AFIP: gastrointestinal carcinoids: imaging features with clinicopathologic comparison. Radiographics 2007;27(1):237–57.

8. Modlin IM, Lye KD, Kidd M. A 5-decade analysis of 13,715 carcinoid tumors. Cancer 2003;97(4):934–59.

9. Rindi G, Bordi C. Highlights of the biology of endocrine tumours of the gut and pancreas. Endocr Relat Cancer 2003;10(4):427–36.

10. Thomas RM, Sobin LH. Gastrointestinal cancer. Cancer 1995;75(Suppl 1):154–70.

11. Crocetti E, Paci E. Malignant carcinoids in the USA, SEER 1992–1999. An epidemiological study with 6830 cases. Eur J Cancer Prev 2003;12(3):191–4.

12. Carter D, Yesner R. Carcinomas of the lung with neuroendocrine differentiation. Semin Diagn Pathol 1985;2(4):235–54.

13. Godwin JD 2nd. Carcinoid tumors. An analysis of 2,837 cases. Cancer 1975;36(2):560–9.

14. Dusmet ME, McKneally MF. Pulmonary and thymic carcinoid tumors. World J Surg 1996;20(2):189–95.

15. Davila DG, Dunn WF, Tazelaar HD, et al. Bronchial carcinoid tumors. Mayo Clin Proc 1993;68(8):795–803.

16. Colby TV, Koss MN, Travis WD. Carcinoid and other neuroendocrine tumors. In: Colby TV, Koss MN, Travis WD, editors. Atlas of tumor pathology: tumors of the lower respiratory tract. Washington, DC: Armed Forces Institute of Pathology; 1995. p. 287–317.

17. Hammar SP. Common neoplasms. In: Dail DH, Hammar SP, editors. Pulmonary pathology. 2nd edition. New York: Springer; 1994. p. 727–845.

18. Marty-Ane CH, Costes V, Pujol JL, et al. Carcinoid tumors of the lung: do atypical features require aggressive management? Ann Thorac Surg 1995; 59(1):78–83.

19. Aronchick JM, Wexler JA, Christen B, et al. Computed tomography of bronchial carcinoid. J Comput Assist Tomogr 1986;10(1):71–4.

20. Shimosato YM, Mukai K. Tumors of the thymus and related lesions. In: Shimosato Y, Mukai K, editors. Atlas of tumor pathology: tumors of the mediastinum. Washington, DC: Armed Forces Institute of Pathology; 1997. p. 158–68.

21. Wick MR, Scott RE, Li CY, et al. Carcinoid tumor of the thymus: a clinicopathologic report of seven cases with a review of the literature. Mayo Clin Proc 1980;55(4):246–54.

22. Bordi C. Gastric carcinoids. Ital J Gastroenterol Hepatol 1999;31(Suppl 2):S94–7.

23. Rindi G, Azzoni C, La Rosa S, et al. ECL cell tumor and poorly differentiated endocrine carcinoma of the stomach: prognostic evaluation by pathological analysis. Gastroenterology 1999; 116(3):532–42.

24. Lehy T, Cadiot G, Mignon M, et al. Influence of multiple endocrine neoplasia type 1 on gastric endocrine cells in patients with the Zollinger-Ellison syndrome. Gut 1992;33(9):1275–9.

25. Binstock AJ, Johnson CD, Stephens DH, et al. Carcinoid tumors of the stomach: a clinical and radiographic study. AJR Am J Roentgenol 2001; 176(4):947–51.

26. Lindberg GM, Molberg KH, Vuitch MF, et al. Atypical carcinoid of the esophagus: a case report and review of the literature. Cancer 1997;79(8): 1476–81.

27. Levy AD, Taylor LD, Abbott RM, et al. Duodenal carcinoids: imaging features with clinical-pathologic comparison. Radiology 2005;237(3):967–72.

28. Modlin IM, Sandor A. An analysis of 8305 cases of carcinoid tumors. Cancer 1997;79(4):813–29.

29. Sweeney JF, Rosemurgy AS. Carcinoid tumors of the gut. Cancer Control 1997;4(1):18–24.

30. Anthony PP, Drury RA. Elastic vascular sclerosis of mesenteric blood vessels in argentaffin carcinoma. J Clin Pathol 1970;23(2):110–8.

31. Burke AP, Thomas RM, Elsayed AM, et al. Carcinoids of the jejunum and ileum: an immunohistochemical and clinicopathologic study of 167 cases. Cancer 1997;79(6):1086–93.

32. Pickhardt PJ, Levy AD, Rohrmann CA Jr, et al. Primary neoplasms of the appendix: radiologic spectrum of disease with pathologic correlation. Radiographics 2003;23(3):645–62.

33. Chang S, Choi D, Lee SJ, et al. Neuroendocrine neoplasms of the gastrointestinal tract: classification, pathologic basis, and imaging features. Radiographics 2007;27(6):1667–79.

34. Nicholls AG. Simple adenoma of the pancreas arising from an Island of langerhans. J Med Res 1902;8(2):385–95.

35. Lam KY, Lo CY. Pancreatic endocrine tumour: a 22-year clinico-pathological experience with morphological, immunohistochemical observation and a review of the literature. Eur J Surg Oncol 1997; 23(1):36–42.

36. De Vita VH, Rosenberg S. Cancer principles and practice of oncology. Philadelphia: JB Lippincott; 1985.

37. Chen H, Hardacre JM, Uzar A, et al. Isolated liver metastases from neuroendocrine tumors: does resection prolong survival? J Am Coll Surg 1998; 187(1):88–92 [discussion: 92–3].

38. Eriksson B, Oberg K. Neuroendocrine tumours of the pancreas. Br J Surg 2000;87(2):129–31.

39. Friesen SR. Tumors of the endocrine pancreas. N Engl J Med 1982;306(10):580–90.

40. Solcia E, Sessa F, Rindi G, et al. Classification and histogenesis of gastroenteropancreatic endocrine tumours. Eur J Clin Invest 1990;20(Suppl 1):S72–81.

41. Kloppel G, Heitz PU. Pancreatic endocrine tumors. Pathol Res Pract 1988;183(2):155–68.

42. Sandelin K, Larsson C, Decker RA. Genetic aspects of multiple endocrine neoplasia types 1 and 2. Curr Opin Gen Surg 1994;60–8.

43. Huai JC, Zhang W, Niu HO, et al. Localization and surgical treatment of pancreatic insulinomas guided by intraoperative ultrasound. Am J Surg 1998;175(1):18–21.

44. Kuzin NM, Egorov AV, Kondrashin SA, et al. Preoperative and intraoperative topographic diagnosis of insulinomas. World J Surg 1998;22(6):593–7 [discussion: 597–8].

45. Buetow PC, Parrino TV, Buck JL, et al. Islet cell tumors of the pancreas: pathologic-imaging correlation among size, necrosis and cysts, calcification, malignant behavior, and functional status. AJR Am J Roentgenol 1995;165(5):1175–9.

46. Van Hoe L, Gryspeerdt S, Marchal G, et al. Helical CT for the preoperative localization of islet cell tumors of the pancreas: value of arterial and parenchymal phase images. AJR Am J Roentgenol 1995; 165(6):1437–9.

47. Somogyi L, Mishra G. Diagnosis and staging of islet cell tumors of the pancreas. Curr Gastroenterol Rep 2000;2(2):159–64.

48. Thoeni RF, Mueller-Lisse UG, Chan R, et al. Detection of small, functional islet cell tumors in the pancreas: selection of MR imaging sequences for optimal sensitivity. Radiology 2000;214(2): 483–90.

49. Cubilla AL, Hajdu SI. Islet cell carcinoma of the pancreas. Arch Pathol 1975;99(4):204–7.

50. Service FJ, McMahon MM, O'Brien PC, et al. Functioning insulinoma–incidence, recurrence, and long-term survival of patients: a 60-year study. Mayo Clin Proc 1991;66(7):711–9.

51. Dizon AM, Kowalyk S, Hoogwerf BJ. Neuroglycopenic and other symptoms in patients with insulinomas. Am J Med 1999;106(3):307–10.

52. Wilder RM, Allan FN, Power MH, et al. Carcinoma of the islands of the pancreas: hyperinsulinism and hypoglycemia. J Am Med Assoc 1927;89: 348.

53. Schindl M, Kaczirek K, Kaserer K, et al. Is the new classification of neuroendocrine pancreatic tumors of clinical help? World J Surg 2000;24(11):1312–8.

54. Boden G. Glucagonomas and insulinomas. Gastroenterol Clin North Am 1989;18(4):831–45.

55. Ectors N. Pancreatic endocrine tumors: diagnostic pitfalls. Hepatogastroenterology 1999;46(26):679–90.

56. Sheppard BC, Norton JA, Doppman JL, et al. Management of islet cell tumors in patients with multiple endocrine neoplasia: a prospective study. Surgery 1989;106(6):1108–17 [discussion: 1117–8].

57. Kaplan EL, Fredland A. The diagnosis and treatment of insulinomas. In: Thompson NW, Vinik AI, editors. Endocrine surgery update. Philadelphia: W.B. Saunders; 1983.

58. Doppman JL, Chang R, Fraker DL, et al. Localization of insulinomas to regions of the pancreas by intra-arterial stimulation with calcium. Ann Intern Med 1995;123(4):269–73.

59. Zeiger MA, Shawker TH, Norton JA. Use of intraoperative ultrasonography to localize islet cell tumors. World J Surg 1993;17(4):448–54.

60. Bottger TC, Junginger T. Is preoperative radiographic localization of islet cell tumors in patients with insulinoma necessary? World J Surg 1993; 17(4):427–32.

61. Wilson SD. Gastrinoma. In: Clark OH, Duh QY, editors. Textbook of endocrine surgery. Philadelphia: W.B. Saunders; 1997. p. 607.

62. Zollinger RM, Ellison EH. Primary peptic ulcerations of the jejunum associated with islet cell tumors of the pancreas. Ann Surg 1955;142(4): 709–23 [discussion: 724–8].

63. Deveney CW, Deveney KE. Zollinger-Ellison syndrome (gastrinoma). Current diagnosis and treatment. Surg Clin North Am 1987;67(2):411–22.

64. Mansour JC, Chen H. Pancreatic endocrine tumors. J Surg Res 2004;120(1):139–61.

65. Norton JA. Neuroendocrine tumors of the pancreas and duodenum. Curr Probl Surg 1994;31(2):77–156.

66. Jensen RT. Pancreatic endocrine tumors: recent advances. Ann Oncol 1999;10(Suppl 4):170–6.

67. Winter TC 3rd, Freeny PC, Nghiem HV. Extrapancreatic gastrinoma localization: value of arterial-phase helical CT with water as an oral contrast agent. AJR Am J Roentgenol 1996;166(1):51–2.

68. Rosch T, Lightdale CJ, Botet JF, et al. Localization of pancreatic endocrine tumors by endoscopic ultrasonography. N Engl J Med 1992;326(26):1721–6.

69. Stabile BE, Morrow DJ, Passaro E Jr. The gastrinoma triangle: operative implications. Am J Surg 1984;147(1):25–31.

70. Gibril F, Reynolds JC, Doppman JL, et al. Somatostatin receptor scintigraphy: its sensitivity compared with that of other imaging methods in detecting primary and metastatic gastrinomas. A prospective study. Ann Intern Med 1996;125(1):26–34.

71. Schillaci O, Corleto VD, Annibale B, et al. Single photon emission computed tomography procedure improves accuracy of somatostatin receptor scintigraphy in gastro-entero pancreatic tumours. Ital J Gastroenterol Hepatol 1999;31(Suppl 2): S186–9.

72. Anderson MA, Carpenter S, Thompson NW, et al. Endoscopic ultrasound is highly accurate and directs management in patients with neuroendocrine tumors of the pancreas. Am J Gastroenterol 2000;95(9):2271–7.

73. Kahan RS, Perez-Figaredo RA, Neimanis A. Necrolytic migratory erythema. Distinctive dermatosis of the glucagonoma syndrome. Arch Dermatol 1977; 113(6):792–7.

74. Mozell E, Stenzel P, Woltering EA, et al. Functional endocrine tumors of the pancreas: clinical presentation, diagnosis, and treatment. Curr Probl Surg 1990;27(6):301–86.

75. Stacpoole PW. The glucagonoma syndrome: clinical features, diagnosis, and treatment. Endocr Rev 1981;2(3):347–61.

76. Aldridge MC, Williamson RC. Surgery of endocrine tumors of the pancreas. In: Lynn JA, Bloom SR, editors. Surgical endocrinology. New York: Butterworth; 1993. p. 503.

77. Wermers RA, Fatourechi V, Kvols LK. Clinical spectrum of hyperglucagonemia associated with malignant neuroendocrine tumors. Mayo Clin Proc 1996;71(11):1030–8.

78. Jensen RT, Norton JA. Endocrine neoplasms of the pancreas. In: Yamada T, editor. Textbook of gastroenterology. Philadelphia: JB Lippincott; 1995. p. 2131.

79. Snow N, Liddle R. Neuroendocrine tumors. In: Rusygi A, editor. Gastrointestinal cancers: biology, diagnosis, and therapy. Philadelphia: Lippincott-Raven; 1995. p. 585.

80. Norton JA. Somatostatinoma and rare pancreatic endocine tumors. In: Clark OH, Duh QY, editors. Textbook of endocrine surgery. Philadelphia: W.B. Saunders; 1997. p. 626.

81. Anene C, Thompson JS, Saigh J, et al. Somatostatinoma: atypical presentation of a rare pancreatic tumor. Am J Gastroenterol 1995;90(5):819–21.

82. O'Brien TD, Chejfec G, Prinz RA. Clinical features of duodenal somatostatinomas. Surgery 1993;114(6):1144–7.

83. Mao C, Shah A, Hanson DJ, et al. Von Recklinghausen's disease associated with duodenal somatostatinoma: contrast of duodenal versus pancreatic somatostatinomas. J Surg Oncol 1995;59(1):67–73.

84. Friesen SR. Update on the diagnosis and treatment of rare neuroendocrine tumors. Surg Clin North Am 1987;67(2):379–93.

85. Verner JV, Morrison AB. Islet cell tumor and a syndrome of refractory watery diarrhea and hypokalemia. Am J Med 1958;25(3):374–80.

86. O'Dorisio TM, Mekhjian HS, Gaginella TS. Medical therapy of VIPomas. Endocrinol Metab Clin North Am 1989;18(2):545–56.

87. Smith SL, Branton SA, Avino AJ, et al. Vasoactive intestinal polypeptide secreting islet cell tumors: a 15-year experience and review of the literature. Surgery 1998;124(6):1050–5.

88. Phan GQ, Yeo CJ, Hruban RH, et al. Surgical experience with pancreatic and peripancreatic neuroendocrine tumors: review of 125 patients. J Gastrointest Surg 1998;2(5):473–82.

89. Yeo CJ, Wang BH, Anthone GJ, et al. Surgical experience with pancreatic islet-cell tumors. Arch Surg 1993;128(10):1143–8.

90. Chu QD, Hill HC, Douglass HO Jr, et al. Predictive factors associated with long-term survival in patients with neuroendocrine tumors of the pancreas. Ann Surg Oncol 2002;9(9):855–62.

91. Lo CY, van Heerden JA, Thompson GB, et al. Islet cell carcinoma of the pancreas. World J Surg 1996;20(7):878–83 [discussion: 884].

92. White TJ, Edney JA, Thompson JS, et al. Is there a prognostic difference between functional and nonfunctional islet cell tumors? Am J Surg 1994;168(6):627–9 [discussion: 629–30].

93. Muller MF, Meyenberger C, Bertschinger P, et al. Pancreatic tumors: evaluation with endoscopic US, CT, and MR imaging. Radiology 1994;190(3):745–51.

94. Thompson GB, van Heerden JA, Grant CS, et al. Islet cell carcinomas of the pancreas: a twenty-year experience. Surgery 1988;104(6):1011–7.

95. Krenning EP, Bakker WH, Breeman WA, et al. Localisation of endocrine-related tumours with radioiodinated analogue of somatostatin. Lancet 1989;1(8632):242–4.

96. Krenning EP, Kwekkeboom DJ, Bakker WH, et al. Somatostatin receptor scintigraphy with [111In-DTPA-D-Phe1]- and [123I-Tyr3]-octreotide: the Rotterdam experience with more than 1000 patients. Eur J Nucl Med 1993;20(8):716–31.

97. Balon HR, Goldsmith SJ, Siegel BA, et al. Procedure guideline for somatostatin receptor scintigraphy with (111)In-pentetreotide. J Nucl Med 2001;42(7):1134–8.

98. Gabriel M, Decristoforo C, Kendler D, et al. 68Ga-DOTA-Tyr3-octreotide PET in neuroendocrine tumors: comparison with somatostatin receptor scintigraphy and CT. J Nucl Med 2007;48(4):508–18.

99. Kwekkeboom DJ, Kam BL, van Essen M, et al. Somatostatin-receptor-based imaging and therapy of gastroenteropancreatic neuroendocrine tumors. Endocr Relat Cancer 2010;17(1):R53–73.

100. Menda Y, Kahn D. Somatostatin receptor imaging of non-small cell lung cancer with 99mTc depreotide. Semin Nucl Med 2002;32(2):92–6.

101. Reubi JC, Waser B, Markusse HM, et al. Vascular somatostatin receptors in synovium from patients with rheumatoid arthritis. Eur J Pharmacol 1994;271(2–3):371–8.

102. Lebtahi R, Cadiot G, Sarda L, et al. Clinical impact of somatostatin receptor scintigraphy in the management of patients with neuroendocrine gastroenteropancreatic tumors. J Nucl Med 1997;38(6):853–8.

103. Gibril F, Reynolds JC, Chen CC, et al. Specificity of somatostatin receptor scintigraphy: a prospective study and effects of false-positive localizations on management in patients with gastrinomas. J Nucl Med 1999;40(4):539–53.

104. Dromain C, de Baere T, Lumbroso J, et al. Detection of liver metastases from endocrine tumors: a prospective comparison of somatostatin receptor scintigraphy, computed tomography, and magnetic resonance imaging. J Clin Oncol 2005;23(1):70–8.

105. Kowalski J, Henze M, Schuhmacher J, et al. Evaluation of positron emission tomography imaging using [68Ga]-DOTA-D Phe(1)-Tyr(3)-Octreotide in comparison to [111In]-DTPAOC SPECT. First results in patients with neuroendocrine tumors. Mol Imaging Biol 2003;5(1):42–8.

106. Kumbasar B, Kamel IR, Tekes A, et al. Imaging of neuroendocrine tumors: accuracy of helical CT versus SRS. Abdom Imaging 2004;29(6):696–702.

Imaging of the Pituitary

Tao Ouyang, MD[a],*, William E. Rothfus, MD[b],
Jason M. Ng, MD[c], Sue M. Challinor, MD[c]

KEYWORDS

- Pituitary • MR imaging • Adenoma • Cushing syndrome
- Sella turcica

Since the advent of magnetic resonance (MR) imaging, imaging has become an integral part of the evaluation of patients with endocrinological abnormalities suspected to be of pituitary etiology. This article discusses normal development and anatomy of the pituitary gland, indications for imaging, and imaging techniques. In addition, imaging characteristics of common pituitary/infundibular lesions are discussed in detail. Juxtasellar/suprasellar pathologies that may mimic primary pituitary lesions are briefly reviewed. The postoperative appearance of sellar and suprasellar contents may be a source of misinterpretation, and this is discussed along with other errors in image interpretation.

DEVELOPMENT AND NORMAL ANATOMY

The pituitary gland is composed of anterior and posterior lobes. The anterior pituitary (adenohypophysis) is the larger part and arises from Rathke's pouch within the fetal nasopharynx. It produces numerous hormones: growth hormone (GH), thyroid-stimulating hormone, adrenocorticotropic hormone (ACTH), prolactin, luteinizing hormone, and follicle-stimulating hormone. The anterior pituitary receives its ample blood supply from the hypophyseal-portal system; blood flows within the infundibulum, which lacks a blood-brain barrier. The posterior pituitary (neurohypophysis) and the median eminence of the hypothalamus arise from neuroectoderm in the floor of the forebrain; the infundibular stalk arises from ventromedial hypothalamus. The pars intermedia separates the anterior gland from the posterior gland; the pars intermedia often contains small colloid cysts. The posterior gland contains two modified glial cell types, the tanycyte and the pituicyte, both of which support the axons of the neurons that produce vasopressin and oxytocin. These hormones are transported directly through the hypophyseal portal system.

The pituitary gland sits within the sella turcica, a cup-shaped bony depression within the basisphenoid. Above the sella is the dural covering known as the diaphragma sellae, and above that lies the suprasellar cistern, the optic chiasm, and the hypothalamus. Posteriorly, the sella is bound by the dorsum sella. The cavernous sinuses form the lateral borders of the pituitary fossa. The gland can be considered to sit within a dural "bag," a thin sheath separating it from the cavernous sinus. The lateral wall is not always a rigid sagittal fold of dura as commonly depicted in anatomic drawings, but may have a more undulating shape, allowing for normal lateral extension of the gland, especially superolaterally over the cavernous carotid.[1] Cranial nerves III, IV, V1, V2, and VI travel through or adjacent to the cavernous sinus, as do the cavernous internal carotid artery (ICA) and venous structures.

The authors have nothing to disclose.
[a] Division of Neuroradiology, Department of Radiology, Penn State Hershey Medical Center, 500 University Drive, H066, Hershey, PA 17033, USA
[b] Division of Neuroradiology, Department of Radiology, University of Pittsburgh Medical Center, 200 Lothrop Street, Pittsburgh, PA 15213, USA
[c] Division of Endocrinology and Metabolism, Department of Medicine, University of Pittsburgh Medical Center, 200 Lothrop Street, Pittsburgh, PA 15213, USA
* Corresponding author.
E-mail address: touyang@hmc.psu.edu

radiologic.theclinics.com

The size and shape of the pituitary gland is dependent on age and gender. The pituitary gland of a neonate is larger than in later childhood. Similarly, the gland is generally larger in women than in men. In pubertal girls and peripartum women, the gland may appear enlarged with a convex upper border. The gland can also become enlarged if exogenous estrogens are present, if there is excess or ectopic hypothalamic releasing factors, and in cases of end-organ failure. The infundibulum tapers normally from superior to inferior. Deviation or tilting of the infundibulum is common and does not always suggest underlying pathology; it may simply reflect a sloping sellar floor. In general, the size of the pituitary gland decreases with age.

In normal adults, the anterior pituitary is isointense to gray matter on T1-weighted and T2-weighted sequences. The posterior pituitary, on the other hand, is typically inherently T1 hyperintense; hyperintensity accounts for the so-called pituitary bright spot, attributed to an antidiuretic hormone neurosecretory granular complex present within the posterior pituitary. In neonates up to 2 months of age and in pregnant women, the anterior pituitary may be as or more hyperintense on T1 as the posterior pituitary. The posterior pituitary generally enhances before the anterior pituitary during dynamic contrast-enhanced imaging. The infundibulum enhances earlier than the remaining gland. Enhancement of the pituitary tuft (the junction of the stalk and gland) follows. Centrifugal enhancement of the remaining gland then occurs (**Fig. 1**). Contrast enhancement varies depending on microscopic anatomy: areas of densely compacted cellularity and/or increased cellular granularity are intermixed with areas of less compacted cellularity and diminished granularity.[2] The normal gland may also appear very heterogeneous because of natural asymmetries of the position of anterior and posterior gland and pars intermedia colloid cyst variability.

INDICATIONS FOR IMAGING

Pituitary imaging is indicated in patients who present with signs and symptoms of either excess or deficiency of pituitary hormone. Imaging is also indicated if a patient presents with symptoms suggestive of a pituitary mass, such as a visual field deficit and/or headaches.

Any disturbance in the hormones that are produced by the adenohypophysis or are a part of the pituitary-hypothalamic axis may cause symptoms that prompt endocrinologic testing. Confirmation of pituitary hormone abnormalities using biochemical testing should be performed before imaging (**Table 1**).

Prolactinoma

One of the most common pituitary hormone abnormalities is hyperprolactinemia, which is caused by an adenoma that secretes excess prolactin. Approximately 40% of all functional adenomas are prolactinomas.[3] Women with hyperprolactinemia will present with galactorrhea and menstrual irregularities whereas men will present with hypogonadism. Stalk compression by a supra- or parasellar lesion may cause hyperprolactinemia as well, although prolactin levels in these patients are usually less than 150 ng/mL, whereas patients with functional prolactinomas usually have prolactin levels greater than 150 ng/mL.[4]

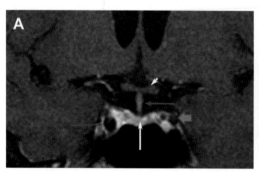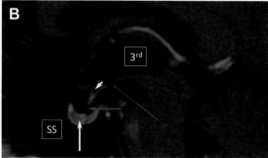

Fig. 1. Normal pituitary anatomy. (*A*) Coronal postcontrast image through the pituitary gland shows the normal position and appearance of the optic chiasm (*white arrowhead*), the infundibulum in the midline (*red arrow*), the homogeneously enhancing pituitary gland (*white arrow*), and the intracavernous ICA flow void (*red arrow*). Note that cranial nerve III is well visualized in the upper outer corner of the cavernous sinus (*blue arrow*). (*B*) Sagittal anatomy. The normal pituitary gland enhances homogeneously (*white arrow*), the infundibulum is wider superiorly and tapers inferiorly (*red arrow*), and the white arrowhead points to the infundibular recess. Behind the infundibulum recess and anterior to the mammillary bodies is the tuber cinereum (*thin blue arrow*), which is the inferior hypothalamus. Note the marked third ventricle (3ʳᵈ) and sphenoid sinus (SS).

Table 1
Common indications for pituitary imaging

Condition	Clinical Considerations
Anterior Pituitary Hyperfunction	
Elevated prolactin	Prolactinoma versus stalk compression or infiltration
Acromegaly and elevated IGF-1	GH-secreting adenoma versus ectopic GHRH syndrome
ACTH-dependent Cushing syndrome	ACTH-secreting adenoma versus ectopic ACTH syndrome
Elevated TFTs with nonsuppressed TSH	TSH-secreting adenoma versus TH resistance syndrome
Elevated LH, FSH (in premenopausal females or males with normal testosterone)	Gonadotroph adenoma
Anterior Pituitary Deficiency	
ACTH deficiency (central adrenal insufficiency) TSH deficiency (central hypothyroidism) GH deficiency, low IGF-1 Hypogonadotropic hypogonadism	Macroadenoma versus empty sella syndrome versus infiltrating stalk or pituitary disease versus pituitary infarction
Posterior Pituitary Deficiency	
Central diabetes insipidus	Suprasellar tumor versus infiltrating stalk or pituitary disease
Visual Field Defect	
eg, Bitemporal hemianopsia or upper/lower quadrantanopia	Sellar versus suprasellar tumor versus optic nerve tumor versus demyelinating disease
Cranial Nerve Palsies	
III, IV, VI	Sellar tumor invading cavernous sinus versus cavernous sinus tumor versus ICA aneurysm

Abbreviations: ACTH, adrenocorticotropic hormone; FSH, follicle-stimulating hormone; GH, growth hormone; GHRH, growth hormone–releasing hormone; ICA, internal carotid artery; IGF-1, insulin-like growth factor 1; LH, luteinizing hormone; TFTs, thyroid function tests; TH, thyroid hormone; TSH, thyroid-stimulating hormone.

Acromegaly

Overproduction of growth hormone leads to acromegaly, manifested by acral overgrowth, soft tissue swelling, prognathism, frontal bossing, diabetes mellitus, hypertension, and osteoarthritis.[5] These patients should undergo an oral glucose tolerance test as well as testing for basal insulin-like growth factor 1 and GH levels. Greater than 90% of patients with acromegaly have a pituitary adenoma as the underlying cause.

Cushing Syndrome

Endogenous Cushing syndrome is the consequence of excess glucocorticoids produced by the adrenal cortex. In 80% to 85% of these cases, the underlying cause is excess ACTH secretion by a pituitary adenoma, termed Cushing disease.[6] Clinical features of Cushing syndrome include central obesity, a cervical fat pad, thin skin, purple striae, proximal muscle weakness, glucose intolerance, acne, hirsutism, supraclavicular fat accumulation, and menstrual irregularities in women. The diagnosis of endogenous Cushing syndrome is made through biochemical testing. Tests include a 24-hour urine free cortisol, a late-night salivary cortisol, and a low-dose dexamethasone suppression test. Second-line testing includes a 2-day low-dose dexamethasone suppression test or a combined dexamethasone suppression–corticotropin-releasing hormone (CRH) stimulation test. Once the diagnosis is established, the endocrinologist will determine the source of excess glucocorticoids by determining if the source is ACTH dependent or independent. Basal ACTH measurements, high-dose dexamethasone suppression, and/or CRH stimulation tests can be performed. If the source of Cushing syndrome is found to be ACTH dependent, imaging of the pituitary is indicated. Depending on results of the MR imaging, inferior petrosal sinus sampling (IPSS) may also be performed (see section on IPSS).

Pituitary Hormone Deficiency

Any lesion involving the sella, infundibulum, or suprasellar region can cause hormonal deficiencies. In addition, diseases that infiltrate the gland or infundibulum, such as sarcoidosis, lymphocytic hypophysitis, or neoplasms, can cause hormonal deficiency. Imaging studies can also show empty sella with total or partial absence of normal pituitary tissue.

IMAGING MODALITIES

MR imaging is the imaging mainstay of the sellar and parasellar regions. MR imaging has better soft tissue resolution than computed tomography (CT) and is not subject to artifacts from surrounding bony structures. In addition, MR imaging allows for direct imaging in all 3 planes. A typical pituitary MR imaging protocol includes high-resolution imaging of the sella and parasellar regions at 3-mm thickness, before and after contrast with fat suppression. Dynamic T1-weighted imaging may be performed when a pituitary adenoma is suspected based on clinical parameters. High-resolution T2-weighted sequences are also usually performed.

In patients who cannot undergo MR imaging (such as patients with non–MR imaging safe metal hardware, pacemakers, or severe claustrophobia), CT can be performed with reformats in coronal and sagittal planes. In addition, CT is better than MR imaging for detecting calcifications, and can be complementary to MR imaging if a primary bony lesion is suspected (eg, chordoma, chondrosarcoma).

Pituitary Adenoma

Pituitary adenomas comprise 10% to 15% of all intracranial neoplasms and are the most common tumor in the sellar region. These adenomas are considered benign and are typically classified based on their size: microadenomas are smaller than 10 mm and macroadenomas are larger than 10 mm. Adenomas can be classified clinically, based their endocrinological activity or lack thereof. Functional pituitary adenomas usually secrete a single hormone, leading to a distinct endocrine syndrome. Prolactin hypersecretion is most common, and may be caused by either hypersecretion of prolactin from the adenoma or any process that disturbs the normal production, storage, and release of prolactin. In general, serum prolactin levels greater than 150 ng/mL are almost always attributable to an autonomously secreting adenoma. The next most common hormonal disturbances are GH and ACTH hypersecretion.

Approximately 60% to 70% of patients with a macroadenoma present with symptoms of hormone disturbance. The rest present with symptoms related to mass effect, such as headache or visual changes.

Microadenoma

MR imaging is the primary imaging modality when a microadenoma is suspected. Most institutions perform dedicated imaging of the pituitary in sagittal and coronal planes. On precontrast T1 images, the lesion may be slightly hypointense to the remainder of pituitary. Some investigators believe that most adenomas can be detected on noncontrast T1 images alone.[7] Intravenous contrast may be selectively used in cases of suspected Cushing disease or when the microadenoma is isointense to pituitary tissue. Many institutions use a half dose of gadolinium contrast (0.05 mmol/kg), finding that the ratio of lesion to gland signal is similar to full-dose. Adenomas and normal pituitary tissue have different patterns of uptake and washout following administration of intravenous contrast; this is thought to be due to the lower vascularity of adenomas compared with normal pituitary (Fig. 2). Dynamic postcontrast imaging takes advantage of differential patterns of uptake and washout to increase the sensitivity of detecting small adenomas. Adenomas hypoenhance relative to normal tissue during the first 60 seconds following contrast administration. Thereafter, adenomas may retain contrast more than surrounding pituitary and may thus be hyperintense on delayed imaging. The pattern of enhancement of adenomas is somewhat inconsistent across various studies, however. One study of the sequential enhancement pattern of the pituitary gland found that some pituitary adenomas enhanced earlier than the anterior lobes, suggesting that adenomas may have a direct arterial supply separate from the anterior pituitary.[8] Studies have also suggested that most adenomas tend to reside in the lateral wings of the gland, and may or may not be surrounded by a pseudocapsule.

Several MR imaging sequences are employed to detect microadenomas. Two methods are typically used—sometimes in conjunction—to image the pituitary in cases of suspected microadenomas. The first is standard spin-echo (SE) T1 precontrast and postcontrast imaging in the coronal plane using a high-resolution technique (thinner slices with smaller intervals). The second method leverages the potential differential enhancement pattern of adenomas versus normal pituitary tissue by using precontrast and dynamic T1 postcontrast images at several small time intervals (10 seconds) after the administration of contrast. Small pituitary lesions, especially ACTH-secreting adenomas, can be difficult to detect with either technique. False-negative rates of 45% to 62% have been reported when only conventional precontrast and postcontrast SE MR imaging is used.[9]

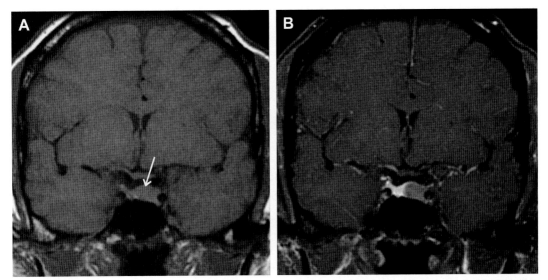

Fig. 2. Classic microadenoma. (A) Lesion is almost isointense to the gland on precontrast T1, although clearly the left aspect of the sella is enlarged and the upper border is convex (arrow), signaling underlying abnormality. (B) Lesion is hypoenhancing on conventional postcontrast T1 image and is located in the left lateral pituitary fossa.

The limitations of both techniques (and the potential added yield when both were applied) were addressed in a study by Bartynski and Lyn[10] of 64 microlesions (3–10 mm) that were studied by dynamic and standard SE sequences. During the first 5 minutes postcontrast, the enhancement characteristics of the gland versus the adenoma were unpredictable. Eleven percent to 14% of lesions were detected only on the dynamic sequences, while 8% to 9% of the lesions were detected only on the standard SE sequences, leading these investigators to conclude that both SE and dynamic imaging are necessary to maximize the likelihood of detection of small lesions.[10] Friedman and colleagues[11] showed that in the clinical setting of Cushing syndrome almost all patients had a lesion on dynamic sequences, although there was a false-positive rate of 16%. These investigators concluded that dynamic MR imaging adds valuable information in cases of suspected Cushing syndrome (Fig. 3). On the other hand, another study of 26 patients with ACTH-dependent Cushing syndrome as well as 10 normal controls found that the sensitivity of dynamic MR imaging is greater than standard MR imaging, 67% versus 52%; however, this came with a loss in specificity, 80% versus 100%. The investigators concluded that dynamic imaging did not improve the usefulness of MR imaging.[12]

Another MR imaging sequence that has recently come into clinical use is the spoiled gradient recalled acquisition in the steady state (SPGR) sequence. It provides excellent soft tissue contrast compared with conventional T1 SE

because thin sections of 1 mm may be obtained. The major drawback of SPGR, however, is lower signal to noise ratio compared with SE. One way to compensate for this loss of signal is to increase the number of excitations (NEX), which increases scan time. Patronas and colleagues[9] studied 50 patients with surgically proven ACTH-secreting microadenomas with both conventional SE MR imaging and SPGR, and found that the sensitivity was higher for SPGR than for conventional SE (80% vs 49%). There was, however, a moderate increase in the false-positive rate (8% vs 4%). The 4% false-positive rate in their study for conventional SE MR imaging is much lower than in studies from other investigators, which report average rates of 18%. Patronas and colleagues speculated that this is due to their more stringent criteria for identification of a microadenoma, therefore accounting for both the lower false-positive rate and the lower sensitivity than has been reported elsewhere. These investigators suggested use of both conventional SE and SPGR sequences in detection of microadenomas, especially if an ACTH-secreting adenoma is suspected. Similarly, Batista and colleagues[13] studied conventional SE MR imaging versus SPGR MR imaging in ACTH-secreting pituitary adenomas in children and adolescents, and found similar results to those of adults. For postcontrast SE, sensitivity was 21% and specificity was 50%. For postcontrast SPGR, the sensitivity of MR for depicting microadenomas was 75% and the specificity was 50%. False-positive rates were higher with SE (28% compared with 10% with SPGR).

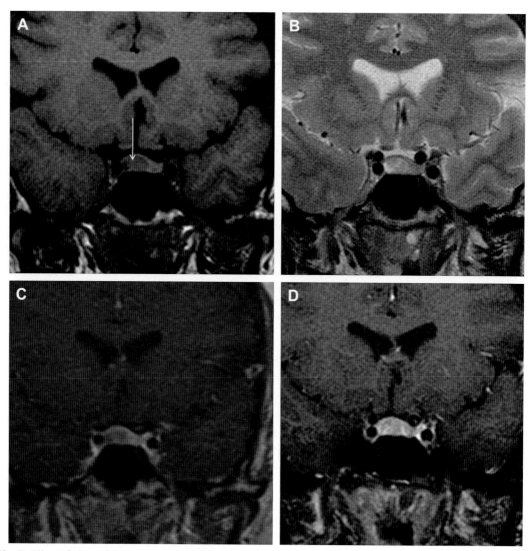

Fig. 3. Microadenoma best seen on precontrast T1 and dynamic scanning. (*A*) Lesion is well seen on noncontrast T1 as an area of hypointensity in the right lateral gland (*arrow*). (*B*) Lesion is slightly hyperintense on T2. (*C*) On dynamic 50-second postcontrast, the lesion is hypoenhancing relative to normal gland. (*D*) However, the lesion is not well delineated from gland on conventional postcontrast image. In this case the precontrast T1 may have sufficed to diagnose the lesion, while the postcontrast delayed image did not give any additional information.

In general, when an endocrinologically active microadenoma is suspected, conventional precontrast and postcontrast imaging with or without dynamic postcontrast imaging continues to be the standard at most institutions. SPGR imaging is promising but is not routinely used. Half-dose contrast is often used, especially with the recent concern regarding gadolinium-based contrast agents and their potential link to nephrogenic systemic fibrosis. The most useful sequences are coronal T1 precontrast, 30- to 50-second dynamic postcontrast images, and conventional postcontrast images.

Small pituitary lesions may also be discovered "incidentally" in a patient without endocrinological or other symptoms. Autopsy series suggest that 5.8% to 8.3% of the adult population may have incidental pituitary lesions larger than 2 mm. These lesions are increasingly discovered because of the wide use of MR imaging for various suspected conditions and improved MR imaging technology. Most of these incidental lesions are nonfunctioning adenomas or Rathke cleft cysts (RCCs). Because small colloid cysts are present in the pars intermedia, images must be scrutinized carefully so that a hypointense lesion between the anterior and posterior glands is not overinterpreted as a microadenoma.

Inferior Petrosal Sinus Sampling

The inferior petrosal sinus (IPS) originates from the posterosuperior aspect of the cavernous sinus (CS), runs along the petroclival fissure, and drains into the jugular bulb. There are variations in the pattern of the IPS–jugular bulb junction; there may be single or multiple connections, a plexiform connection, no connection, or a connection with the cervical venous plexus.[14] IPSS plays a role in defining the origin of ACTH secretion in patients with Cushing syndrome. Approximately 80% of these patients have Cushing disease, that is, ACTH-secreting pituitary adenoma, another 10% have an adrenal lesion, and the remainder ectopic ACTH secretion. In cases of Cushing syndrome when MR imaging is nonrevealing or when there is an incidental pituitary lesion as well as another ectopic source of ACTH, IPSS can differentiate between pituitary and ectopic ACTH secretion.

In IPSS, catheters are used to access the IPSs via the femoral veins and jugular veins. Blood ACTH levels are then measured from each sinus at regular intervals and compared with levels from peripheral blood samples that are obtained concurrently. ACTH secretion can be episodic; therefore CRH is used as a stimulating agent. Samples are obtained before and after CRH administration. Earlier studies reported sensitivity and specificity of 100% for bilateral IPSS, but more recent studies dispute this. Swearingen and colleagues[15] demonstrated a sensitivity of up to 90% with CRH stimulation and a very high positive predictive value (99%). On the other hand, a false-negative rate of bilateral IPSS (BIPSS) of up to 20% suggests that a negative IPSS does not rule out a pituitary source of ACTH, especially if other findings such as MR imaging or reactions of peripheral ACTH levels to CRH are suggestive. Kaskarelis and colleagues[16] compared MR imaging with BIPSS, and reported a 50% accuracy rate for MR imaging compared with 88% for BIPSS (with CRH or CRH and desmopressin stimulation). IPSS for lateralization of the adenoma within the gland is less reliable; one study showed higher levels of ACTH on the side of the tumor 70% of the time and opposite of the tumor 23% of the time.[7] One pitfall of BIPSS for lesion localization is anatomic variation in the size of the sinus from side to side: measurements taken from a dominant sinus may be artificially elevated compared with the hypoplastic side (**Fig. 4**).

Macroadenoma

Conventional SE precontrast and postcontrast MR imaging suffices for identification of macroadenomas which, by definition, are always identified because of their larger size.[9] Macroadenomas have many of the same imaging characteristics as microadenomas. In many cases, the lesion is

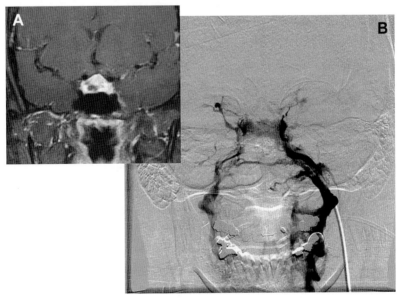

Fig. 4. Microadenoma and bilateral inferior petrosal sinus sampling (BIPSS). (*A*) Postcontrast T1 image shows a microadenoma in the right aspect of the gland (*arrow*). (*B*) Characteristic appearance of IPSS; in this case the left IPS is dominant. This situation led to localization of the lesion to the left, probably due to caliber difference. Surgery confirmed that the lesion is on the right, as predicted on MR imaging.

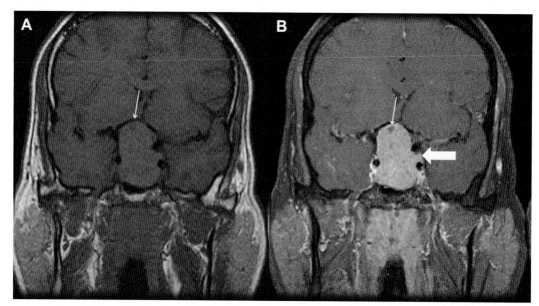

Fig. 5. Macroadenoma. (*A, B*) Precontrast and postcontrast coronal images show a large sellar/suprasellar mass. The sellar floor is bowed inferiorly, the sella is enlarged, and no normal pituitary tissue can be identified, all suggesting that the mass is sellar in origin. Note the small area of hypointensity and nonenhancement in the most cranial portion of the mass (*small arrows*), likely cystic degeneration. Note left cavernous sinus invasion (*large arrow*) with enhancing tumor extending to the lateral intercarotid line.

so large that no normal pituitary tissue can be identified confidently. Macroadenomas may expand to involve adjacent structures; they often grow superiorly into the suprasellar cistern and compress the optic chiasm or nerves. The pattern of compression is largely dependent on the position of the chiasm (directly above, prefixed, or postfixed) relative to the sella. Inferiorly, macroadenomas can extend into the sphenoid sinus and posteriorly they extend into the dorsum sella. Laterally, they can invade the cavernous sinuses (**Fig. 5**). Unfortunately, cavernous sinus invasion can be difficult to detect with certainty on preoperative imaging. Given the thin medial cavernous wall, tumors may project well laterally and compress cavernous sinusoids without actually invading the sinus. Complete encasement of the ICA or presence of tumor between the lateral wall of the cavernous sinus and the carotid artery is the most reliable sign of cavernous sinus invasion. In cases where there is incomplete encasement of the ICA, Cottier and colleagues[17] suggest certain criteria that may be helpful for identifying or excluding cavernous sinus invasion (**Table 2**). Another study by Vieira and colleagues[18] reported similar findings that exclude cavernous sinus invasion, but suggested that 30% encasement of the ICA suggests CS invasion, rather than the 67% suggested by Cottier. There are preliminary data suggesting that higher field

MR imaging (3 T) can potentially increase sensitivity and specificity for prediction of invasion of adjacent structures by pituitary adenomas and can assist in surgical planning.[19,20]

Table 2	
Summary of most useful criteria for diagnosis of invasion or absence of invasion of the cavernous sinus (CS) by pituitary adenoma	
CS Invasion	**Absence of CS Invasion**
Percentage of ICA encasement equal or greater than 67%	Presence of normal pituitary tissue between tumor and CS
Obliteration of carotid sulcus venous compartment[a]	Percentage of ICA encasement less than 25%
Lateral intercarotid line crossed[c]	Intact medial venous compartment[b]
	Medial intercarotid line not crossed

[a] Carotid sulcus compartment is defined as the space between the ICA and the carotid sulcus of the sphenoid bone.
[b] Medial venous compartment is the space between the ICA and the pituitary fossa.
[c] Medial and lateral intercarotid lines are lines joining the medial and lateral walls of the intracavernous and supracavernous portions of the ICA.

Adenomas, especially macroadenomas, can hemorrhage or undergo cystic change. Hemorrhage within an adenoma often is manifested as a T1 hyperintense mass, with or without fluid-blood levels. Hemorrhage with infarction may result in the clinical syndrome of apoplexy, but hemorrhage itself is often subclinical and detected incidentally (**Fig. 6**). The incidence of hemorrhage is higher in patients receiving bromocriptine or similar agents. About half of prolactin-secreting adenomas treated medically with these D2 agonists will decrease in size, undergoing involution and fibrosis. Imaging may demonstrate a smaller area of hypointensity and variable enhancement.

Blood products may bloom on gradient echo (GRE) sequences, but susceptibility artifact induced by air in the paranasal sinuses and bony structures limits the utility of GRE in this scenario. A hemorrhagic adenoma presenting de novo may be difficult to distinguish from an RCC, which classically has inherent T1 hyperintense signal because of its proteinaceous content. Cystic degeneration can also occur spontaneously or after medical treatment, surgery, or radiation. On imaging, cystic degeneration is manifested by well-defined areas of T2 hyperintensity and relative T1 hypointensity. The size of the hemorrhagic cyst may change over time as well. These cysts are often heterogeneous; heterogeneity is attributable to varying compositions of tumor, protein content, and/or hemorrhage. On the other hand, colloid cysts are usually uniform, with well-defined borders and minimally enhancing walls.

Invasive Macroadenoma and Apoplexy

Macroadenomas that show unusual growth characteristics may be termed "invasive." Such behavior involves aggressive growth superolaterally into the frontal or temporal lobes, inferiorly into the sphenoid, clivus, and nasal cavity, posteriorly into the interpeduncular cistern, or anteriorly into the orbit or ethmoid (**Fig. 7A**).

Pituitary apoplexy is a clinical syndrome consisting of headache, visual changes, ophthalmoplegia, and mental status changes. Apoplexy

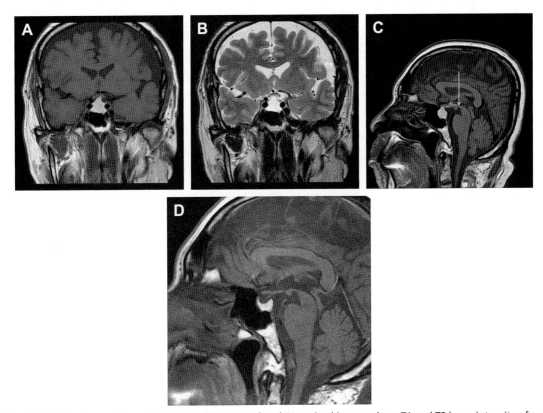

Fig. 6. Pituitary hemorrhage. (*A–C*) T1 and T2 coronal and T1 sagittal images show T1 and T2 hyperintensity of an enlarged sella with mass effect on the optic chiasm. T1 hyperintensity extends long floor of third ventricle (*arrow*). This patient presented with headache after initiation of anticoagulation for atrial fibrillation. (*D*) Follow-up noncontrast T1 image several months later shows decreased hemorrhage and decreased size of the sella, with resolution of suprasellar and intraventricular extension, although the gland continues to be entirely hyperintense on T1, probably due to residual blood products.

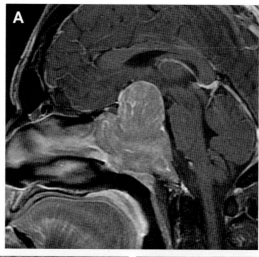

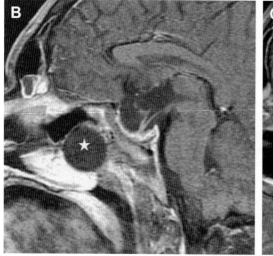

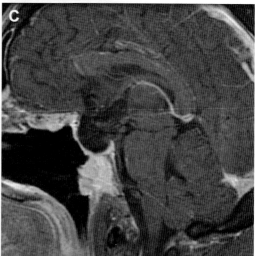

Fig. 7. Invasive pituitary macroadenoma then treated with expanded endonasal approach (EEA). (*A*) Preoperative sagittal postcontrast T1 image shows a large enhancing solid sellar mass with invasion of the sphenoid sinus, clivus, and extension into the suprasellar cistern. The optic chiasm is not discernible and is compressed by the mass. (*B*) Immediate post-EEA appearance with heterogeneous postoperative material in the sphenoid sinus and an inflated Foley catheter balloon (*star*). Enhancing posterior nasal septal graft sits behind the balloon and in this case enhances only modestly. (*C*) Four months post-EEA appearance shows resolution of much of the postoperative changes and no residual mass in the expanded, empty-appearing sella tursica. The graft has contracted and remains continuous along the sellar face.

represents acute infarction of the pituitary gland, which may or may not be hemorrhagic. An underlying adenoma may often be present. Imaging may show blood products if the lesion is hemorrhagic, which would be hyperdense on CT and of variable signal on MR imaging, depending on acuity of blood. Peripheral enhancement has been described as a classic feature with apoplexy (**Fig. 8**), but some investigators suggest that peripheral enhancement is nonspecific and have found diffusion-weighted imaging (DWI) to be useful. In a report of 2 patients, restricted diffusion within an enlarged pituitary gland with absolute or

relatively decreased apparent diffusion coefficient (ADC) values correlated with apoplexy and led to early surgical intervention, with good outcomes.[21] A potentially helpful ancillary finding is thickening of the sphenoid sinus mucosa. Thickening is thought to correlate with higher grades of apoplexy and worse outcomes.[22] This finding is thought to be due to regional venous engorgement and does not indicate sinus infection. Mucosal thickening does not preclude a transsphenoidal surgical approach.[23]

Sheehan syndrome refers to postpartum apoplexy within a nontumorous gland. The

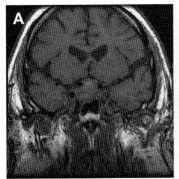
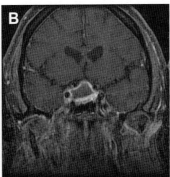
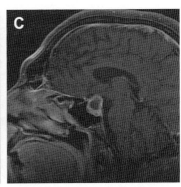

Fig. 8. Pituitary apoplexy. (*A, B*) Precontrast and postcontrast coronal images show enlarged sellar mass with suprasellar extension and mass effect on the optic chiasm. The lesion is centrally nonenhancing, characteristic for pituitary infarction. (*C*) Sagittal postcontrast image shows the same lesion with adjacent sphenoid sinus mucosal thickening.

syndrome typically occurs in women who have suffered significant postpartum hemorrhage and hypovolemia. It is hypothesized that as the pituitary gland normally hypertrophies during pregnancy, it becomes more susceptible to infarction from hypoperfusion. Sheehan syndrome is sometimes diagnosed retrospectively, when the patient develops amenorrhea after the peripartum period.

SURGICAL TREATMENT AND POSTOPERATIVE IMAGING

Surgical treatment of microadenomas and macroadenomas involves resection of the adenoma. At present, this is done with an endoscopic, transsphenoidal approach via the nose. The sella as well as the sphenoid sinus may be packed at the end of the resection with either Gelfoam or fat packing to prevent or treat cerebrospinal fluid (CSF) leak. The imaging appearance of the sella after "traditional" transsphenoidal surgery depends on the amount of time that has lapsed since surgery. Initially the operative bed maybe filled with debris, blood products, and fat packing, giving a very heterogeneous appearance with inherently T1 hyperintense material. It may be difficult to discern residual pituitary tissue. In subsequent studies, the fat packing and blood products usually are resorbed, and normal pituitary tissue may reexpand (**Fig. 9**).[24] Enhancing soft tissue in the operative bed may be granulation tissue, but is difficult to distinguish this from a residual or recurrent adenoma, especially in the first 6 months following surgery. Precontrast and postcontrast high-resolution imaging with SPGR sequences may play a role. Endocrinologic correlation and serial postoperative imaging is most helpful. Progressive growth of a soft tissue mass

or nodule is the best sign of recurrence with the caveat that most adenomas are, in fact, slow-growing tumors and therefore change may not be apparent for many months.

In the last decade, the expanded endonasal approach (EEA) has been pioneered to reach parasellar and intracranial lesions. This method can be used to treat large or invasive adenomas, as well as other sellar/parasellar lesions (see later discussion on adenoma mimics) (**Fig. 7**B, C). It has even been used to treat clival lesions and lesions at the craniocervical junction. More extensive tumor resection is possible because the approach provides a larger window to the sella, and suprasellar and parasellar regions. The expanded endonasal approach requires the combined expertise of neurosurgeons and ear/nose/throat surgeons, and can be divided into 4 "corridors": transcribriform, transplanum, transsellar, and transclival. The initial approach for all 4 of these approaches is a nasal corridor, with unilateral turbinectomy, bilateral sphenoidotomies, and posterior septotectomy. Because of the wider exposure a multilayer reconstruction, including a vascularized nasoseptal flap, is placed in the surgical bed, either directly over dura or over fat. This reconstruction appears C-shaped and is of variable thickness on postoperative imaging. It enhances because of its vascularity, but the degree of enhancement is variable. The thickness of the flap may also change over time because of resorption of fat packing underneath it or formation of granulation tissue. On postoperative studies, it is important to look for flap migration and devascularization as potential causes of flap failure.[25] It is essential to communicate with the local surgical team to understand their techniques when interpreting postoperative imaging studies.

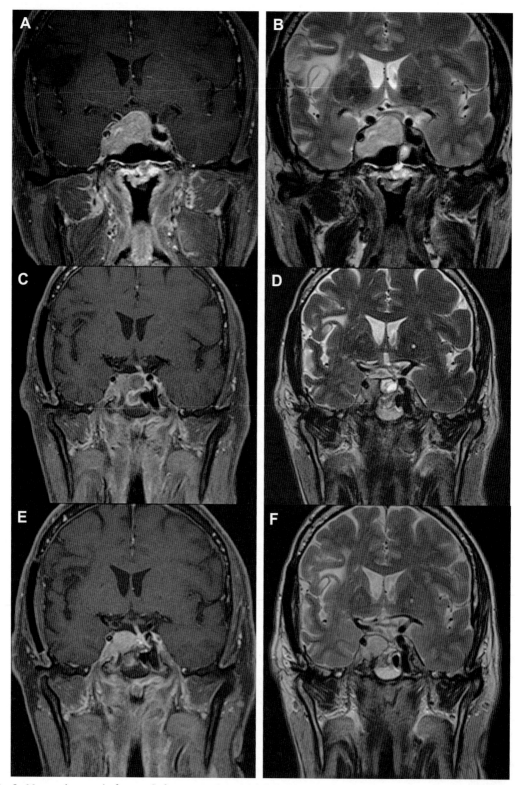

Fig. 9. Macroadenoma before and after transsphenoidal debulking. (*A, B*) Coronal T1 postcontrast and T2 images preoperatively of a large macroadenoma with right cavernous sinus invasion and mass effect on the optic chiasm. (*C, D*) Short-term follow-up appearance after transsphenoidal debulking shows heterogeneous material in the sphenoid sinus, residual tumor in the right sella and cavernous sinus, and a central cystic cavity from debulking. The mass effect on optic chiasm has resolved and the infundibulum is now visible, although deviated to the left. (*E, F*) Ten-month follow-up appearance shows resolution of the surgical cavity in the gland, persistent material in the sphenoid sinus, and residual tumor. The patient subsequently underwent radiation treatment to the remaining tumor.

Pituitary Hypoplasia/Hyperplasia

True pituitary hypoplasia is a congenital abnormality, often associated with midline anomalies of the optic apparatus, septum pellucidum, skull base, and palate. The gland, infundibulum, and sella turcica are small. Patients usually present in childhood or adolescence with pituitary-hypothalamic dysfunction and are clinically recognized by manifestations of GH deficiency: MR imaging findings include small sella tursica, small anterior pituitary gland, absence of the usual posterior pituitary bright spot, infundibular hypoplasia, and sometimes an abnormal hyperintense focus in the region of the primal infundibulum (**Fig. 10**). Not unexpectedly, on formal testing these patients often have multiple hormone deficiencies in addition to GH deficiency. Prior radiation to the sella region or pituitary infarction may also lead to acquired pituitary insufficiency.

It is important to be aware that the commonly seen "empty sella" is not equivalent to hypoplasia. In the former entity, the superior portion of the sella turcica appears devoid of tissue and is instead filled with CSF. In many cases the overall volume of sella turcica is expanded. The "empty sella" is thought to be due to the thinning or absence of the diaphragma sella. The suprasellar cistern herniates into the sella, and the sella enlarges because of chronic CSF pulsation. This process is often of no or little clinical significance, as the normal pituitary tissue exists but is flattened to the floor of the sella. When symptomatic, patients present with nonspecific complaints such as headache and dizziness. The finding has been described in patients with increased intracranial CSF pressure (pseudotumor cerebri).

Occasionally the pituitary gland appears large and may have a convex superior border, but no discrete lesions are identified. Hyperplasia of the gland is normally seen in puberty and in pregnant or postpartum females. In addition, apparent hyperplasia of the gland can be seen in the setting of intracranial hypotension (in cases of CSF leak or overshunting). Other imaging findings such as smooth diffuse dural enhancement and brainstem sagging are usually present to suggest this diagnosis.

Hyperplasia of the pituitary gland has also been described in patients with primary hypothyroidism.[26] However, in general these patients will not be referred by endocrinology for pituitary imaging. An enlarged gland may be seen incidentally, however, and caution should be exercised before calling it an adenoma.

Adenoma Mimics

Many other entities may arise in the sellar and parasellar regions, including aneurysms, RCCs, craniopharyngiomas, gliomas of the optic chiasm or hypothalamus, meningiomas, germ cell tumors, hamartomas, lipomas, and epidermoid/dermoid cysts. Metastases and granulomatous disease

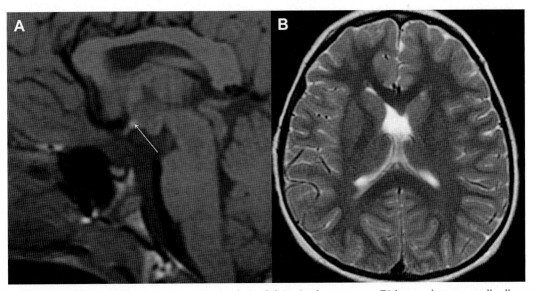

Fig. 10. Pituitary hypoplasia and septo-optic dysplasia. (*A*) Sagittal precontrast T1 image shows a small sella, no distal infundibulum, and a hyperintense spot in the region of the proximal infundibulum (*arrow*). Note that the optic chiasm is also not well seen and likely hypoplastic. (*B*) Axial T2 image shows absence of the septum pellucidum.

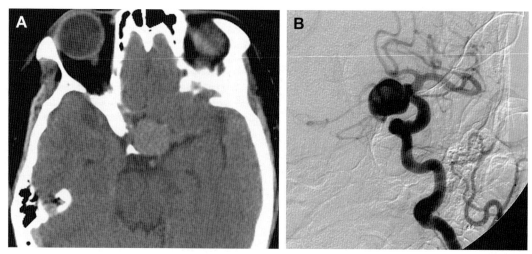

Fig. 11. Aneurysm. (A) Noncontrast CT image through the suprasellar cistern shows a round, slightly hyperdense lesion, the density being equivalent to adjacent blood vessels. (B) Carotid angiogram image shows a large supraclinoid ICA aneurysm.

can also occur, but these entities generally affect the posterior pituitary and the infundibulum more so than the anterior pituitary. Adenomas arise from the gland, whereas other entities listed within the differential diagnosis are centered elsewhere and may be discernible from the gland with careful examination.

The circle of Willis is in close proximity to the sella turcica and suprasellar cistern. It is the most frequent location of intracranial aneurysms. However, aneurysms arising from the cavernous and supraclinoid ICA are the most likely to present as a mass in the sellar/parasellar region (**Fig. 11**). Aneurysms have variable MR imaging characteristics depending on whether they are patent or thrombosed. Patent aneurysms will appear hypointense, due to flow on T2-weighted images. However, thrombosed aneurysms may be T1 hyperintense and be of mixed intensity on T2-weighted imaging.[27] Pulsation artifact, occurring in the phase-encoding direction, favors an aneurysm over other sellar/juxtasellar masses.

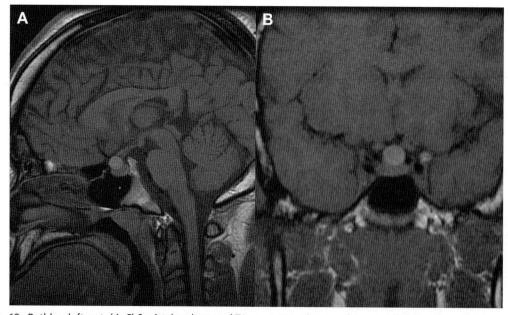

Fig. 12. Rathke cleft cyst. (A, B) Sagittal and coronal T1 precontrast images show a well-defined, small, inherently T1 hyperintense suprasellar mass. It is clearly separate from and hyperintense relative to the pituitary gland that sits beneath it.

Noninvasive angiography (CT angiography or MR angiography) should be performed before surgical intervention if this diagnosis is considered.

RCCs arise from the Rathke pouch; the pouch is a precursor of the anterior and intermediate lobes of the pituitary gland. RCCs can be purely sellar or have sellar and suprasellar components, and are often incidentally identified in adults. RCCs classically are well-defined cystic lesions, which often are hyperintense on T1 because of their proteinaceous content (**Fig. 12**); they may contain an intracystic nodule. In fact, a nonenhancing, T2 hypointense nodule within a cystic sellar lesion in a relatively asymptomatic patient is highly suggestive of this diagnosis (**Fig. 13**).[28] RCCs are usually related to the midline pars intermedia. RCCs may less frequently be eccentric and imbedded in the anterior gland. Unlike craniopharyngiomas, RCCs are more homogeneous, less enhancing, and rarely calcify. Purely sellar

RCCs can be difficult to distinguish from cystic and/or hemorrhagic adenomas and pituitary cysts.

Craniopharyngioma is another relatively common suprasellar mass, but these lesions often extend beyond the sella; up to 10% may be confined to the sella. Craniopharyngioma has two distinct histologies: adamantinomatous and papillary. The former is more common and has a bimodal age distribution, presenting in late childhood to early adolescence and again in the fifth to seventh decades.[7] In general they are heterogeneous-appearing masses containing solid and cystic areas, as well as calcifications. The cystic areas are often proteinaceous and therefore T1 hyperintense (**Fig. 14**). The adamantinomatous entity is one for which CT may be helpful in identifying calcifications, which would favor this diagnosis over the others. The papillary variety is seen in older patients, and is more uniform and

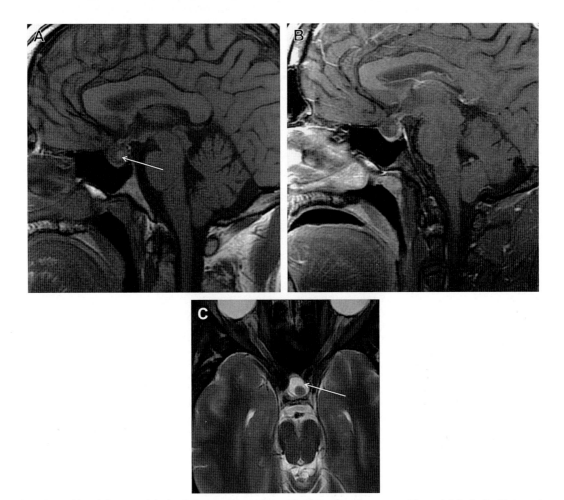

Fig. 13. Rathke cleft cyst with classic intracystic nodule. (*A, B*) Small sellar mass with an intrinsically T1 hyperintense nodule (*arrow*). (*C*) Axial T2 image shows that the lesion is cystic and hyperintense while the nodule is hypointense (*arrow*). These imaging findings are classic for Rathke cleft cyst.

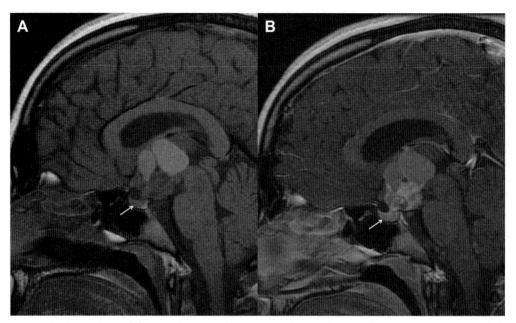

Fig. 14. Craniopharyngioma. (*A*) Precontrast T1 sagittal image shows a large, heterogeneous midline mass in the suprasellar cistern, clearly separate from pituitary, which appears normal in size and configuration (*arrow*) but inseparable from the infundibulum. There are areas of inherent T1 hyperintensity. (*B*) Postcontrast image shows enhancement within portions of this mass (*arrow*), noting that the cystic areas that were inherently T1 hyperintense on image *A* do not enhance; rather, the solid portions do. Calcifications are not well appreciated by MR imaging.

solid. Often it is found solely in the third ventricle. On MR imaging, the papillary form enhances but the appearance is otherwise nonspecific, without the characteristic T1 hyperintensity or heterogeneity of the adamantinomatous variety. The adoption of EEA surgery for suprasellar and parasellar lesions has prompted a newly proposed classification based on the relationship of the mass to the infundibulum: type I is preinfundibular, type II involves the infundibulum, type III is retroinfundibular, and type IV is isolated in the third ventricle and/ or optic recess and is not amenable to endonasal resection.[29] This classification is useful to the skull base surgeon for planning, and should be familiar to radiologists at centers where EEA is used.

Meningiomas can arise in and around many structures in the anterior cranial fossa, including the planum sphenoidale, the clinoid processes, olfactory groove, tuberculum sellae, or diaphragma sellae. Meningiomas are generally homogeneous, T1 isointense, and T2 iso-hyperintense masses that enhance avidly, often having a broad base with a dural surface. Meningiomas in the sella/parasellar regions can usually be distinguished from macroadenomas by the normal size of the sella turcica and identification of normal pituitary tissue separate from the mass (**Fig. 15**). Growth is often anterior and superior to the pituitary, and is centered along the tuberculum sella.

Like macroadenomas, meningiomas can invade the cavernous sinus; narrowing or occlusion of the cavernous ICA suggests a meningioma rather than adenoma. CT maybe helpful for identification of hyperostosis, although MR imaging is often sufficient for diagnosis.

Gliomas of the optic chiasm are tumors of childhood. The majority are considered benign and slow growing. Gliomas often occur in the setting of neurofibromatosis type 1. Hypothalamic gliomas tend to be more aggressive and present in adulthood. These tumors have variable signal characteristics on MR imaging, and may or may not enhance. Sometimes the exact site of origin may be difficult to determine when they are large, but the pituitary gland will usually be discernible from the tumor, indicating that the mass is not sellar in origin.

Germ cell tumors are midline lesions of childhood and adolescence. The most common cell type is a germinoma, of which 20% arise in the sellar/suprasellar region and the remainder from the pineal region. Imaging shows a large midline mass with homogeneous avid enhancement, often in combination with pineal region mass and with similar characteristics (**Fig. 16**). Again, this mass is generally separate from the pituitary gland, and the size of the sella is normal.

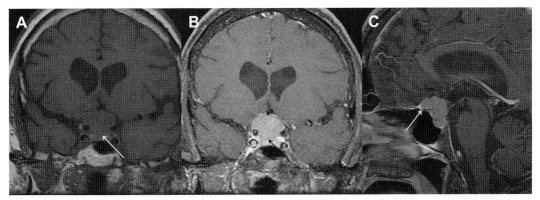

Fig. 15. Meningioma. (*A, B*) Large suprasellar mass, hypointense relative to normal pituitary tissue, which is seen inferior to the mass with a thin line separating the pituitary tissue from mass, likely the diagphragma sella, a dural covering (*arrows*). (*C*) Sagittal postcontrast image again shows the mass to be separate from pituitary; note that the sella tursica is normal sized and the broad base with dura along planum sphenoidale (*arrow*), all favoring meningioma.

Epidermoids, dermoids, lipomas, and arachnoid cysts can all arise in the suprasellar region, but again are usually easily distinguished from sellar lesions. Lipomas are benign fatty tumors and are usually incidental; they cause symptoms only when they are large. Lipomas are homogeneously hypodense on CT and hyperintense on T1 images. Usually they are well defined and do not enhance. Fat-suppressed sequences confirm fat content and distinguish them from hemorrhagic or

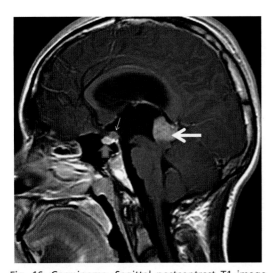

Fig. 16. Germinoma. Sagittal postcontrast T1 image shows a larger enhancing mass "engulfing" the pineal gland (*large arrow*) and downwardly displacing the tectal plate. A smaller enhancing mass is in the suprasellar region (*small arrow*), just above and posterior to the normal-appearing pituitary gland (*blue arrow*). Note the obstructive hydrocephalus due to the pineal mass.

proteinaceous lesions. Dermoids also contain fat, but are less homogeneous and appear hyperintense on T1. Rupture can cause chemical meningitis. Epidermoids appear similar to CSF signal intensity but show restricted diffusion, that is, DWI hyerintensity and corresponding hypointensity on ADC maps (**Fig. 17**). Arachnoid cysts follow CSF signal on all pulsing sequences and do not show restricted diffusion.

Another common bony lesion of the juxtasellar sphenoid and clivus is fibrous dysplasia. Its signal intensity depends on the fibrous, calcific, and vascular content of the lesion. Marked contrast enhancement may give fibrous dysplasia an aggressive MR appearance. CT, however, can confirm benign bony expansion, intact cortical margins, and a characteristic ground-glass internal matrix, which frequently has interspersed lucent regions.

Hamartomas of the tuber cinereum are rare but fascinating lesions, which classically cause precocious puberty and gelastic (laughing) seizures. The tuber cinereum is a small structure anterior to the mammillary bodies and behind the optic chiasm. Hamartomas in this region appear as nonenhancing sessile masses that are similar to gray matter in signal intensity. Hamartomas are not true neoplasms but they can grow in time. Their location is characteristic and differentiates them from other sellar lesions (**Fig. 18**).

Metastatic lesions tend to affect the stalk and the posterior lobe more than the anterior lobe; however, involvement of the entire gland is possible. Metastasis can occur from CSF seeding or hematogenous spread. Therefore, primary central nervous system (CNS) tumors with a propensity for CSF seeding, breast cancers,

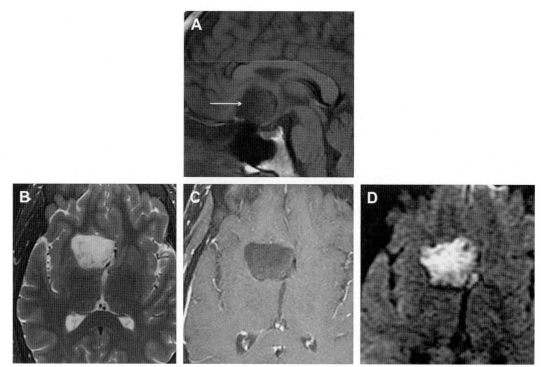

Fig. 17. Epidermoid. (*A*) Precontrast T1 sagittal image shows a hypointense mass above the optic chiasm (*arrow*), clearly separate from the pituitary gland, which is normal. (*B–D*) Axial T2, postcontrast, and DWI images show that the lesion is T2 hyperintense, nonenhancing, and hyperintense on diffusion, characteristic of epidermoid.

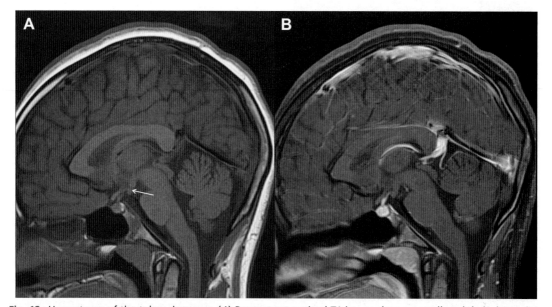

Fig. 18. Hamartoma of the tuber cinereum. (*A*) Precontrast sagittal T1 image shows a small nodule isointense to brain just anterior to the mammillary bodies (*arrow*). The infundibulum and pituitary gland are normal for this 10-year-old patient. (*B*) The nodule does not enhance after contrast, in keeping with the diagnosis of a hamartoma. The patient presented with precocious puberty.

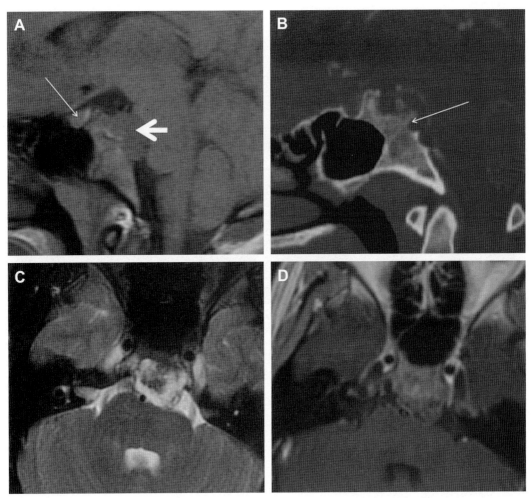

Fig. 19. Chordoma. (*A*) Sagittal precontrast T1 image shows a mass in the prepontine cistern along the back of the clivus (*large arrow*). It is clearly separate from the pituitary gland (*small arrow*). (*B*) Sagittal CT in bone window shows erosion of the posterior margin of the clivus (*arrow*). (*C, D*) T2 and postcontrast T1 axial images of the same lesion show that it is characteristically T2 hyperintense and moderately enhancing.

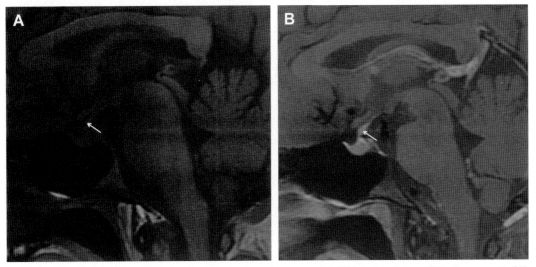

Fig. 20. Lymphocytic hypophysitis. (*A, B*) Precontrast and postcontrast T1 images show mild enlargement of the mid-inferior infundibulum (*arrows*) in a patient with diabetes insipidus. Note that the normal hyperintense posterior pituitary is not seen.

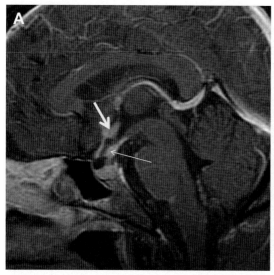
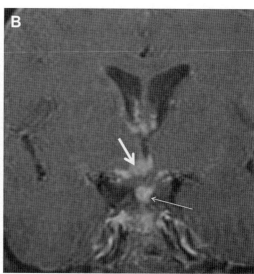

Fig. 21. Sarcoid. (*A, B*) Sagittal and coronal postcontrast images show thickening of the infundibulum (*thin arrows*) and nodular enhancement of the hypothalamus (*thick arrows*). In the absence of patient history or concurrent pulmonary disease, the appearance is not specific for sarcoid. The differential diagnosis includes other granulomatous conditions, lymphoma, and metastasis.

and lung cancers are the primary origins. The imaging appearance of pituitary metastases is nonspecific, but knowledge of the patient's history and the presence of other intracranial lesions/leptomeningeal involvement may suggest this diagnosis. Bony erosion (due to a metastasis) rather than bony remodeling (due to an adenoma) is another feature that may help in diagnosis.

Two other lesions that may arise in the parasellar region are chordomas and ecchordosis. Chordomas arise from primitive notochord remnants, and are generally associated with the clivus when they occur intracranially. These tumors present in middle age and, although histologically benign, they are locally invasive and destructive. Chordomas are isointense to hypointense on T1 and characteristically hyperintense on T2, may appear lobulated because of thick fibrous connective tissue, and may extend into the marrow space of the clivus. CT shows clival destruction well (**Fig. 19**). Ecchordosis is a nodule of cells also of notochord origin but, as opposed to chordoma, it is not a neoplasm. Ecchordosis is usually small and occurs in or is attached to the clivus.

Infundibular Lesions

Infundibular lesions fall into 3 broad categories: congenital/developmental, inflammatory/infectious, and neoplastic.

In a recent retrospective series of 65 infundibular lesions of adults and children, the most common congenital/developmental abnormality was pituitary hypoplasia. Hypoplasia typically presents in

childhood with dwarfism or GH deficiency. On imaging, the infundibulum appears hypoplastic or absent with ectopic posterior pituitary.[30] Rarely, nonenhancing cystic masses can be confined to the infundibulum; these are thought to represent either RCCs or pars intermedia cysts.

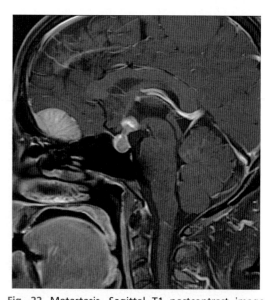

Fig. 22. Metastasis. Sagittal T1 postcontrast image shows sellar/infundibular and hypothalamic solid enhancing mass in a patient with breast cancer and new-onset diabetes insipidus. The lesion was not present on prior MR imaging 1 year previously. Note incidental frontal meningioma.

Inflammation of the hypophysis, either the anterior or posterior gland, occurs in adults and is typically described in women late in pregnancy or postpartum. It has also been described in children and elderly patients. This entity has been called lymphocytic hypophysitis or infundibuloneurohypophysitis. Histologically it is characterized by chronic inflammatory changes, hyaline fibrosis, and infiltration by plasma cells or lymphocytes. Imaging features include mass-like thickening of the infundibulum, although in some cases there may be mass-like thickening of the pituitary gland itself (**Fig. 20**). This entity is thought to be the underlying cause of many cases of central diabetes insipidus. The clinical history, the patient's age and gender, and any history of autoimmune disease help in this diagnosis.

Langerhans cell histiocytosis (LCH), a disease of children, can also present with infundibular thickening and central diabetes insipidus. There is some controversy regarding the classification of LCH; it has been classified as either a neoplastic

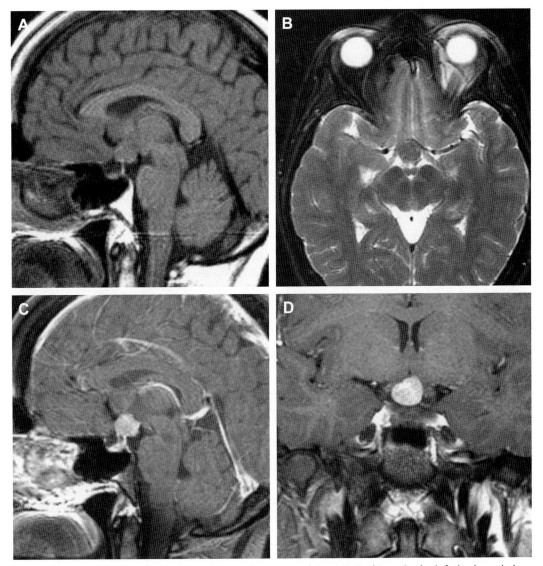

Fig. 23. Granular cell tumor. (*A*) Precontrast sagittal T1 image shows a round mass in the inferior hypothalamus involving the superior infundibulum that is isointense to brain. Note that the inferior infundibulum and the pituitary gland are normal in size and configuration. (*B*) The mass is isointense to brain on axial T2 as well. (*C, D*) Postcontrast sagittal and coronal images show homogeneous, avid enhancement. Appearance is not specific for this histology; however, it should be clearly noted to be separate from the anterior pituitary. This appearance was histologically proven to be a granular cell tumor at surgery.

Table 3
Common misinterpretations in pituitary imaging

Misinterpretation	Consider
Physiologic hypertrophy misinterpreted as macroadenoma	Consider age, sex, pregnancy, and depth of sellar floor. Gland is homogeneous
Pars intermedia cyst or normal pituitary heterogeneity misinterpreted as microadenoma	Consider location between the anterior and posterior pituitary. Secondary gland convexity is lacking
Rathke cleft cyst misinterpreted as hemorrhagic macroadenoma	Rathke cleft cyst is usually smaller, uniform, and thin-walled. T_1 hyperintensity and T_2 hyperintensity or hypointensity reflect high protein content
Pituitary metastasis misinterpreted as macroadenoma	An atypical growth pattern with bony erosion of the tuberculum, sellar floor, or dorsum/clivus suggests metastasis
Suprasellar tumor misinterpreted as macroadenoma with suprasellar extension	Precontrast images may better demonstrate pituitary and tumor separated by the diaphragma sellae
Fibrous dysplasia misinterpreted as skull base tumor	Whereas fibrous dysplasia may be heterogeneous and enhance, CT will show typical expansile lesion with preserved cortical margins and areas of ground-glass density
Postoperative heterogeneity misinterpreted as residual/recurrent tumor	Hemorrhagic mixed intensity material is commonly seen filling the operative bed and may take weeks to months to resolve. Pituitary tumors are generally slow growing

or granulomatous process. In LCH, the normal T1 hyperintense signal of the posterior pituitary is absent and the stalk is thickened.

In adults, the primary granulomatous disease that involves the infundibulum is sarcoidosis. Other entities include tuberculosis and Wegener disease. Sarcoidosis involving the stalk has a nonspecific appearance, and is rarely the only manifestation of the disease (**Fig. 21**). Imaging alone cannot differentiate among the granulomatous diseases that can involve the stalk; other signs such as meningeal involvement, cranial nerve involvement, and disease outside the CNS can be helpful.

Neoplasms (primary and metastatic) accounted for 37% of infundibular lesions in a recent review.[30] In children, germinomas were most common. These lesions manifested as stalk thickening. CSF seeding and pineal region lesions may help in narrowing the differential diagnosis. In adults, metastatic disease was the most common, with breast and lung being the most common primaries (**Fig. 22**). Leukemia and lymphoma can also involve the infundibulum. Hypothalamic-chiasmatic glioma may involve the infundibulum by secondary extension.

Primary glial tumors can occur in the infundibulum, but several neurohypophyseal-specific glial tumors exist and deserve special mention: these include pituicytomas, granular cell tumors, and choristomas. These tumors are isodense to normal brain and enhance homogeneously. The tumors are centered in the stalk and/or posterior pituitary, can grow into the suprasellar cistern, and may be highly vascular (**Fig. 23**). The sella is not enlarged. This observation can help to differentiate them from adenomas, although the most common tumor overall of the sella remains adenoma. Tanycytomas often present as a large suprasellar mass that is often indistinguishable from the stalk.

SUMMARY

Knowledge of the normal anatomy and pathologic imaging appearance of pituitary lesions is essential in the interpretation of MR imaging of brain and pituitary. There are many pitfalls of interpretation, some of which can be avoided by soliciting detailed clinical histories. Some of the common interpretation mistakes are listed in **Table 3**. Careful consideration of the anatomy and location of the lesion as well as correlation with the clinical situation and previous medical/surgical treatment are essential in the imaging diagnosis of pituitary masses.

REFERENCES

1. Destrieux C, Kakou MK, Velut S, et al. Microanatomy of the hypophyseal fossa boundaries. J Neurosurg 1998;88:743–52.

2. Roppolo HM, Latchaw RE. Normal pituitary gland: 2. Microscopic anatomy-CT correlation. AJNR Am J Neuroradiol 1983;4:937–44.

3. Casanueva FF, Molitch ME, Schlechte JA, et al. Guidelines of the pituitary society for the diagnosis and management of prolactinomas. Clin Endocrinol 2006;65:265–73.

4. Molitch ME. Prolactinoma. In: Melmed S, editor. Pituitary. Cambridge (UK): Blackwell Science; 1995. p. 433–77.

5. Colao A, Ferone D, Marzullo P, et al. Systemic complications of acromegaly: epidemiology, pathogenesis, and management. Endocr Rev 2004;25:102–52.

6. Arnaldi G, Angeli A, Atkinson AB, et al. Diagnosis and complications of Cushing's syndrome: a consensus statement. J Clin Endocrinol Metab 2003;88: 5593–602.

7. Symons SP, Aviv RI, Montanera WJ, et al. The sellar turcica and parasellar region. In: Atlas SW, editor. Magnetic resonance imaging of the brain and spine. 4th edition. Philadelphia: Lippincott Williams & Wilkins; 2009. p. 1120–92.

8. Yuh WT, Fisher EJ, Nguyen HD, et al. Sequential MR enhancement pattern in normal pituitary gland and in pituitary adenoma. AJNR Am J Neuroradiol 1994;15:101–8.

9. Patronas N, Bulakbasi N, Stratakis CA, et al. Spoiled gradient recalled acquisition in the steady state technology is superior to conventional postcontrast spin echo technique for magnetic resonance detection of adrenocorticotropin-secreting pituitary tumors. J Clin Endocrinol Metab 2003;88:1565–9.

10. Bartynski WS, Lin L. Dynamic and conventional spin-echo MR of pituitary microlesions. AJNR Am J Neuroradiol 1997;18:965–72.

11. Friedman TC, Zuckerbraun E, Lee ML, et al. Dynamic pituitary MRI has high sensitivity and specificity for the diagnosis of mild Cushing's syndrome and should be part of the initial workup. Horm Metab Res 2007;39:451–6.

12. Tabarin A, Laurent F, Catargi B, et al. Comparative evaluation of conventional and dynamic magnetic resonance imaging of the pituitary gland for diagnosis of Cushing's disease. Clin Endocrinol 2008; 49:293–300.

13. Batista D, Courkoutsakis NA, Oldfield EH, et al. Detection of adrenocorticotropin-secreting pituitary adenomas by magnetic resonance imaging in children and adolescents with Cushing disease. J Clin Endocrinol Metab 2005;90:5134–40.

14. Tanoue S, Kiyosue H, Sagara Y, et al. Venous structures at the craniocervical junction: anatomic variations evaluated by multidetector row CT. Br J Radiol 2010;83:831–40.

15. Swearingen B, Katznelson L, Miller K, et al. Diagnostic errors after inferior petrosal sinus sampling. J Clin Endocrinol Metab 2004;89:3752–63.

16. Kaskarelis IS, Tsatalou EG, Benakis SV, et al. Bilateral inferior petrosal sinuses sampling in the routine investigation of Cushing's syndrome: a comparison with MRI. AJR Am J Roentgenol 2006;187:562–70.

17. Cottier JP, Destrieux C, Brunereau L, et al. Cavernous sinus invasion by pituitary adenoma: MR imaging. Radiology 2000;215:463–9.

18. Vieira JO Jr, Cukiert A, Liberman B. Evaluation of magnetic resonance imaging criteria for cavernous sinus invasion in patients with pituitary adenomas: logistic regression analysis and correlation with surgical findings. Surg Neurol 2006;65:130–5.

19. Pinker K, Ba-Ssalamah A, Wolfsberger S, et al. The value of high-field MRI (3T) in the assessment of sellar lesions. Eur J Radiol 2005;54:327–34.

20. Wolfsberger S, Ba-Ssalamah A, Pinker K, et al. Application of three-tesla magnetic imaging for diagnosis and surgery of sellar lesions. J Neurosurg 2004;100: 278–86.

21. Rogg JM, Tung GA, Anderson G, et al. Pituitary apoplexy: early detection with diffusion weighted MR imaging. AJNR Am J Neuroradiol 2002;22:1240–5.

22. Liu JK, Couldwell WT. Pituitary apoplexy in the magnetic imaging era: clinical significance of sphenoid mucosal thickening. J Neurosurg 2006;104: 892–8.

23. Arita K, Kurisu K, Tominaga A, et al. Thickening of the sphenoid sinus mucosa during the acute stage of pituitary apoplexy. J Neurosurg 2001;95:897–901.

24. Yoon PH, Kim DI, Jeon P, et al. Pituitary adenomas: early postoperative MR imaging after transsphenoidal resection. AJNR Am J Neuroradiol 2001;22:1097–104.

25. Kang MD, Escott E, Thomas AJ, et al. The MR imaging appearance of the vascular pedicle nasoseptal flap. AJNR Am J Neuroradiol 2009;30:781–6.

26. Shimono T, Hatabu H, Kasagi K, et al. Rapid progression of pituitary hyperplasia in humans with primary hypothyroidism: demonstration with MR imaging. Radiology 1999;213:383–8.

27. Bonneville F, Cattin F, Marsot-Dupuch K, et al. T1 hyperintensity in the sellar region: spectrum of findings. Radiographics 2006;26:93–113.

28. Binning MJ, Gottfried ON, Osborn AG, et al. Rathke cleft cyst intracystic nodule: a characteristic magnetic resonance imaging finding. J Neurosurg 2005;103:837–40.

29. Kassam AB, Gardner PA, Snyderman CH, et al. Expanded endonasal approach, a fully endoscopic transnasal approach for the resection of midline suprasellar craniopharyngiomas: a new classification based on the infundibulum. J Neurosurg 2008;108:715–28.

30. Hamilton BE, Salzman KL, Osborn AG. Anatomic and pathologic spectrum of pituitary infundibulum lesions. AJR Am J Roentgenol 2007;188:W223–32.

Index

Note: Page numbers of article titles are in **boldface** type.